Contents

Preface

This book is designed to help nurses learn how to teach. Whether they are teaching patients, staff, or students in an academic setting, nurses who are in the educator role need a theory base from which to work. They also must develop an understanding of educational issues and innovations like literacy and distance learning. They especially need to develop a wide repertoire of teaching strategies.

In my 30 years of experience as an educator and my last 4 years of teaching a teaching strategies course to graduate students, I have developed a keen appreciation of the commonalities of teaching across settings. In my graduate classes, some students are employed in staff development, some are preparing to be advanced practice nurses, some are functioning as clinical preceptors, and some aim toward a future in academia. Yet they can all give examples of how the concepts in this book are applied in their work settings.

Some of the chapters in this book apply more to one setting than another. In such cases, that fact is pointed out. For example, Chapter 6, Literacy and Readability, applies primarily to patient teaching. Chapter 12, Promoting and Assessing Critical Thinking, applies primarily to academic and staff development settings. However, even these topics apply to some degree to all forms of nursing education.

The book is divided into three sections. Part I, Teaching and Learning, includes Chapter 1, which focuses on "good teaching." Research on evidence of good teaching and the principles for good practice in teaching are highlighted. Chapter 2 is about learning theories and concepts, with application to nursing and health education. Chapter 3 explicates how to plan and conduct classes, regardless of the setting of those classes. It includes writing objectives, selecting content and teaching methods, planning assignments, and conducting the class.

Part II, The Learner, incorporates information about patients, students, and nurses as learners. Chapter 4, written by Dr. Joanna Hayden, focuses on motivation and readiness for learning, with application of additional theories, and a discussion of the effectiveness of patient teaching. Chapter 5, authored by Dr. Kem Louie, discusses multicultural and gender aspects of learning. Chapter 6 is about literacy and readability, with focus on the impact of low literacy and the development of printed educational materials.

Part III, Teaching Strategies, covers advantages and disadvantages, purposes and uses of the methods, and research on the strategies that are discussed. Chapter 7 includes the traditional teaching strategies of lecture, discussion, questioning, and audiovisual technology. Chapter 8 highlights activity-based teaching strategies, with emphasis on collaborative learning, simulations, games, case studies, problem-based learning, and self-learning modules. Chapter 9 is about computer teaching strategies, including virtual reality. Chapter 10 explains what distance learning is and how it is expanding in all settings today. Chapter 11 discusses how to teach psychomotor skills. Chapter 12, authored by Dr. Terry Valiga, focuses on promoting critical thinking and includes evaluating and measuring critical thinking. Chapter 13 sets forth principles and practices of clinical teaching, including precepting. Finally, Chapter 14 is about assessing and evaluating learning.

Each chapter includes **three features** that are useful as teaching strategies in themselves. They are:

- **Case Study.** The case applies the information in the chapter and gives the students an opportunity to actively manipulate some of the chapter content. Students will learn the information better if they can apply it to a real-life situation. The Case Studies can be used as group exercises or can first be completed by individual learners and then discussed in class.

- **Critical Thinking Exercises.** Key concepts in the chapters are the focus of these exercises. Learners are asked to consider the validity of assumptions, reflect on issues, rethink points of view, apply information in new contexts, and make reasoned judgments. The Exercises serve as a model of the types of questions that nurse educators should be asking learners to deal with.

- **Ideas for Further Research.** The research suggestions are designed primarily for graduate students. The research ideas can be used as trigger points for graduate research in the form of master's theses and doctoral dissertations. Faculty may also find that some of the ideas stimulate their own desire to conduct research on these worthy topics.

Too often new educators teach as they were taught without questioning their methods or rationale. It is my hope that after studying this text, the new (or renewed) nurse educator will teach with a sound understanding of basic learning theory and an excitement about the many approaches she or he can use to achieve desired learning outcomes.

Sandra DeYoung

Acknowledgments

Many people have contributed their expertise to the writing and publication of this book. I am indebted to the three chapter authors, Joanna Hayden, Kem Louie, and Theresa Valiga for sharing their expertise with me and the learners who will study this book. All three of them are master teachers with much to share.

The reviewers who spent time reading drafts and making suggestions for improvements of the text are also experts whose efforts are much appreciated.

Finally, I extend my thanks to the editorial teams at Prentice Hall Health and Rainbow Graphics for helping us to create a book that I hope will be a helpful resource to all readers.

Sandra DeYoung

Contributing Authors

Chapter 4 Motivation and Behavior Change
Authored by: **Joanna Hayden,** PhD, RN, CHES
Professor of Community Health
William Paterson University
Wayne, NJ

Chapter 5 Multicultural Aspects of Learning
Authored by: **Kem Louie,** PhD, RN, FAAN
Associate Professor of Nursing
William Paterson University
Wayne, NJ

Chapter 12 Promoting and Assessing Critical Thinking
Authored by: **Theresa M. Valiga,** EdD, RN
Director of Research and Professional Development
National League for Nursing
New York, NY

Reviewers

Ann Marriner Tomey, BS, MS, RN, FAAN, PhD in Higher Education
Indiana State University
School of Nursing
Terre Haute, IN

Claudia Barone, EdD, RN
Clinical Assistant Professor, Specialty Coordinator
Acute Care Practitioner Program
University of Arkansas for Medical Sciences
College of Nursing
Little Rock, AR

Linda A. Howe, PhD, RN, CS
Critical Care Clinical Nurse Specialist
Clemson University
School of Nursing
Clemson, SC

Betty J. Beard, RN, PhD
Professor of Nursing
Eastern Michigan University
Department of Nursing
Ypsilanti, MI

Part I

Teaching and Learning

1

Good Teaching

Learners can easily identify their "best" teachers and "worst" teachers. After all, we have been students, or at least informal learners, for years. As consumers, we have learned to identify the differences between effective and ineffective teaching. We may even be able to distinguish some of the factors that make up those differences. Yet if these same learners become teachers themselves, they may not find it so easy to follow in the footsteps of their good role models. Different skills are required for subjectively evaluating a teacher than for *being* a good teacher, just as different skills are needed to be a theater critic than to be a good actor.

The effective teacher does not become so just by imitating former good teachers, although following a good role model can be helpful. The process also involves a knowledge of educational theory and research, a willingness to learn new roles and teaching methods, and the ability to reflect on one's own performance. Some people have inherent qualities that increase the likelihood of their being good teachers, and they can improve on their natural abilities to make themselves excellent teachers. Those less well endowed with natural talent can still become good teachers, given the proper education, support, and desire to succeed. If it were not possible for "weak" teachers to become better and "good" teachers to become excellent, education courses and texts such as this would be a waste of time.

Hallmarks of Good Teaching

Considerable research has been devoted to the question of what constitutes good teaching. While some research has involved asking faculty about good teaching practices, most studies have surveyed students to ask their opinions—a logical method of asking the consumer to evaluate the quality of a product or service. Student surveys have inherent weaknesses, however. Although the majority of students in a class may agree on the qualities of a good teacher, some students have different opinions based on their individual learning styles, goals, and personal needs. Despite the weaknesses of survey methods, such research provides useful insights into the components of good teaching. Following is first a discussion of behaviors that both nursing students and faculty generally agree contribute to effective teaching in nursing, especially clinical teaching. Second will be a discussion of effective teaching in more general terms.

Effective Teaching in Nursing

In 1966, Jacobson, in a classic article, delineated six major categories of effective teaching in nursing: professional competence, interpersonal relationships, teaching practices, personal characteristics, evaluation practices, and availability to students. Many researchers since that time have studied effective teaching in nursing, especially clinical teaching, and have found that the behaviors that emerged fit fairly well into those categories.

PROFESSIONAL COMPETENCE

The teacher who enjoys nursing, shows genuine interest in patients, and displays confidence in his or her professional abilities is rated high. The teacher who is creative and stimulating, can excite student interest in nursing, and can demonstrate clinical skills with expertise is also valued (Benor & Leviyof, 1997; Bergman & Gaitskill, 1990; Brown, 1981; Dixon & Koerner, 1976; Jacobson, 1966; Kiker, 1973; Knox & Mogan, 1987; Kotzabassaki et al., 1997; Nehring, 1990; O'Shea & Parsons, 1979).

Professional competence has several aspects. The teacher who aims at excellence develops a thorough knowledge of subject matter and polishes skills throughout his or her career. He or she maintains and expands this knowledge through reading, research, clinical practice, and continuing education. Learners need to know that they can trust the clinical expertise of the teacher, that information given is accurate, and skills are being demonstrated correctly. A teacher who portrays excellent clinical skills and judgment becomes a positive role model for learners.

INTERPERSONAL RELATIONSHIPS WITH STUDENTS

An effective teacher is skillful in interpersonal relationships. This skill is demonstrated by taking a personal interest in learners, being sensitive to their feelings and problems, conveying respect for them, alleviating their anxieties, being accessible for conferences, being fair, permitting learners to express differing points of view, creating an atmosphere in which they feel free to ask questions, and conveying a sense of warmth (Brown, 1981; Fairbrother, 1996; Griffith & Bakanauskas, 1983; Karns & Schwab, 1982; Kiker, 1973; Li, 1997; Mogan & Knox, 1987; Nehring, 1990; O'Shea & Parsons, 1979; Van Ort, 1983; Wong, 1978; Zimmerman & Westfall, 1988).

Many teachers with well-developed interpersonal skills find that good relationships with students evolve almost automatically. Others have to become aware of their deficiencies and work on improvement. Novice teachers in academia sometimes express misgivings about "getting too involved with students." They are afraid they will not be able to maintain a professional distance that will be necessary when it comes time to evaluate the student, or they feel it is not their role to consider students' personal problems, since they are not trained to be counselors. Some teachers believe that showing concern for and interest in students leads to lack of discipline in the classroom, with students taking advantage of their relationship with the teacher. There is no evidence that this belief is accurate; in fact, there is considerable evidence that good student–teacher relationships enhance learning. Carl Rogers (1969) summarized a collection of studies indicating that students actually learn more in classrooms where teachers are student oriented and empathic. With experience, teachers learn how to balance the professional role with showing sincere concern for students' welfare. The relationship is not unlike the one nurses develop with patients, where professional boundaries must be drawn, but an interpersonal relationship is a requisite to helping the patient. Viewing students as worthwhile individuals who have something to offer the nursing profession helps to keep relationships with them in perspective. It is also helpful to remember the old adage, "Today's student is tomorrow's colleague."

Nursing students and patients are often plagued by lack of self-confidence and by fear of making mistakes while learning, which leads them to experience high levels of stress. While some anxiety contributes to learning, too much anxiety interferes with the ability to learn. Educators can help learners maintain self-esteem and minimize anxieties by using three basic therapeutic approaches of empathic listening, acceptance, and honest communication.

As in all relationships, it is important that teachers listen to learners and try to see the world through their eyes. This approach requires teachers to respect learners and care about their concerns and try to understand the world as learners experience it.

The second approach is to accept learners as they are, whether or not you like them. Affirming the fact that learners are worthwhile people, even though different from yourself, enhances their self-esteem and convinces them that you have faith in their desire and ability to learn. This faith is often rewarded by the learner's attempts to live up to the teacher's expectations.

Honest communication is the third ingredient contributing to healthy relationships with learners. Learners need to know something about the teacher's thoughts regarding the topic and regarding the learner's abilities and performance. It is disconcerting for learners to be in the dark about what the teacher is thinking. Openness between educator and students creates a relaxed atmosphere in which students are able to see the teacher as a role model. Students are also better able to handle and accept criticism of their work if the teacher has established an honest and caring relationship with them.

Another aspect of honest communication is clearly identifying the learners' responsibilities in the learning process. If learners know exactly what is expected of them and what they have to do to succeed, their anxieties will be lessened and the teacher's frustrations will be minimized.

These basic necessities for establishing good relationships with learners are not unique to education or to nursing—they are the same components needed for all interpersonal relationships. If students experience them in the teacher–student relationship, they may learn how to incorporate them into other relationships, especially with their patients.

It is easy to understand why students often rate the interpersonal and social aspects of teaching as most important in the learning process. They realize that they are more comfortable with and learn better from teachers who have good interpersonal skills.

PERSONAL CHARACTERISTICS

Qualities such as personal magnetism, enthusiasm, cheerfulness, self-control, patience, flexibility, a sense of humor, a good speaking voice, self-confidence, willingness to admit errors, and a caring attitude are all desirable personal characteristics of teachers (Brown, 1981; Fairbrother, 1996; Griffith & Bakanauskas, 1983; Kiker, 1973; Kotzabassaki et al., 1997; Nehring, 1990; Van Ort, 1983). Students value these personal qualities because they make learning more interesting, fun, or pleasant.

Are there any paragons in the field of education who can lay claim to all of these qualities? Probably not. Maybe over the course of a day or a week an individual can maintain that level of behavior, but over the long haul everyone crumbles under the pressure of teaching and of life. That doesn't mean that teachers should not aim for these high standards of personal behavior because they should, and they as well as their students will benefit from these efforts.

TEACHING PRACTICES

Jacobson (1966) defined teaching practices as the mechanics, methods and skills in classroom and clinical teaching. Students and colleagues value a teacher who has a thorough knowledge of the subject matter and can present material in an interesting, clear, and organized manner (Dixon & Koerner, 1976; Fairbrother, 1996; Gignac-Caille & Oermann, 2001; Kotzabassaki et al., 1997; Mogan & Knox, 1987; Van Ort, 1983). Presenting subject matter in such a way is a skill that can be learned. This topic is addressed in Chapter 3 but deserves a few words here. Organization of subject matter requires careful planning to ensure that material is presented logically.

Teaching subject matter in a stimulating way and inspiring learner interest hinge on several factors, including the teacher's style, personality, personal interest in the subject, and use of a variety of teaching strategies. We have all been subject to teachers who, while brilliant, organized, and even clear, lack the ability to present the class material in anything but a boring manner. The content of this book is geared toward helping teachers become more interesting as well as more effective.

EVALUATION PRACTICES

Evaluation practices valued by students include clearly communicating expectations, providing timely feedback on student progress, correcting students tactfully, being fair in the evaluation process, and giving tests that are pertinent to the subject matter (Benor & Leviyof, 1997; Bergman & Gaitskill, 1990; Brown, 1981; Gignac-Caille & Oermann, 2001; Knox & Mogan, 1985; Krichbaum, 1994; Lowery, Keane & Hyman, 1971; Nehring, 1990; O'Shea & Parsons, 1979; Zimmerman & Waltman, 1986; Zimmerman & Westfall, 1988).

At the beginning of a teaching/learning relationship, expectations should be clearly expressed (Sufka & George, 2000). The teacher should let the students know if they are expected to read assignments before class and what will happen if they don't. If there are expectations about attendance and being on time, handing in assignments on time, or what resources may and may not be used, all of these should be clearly communicated. The issues of whether nursing students in the clinical laboratory may seek assistance from staff nurses, or whether they may take coffee breaks, or may consult with other students on care plans and documentation should all be expressed at the beginning of the learning experience. Criteria for evaluation of clinical performance should also be made explicit and put in writing or available on the course Web site.

If learners are not meeting a teacher's expectations, they should know it as soon as possible. No learner should progress through an entire teaching session, inservice program, or semester, to be told at the end that he or she is not doing well. On the other hand, learners who are doing a superior job should be told so; it is not necessary to search for weaknesses to write on an evaluation if they do not exist.

Fairness in evaluation is a rather subjective phenomenon. What is fair to me may not seem so to you. However, complaints of unfairness can be minimized if evaluation is based on published criteria and if those criteria are pertinent to the learning objectives. Further information on evaluation principles may be found in Chapters 13 and 14.

AVAILABILITY TO STUDENTS

Nursing students, especially those taking clinical courses, expect the instructor to be available to them when needed. This may take the form of being there in stressful clinical situations, physically helping students give nursing care, giving appropriate amounts of supervision, freely answering questions, and acting as a resource person during clinical learning experiences (Fairbrother, 1996; Jacobson, 1966; Kotzabassaki et al., 1997; O'Shea & Parsons, 1979; Wong, 1978; Zimmerman & Waltman, 1986; Zimmerman & Westfall, 1988).

One of the great stressors for teachers in nursing is trying to be available to students or patients who need instruction, at the precise time they need it. The reality is that teachers usually have many other students or patients they are working with, and they cannot be in six places at once. Learners should be told at the beginning of instruction what they should do if they need assistance and the instructor is not available at the time. The teacher should have a back-up plan for assistance by a staff nurse, another instructor, or head nurse who can be "on call" when the need arises.

Effective Teaching Identified by Non-Nursing Studies

The literature outside of the field of nursing corroborates many of the above characteristics of good teaching (McKeachie, 1999). Because non-nursing studies primarily involve classroom rather than clinical teaching, a few other characteristics are identified. They include teacher clarity, time on task, and class time being well used (Cruickshank, 1992; Pascarella, Edison, Nora, Hagedorn, & Braxton, 1996).

Teacher clarity is a quality worth focusing on. It is defined by Cruickshank (1992) as "a mosaic of behaviors that teachers use in order to make what is to be learned intelligible, comprehensible, and learnable" (p. 312). Researchers have found that the clear teacher is one who logically organizes instruction, explains what is to be learned, uses simple terms to present new material, constantly assesses whether students are understanding and can follow the teacher's train of thought, uses examples whenever possible, allows students time to think about what is being taught, and uses repetition and summarization (Civikly, 1992; Cruickshank, 1992). Students appreciate clarity, and studies have demonstrated that teacher clarity is positively correlated with student achievement and student attitudes toward a class (Civikly, 1992; Pascarella et al., 1996). The good news is that clarity of instruction can be taught by helping teachers focus on and practice the characteristics of clarity listed above (Cruickshank, 1992). Because it is such an important quality, new teachers should ask students periodically if they are being clear, and clarity should be an item on any teacher assessment form. Videotaping a teaching session and then watching it afterward can help a teacher assess his or her own clarity of teaching.

Additional characteristics of effective teaching were identified in a qualitative study of physician-teachers conducted by Crandall in 1993. Thirteen teachers who were identified as above average by the students were interviewed to determine if they had common characteristics of excellence. Several commonalities were identified. The first was viewing learners as collaborators, which led to the teachers being very respectful and supportive of the learners. The second quality these excellent teachers shared was admitting weaknesses. They made themselves somewhat vulnerable when they admitted to students that they did not know an answer or had no experience in a certain field of knowledge, but students seemed to benefit by seeing the humanness of their role models. Third, these teachers said they recognized when their students were having difficulty and were able to figure out what to do to help.

Some of these same qualities were revealed by Carnegie Professors of the Year when they wrote essays on good teaching (Rodgers, Cross, Tanenbaum, & Tilson, 1997). Each year the Carnegie Foundation identifies a few college professors who are said to be excellent in their fields. These professors wrote about many of the qualities already discussed. In addition, one teacher said that to be a good teacher you have to really have the desire to be good because it takes a lot of work to succeed in every aspect of teaching. He also wrote that good teaching is a form of parenting—caring about students, knowing when to set boundaries, and knowing students' potential. One of the award-winning professors was a nurse. She added that a good teacher is concerned with more than just what students know; he or she should also be concerned with students' beliefs, values, and relationships. In other words, a good teacher cares.

Flowers (2000) adds that effective teachers are committed and creative. They are committed in that they don't watch the clock, often working long hours. They are creative in their attempts to stimulate intellectual inquisitiveness in their students and to help students explore their world. In a tribute to a few of his former teachers, Rodden (2000) wrote:

> Ultimately, what distinguishes the great teachers is what I can only call their unsparing gift of self, their capacity for caring about students. Not pseudo-care via maudlin gestures or gushy words. Perhaps even a bracing care, laced with stern affection or bolstered by an impersonal rigor. But their aim is always to awaken students to an awareness of their greater potential (p. 40).

Teacher Style

The interpersonal, professional, and personal aspects of good teaching are all important. But more is involved in being a good teacher than just the skills, techniques, and attributes mentioned thus far. Effective teaching involves another phenomenon sometimes referred to as *teacher style*. Style can be considered a blending of form and content. Eble (1980) believes that style in teaching is an outgrowth of the teacher's personality and character, which is undoubtedly true. For a distinctive style to emerge, it must emerge from something, and that something is probably not just the intellect, but the essential personality. It is style that makes a teacher memorable, interesting, and worth listening to. It is style that makes good teachers into inspired teachers.

Style goes beyond having certain skills and behaviors. It goes beyond carrying out handy hints in a teacher's handbook. Style is a blending of certain ways of talking, moving, relating, and thinking. It is more than the ability to entertain or a sense of humor, although these qualities may play a part in a teacher's style.

If you think back to the memorable and inspiring teachers you have had (probably very few), you may be able to recognize style as an important part of their effectiveness. One professor who stands out in my memory had a unique style. He would often sit on the front of his desk, tell a story related to the topic for the day, then relate the story to the class material. He had a homespun appearance and down-to-earth manner, and he conveyed warmth and enthusiasm. Yet for all his folksy style, his scholarliness, intelligence, and sincerity were clearly evident.

Parini (1997) uses the term *teaching persona* instead of style. His example of a distinct persona is a professor named Jim.

> Jim didn't enter a classroom, he swept into it. His eyes were intense; he was somehow pregnant with the material at hand, preparing to give birth. We sat up, eager; we knew that what was coming was going to be good. After a brief pause, he would catch someone's eye. At that moment, everyone in the room felt caught. It was uncanny . . . he conducted the class a bit like a conductor might work an orchestra (p. A92).

Some teachers develop a humorous style and use cartoons, jokes, and funny stories, not just to entertain students but to stimulate their interest and enthusiasm for the subject. Of course, if humor and laughing also helps to keep students awake, few would complain.

You may not be able to label a particular teacher's style, but you can see that it is there. It may manifest itself in a pleasant speaking voice and animated gestures. It may be observable in the teacher's skill at timing—knowing how to adapt speed of delivery for individual learners or a whole class, knowing when they are ready for new material, and knowing when to shift gears or stop. Humor is often a part of style. It may involve telling funny stories, pointing out the ridiculous in certain human situations, laughing with the students, or laughing at oneself, even in front of a class. Using a variety of teaching strategies is a part of style. A personal style may include willingness to share stories from one's professional experience to illustrate certain points; it may be the ability to evoke emotion in students. All these aspects of style blend with the personal and professional attributes already discussed to make the teacher what he or she is. If the blend is just right, the teacher will be hard to forget.

Can style be taught? And once established, can it be changed? Tuckman and Yates (1980) found that a teacher's style could be shaped by student feedback, although their sample consisted of student teachers whose beginning style might well have been malleable. But even veteran teachers whose habits are set can modify their teaching style if they see the need to do so.

Perhaps the most effective means of changing your style is to discuss your teaching with a knowledgeable peer or consultant who has seen you in action or who has reviewed videotapes of your teaching. Discussion of your style can raise your awareness of it and help you examine it more objectively. Reading books on teacher style can help if you discuss the contents with someone and consider ideas on how to implement what you have read.

Kenneth Eble (1980) has said that an admirable style develops only after years of teaching. There is some truth in this. Style does develop slowly in response to results (or lack of them) in your teaching and in response to learner and peer evaluations. But because style is also a function of personality and character, for some teachers an admirable style may develop early and continue to evolve into something even better over the years.

Seven Principles of Good Practice in Undergraduate Education

Another way of looking at the elements of good teaching is through the framework of what are generally known as the Seven Principles. In 1987, Chickering and Gamson described the

Seven Principles of Good Practice in Undergraduate Education. Although the principles were written in reference to college settings, clearly they apply to all adult education settings. In summary, the seven principles are:

1. Encourage student–faculty contact.
2. Encourage cooperation among students.
3. Encourage active learning.
4. Give prompt feedback.
5. Emphasize time on task.
6. Communicate high expectations.
7. Respect diverse talents and ways of learning.

These elements refer to effective teacher characteristics and to what teachers do in the learning environment. Some of the practices have already been discussed, but, in addition, some new ideas have appeared.

Encouraging cooperation among students refers to collaborative learning, study groups, and a variety of group projects. This subject will be discussed in more detail in Chapter 8. There is a large body of research indicating that most students learn better collaboratively than they do competitively.

Using active learning techniques refers to enabling students to actively manipulate the content they are learning. It may include students talking about the material, writing about it, outlining it, applying it, asking questions about it, acting it out, or just reflecting on it. Many of the teaching strategies discussed in this book are designed to encourage active rather than passive learning.

Emphasizing time on task means ensuring that students know how much time they should spend learning particular material and encouraging them to take studying and practice seriously. It also means using time efficiently by knowing how to study, do library research, and write a paper.

Communicating high expectations refers to the challenge that teachers hold out to learners. Learners should be told that they are expected to work hard, and specific expectations should be clearly stated. Learners rise to meet the high expectations if they are motivated and are given the support and encouragement they need.

The last principle is that of respecting diverse talents and ways of learning. A skilled teacher considers the fact that learners have different learning styles (see Chapter 2). The teacher uses a variety of teaching strategies and assignments to meet the needs of diverse learners (Duck, 2000). Consideration is also given to the various talents or "seven types of intelligence" written about by Gardner (1992). He identified the following types of intelligence: linguistic, logical–mathematical, spatial, musical, bodily kinesthetic, interpersonal, and intrapersonal. The intuitive teacher sees the degree to which these different types of intelligence have developed in students as he or she gets to know them and builds on students' strengths.

One important fact must be kept in mind when evaluating teaching effectiveness. There is no one style, technique, or skill that is effective for all learners and all teaching situations. Teachers hope that their skill helps most of the learners and that their style is pleasing and stimulating for the majority. But teachers have to be flexible, modifying their techniques and style to best meet the requirements of the situation.

Nurses as Teachers

Nurses take on the teaching role in many settings. They may be patient or client teachers, school nurses, staff development instructors, or collegiate educators. In any nursing position, it is safe to say that the nurse will be teaching.

In a survey of staff nurses, nurse administrators, and nurse educators, 74 percent of the sample (n = 549) believed the nurse should assume primary responsibility for patient education, and 97 percent believed the nurse's responsibility for patient teaching would be greater in the future (Kruger, 1991). With shorter hospital stays, increase in community-based care, and the growth of health care consumerism, we can expect that staff nurses will have to be skilled teachers. They will need to learn the basic principles of teaching included in this text and how to apply them in diverse settings.

Nurses who spend the majority of their time in the educator role such as staff development instructors or educators in collegiate settings have more formal preparation for the educator role and need to become expert teachers in order to prepare the next generation of patient educators.

In all cases, the characteristics of the effective teacher as outlined in this chapter should be studied and applied to the educator role if we are to fulfill our professional responsibility for providing high-quality care and high-quality education.

CASE STUDY

A staff development manager writes on a new staff member's yearly evaluation that she needs to improve her teaching skills. Her teaching needs to be more organized and clear, and she must express more enthusiasm in her classes.

1. Where can this new educator go for help?
2. What resources are available to help her?
3. If you were asked to help her, how would you begin?

CRITICAL THINKING EXERCISES

1. Identify a teacher you might have had in the past who you think was a good teacher but who did not exhibit many of the "hallmarks of good teaching" listed in the chapter. Why do you consider this teacher to be a "good" one?
2. You are a new part-time clinical faculty member. A faculty colleague says to you, "You should be careful about becoming too chummy with the students. That can be a problem." Can being very friendly with students ever become a problem? How

can being friendly (and human) with students coexist with a professional relationship?

3. Do you agree with Gardner (1992) that there are different types of intelligence? Why or why not?

Ideas for Further Research

1. Interview staff nurses about their patient and family teaching. Do they feel prepared to do a good job? Do they feel effective as teachers? What is the most common area of teaching that they do?

2. Observe clinical nurse educators. What strategies do they use that enhance student learning? What do they do that obstructs student learning? What strategies do they use to make themselves available to all students during the learning period?

3. Survey or interview nursing faculty regarding their understanding of Chickering and Gamson's (1997) principle of "emphasizing time on task." Does the principle apply to both classroom and clinical learning? If so, can it be used in both settings?

4. Research whether Jacobsen's (1966) categories of effective teaching apply to staff development teaching. You may survey participants in staff development classes using one of the measurement tools published in the studies listed in the References.

References

Benor, D. E., & Leviyof, I. (1997). The development of students' perceptions of effective teaching: The ideal, best and poorest clinical teacher in nursing. *Journal of Nursing Education, 36*(5), 206–211.

Bergman, K., & Gaitskill, T. (1990). Faculty and student perceptions of effective clinical teachers: An extension study. *Journal of Professional Nursing, 6*(1), 33–44.

Brown, S. T. (1981). Faculty and student perceptions of effective clinical teachers. *Journal of Nursing Education, 20*(9), 4–15.

Chickering, A. W., & Gamson, Z. F. (1987). Seven principles for good practice in undergraduate education. *AAHE Bulletin, 45*(8), 3–7.

Civikly, J. M. (1992). Clarity: Teachers and students making sense of instruction. *Communication Education, 41*(2), 138–152.

Crandall, S. (1993). How expert clinical educators teach what they know. *Journal of Continuing Education in the Health Professions, 13*, 85–98.

Cruickshank, D. (1992). Be good! Start by being clear. *The Clearing House, 65*(5), 311–314.

Dixon, J. K., & Koerner, B. (1976). Faculty and student perceptions of effective classroom teaching in nursing. *Nursing Research, 25*(4), 300–305.

Duck, L. (2000). The ongoing professional journey. *Educational Leadership, 57*(8), 42–45.

Eble, K. E. (1980). *Improving teaching styles.* San Francisco: Jossey-Bass.

Fairbrother, P. (1996). Recognition and assessment of teaching quality. *Nurse Education Today, 16,* 69–74.

Flowers, L. (2000). The four C's of an effective college teacher: A commentary on exceptional college teaching. *TC Record.org,* Article 10530. Retrieved November 2, 2001 from *http://www.tcrecord.org/indexing.asp?*

Gardner, H. (1992). *Multiple intelligences: The theory in practice.* New York: Basic Books.

Gignac-Caille, A. M., & Oermann, M. H. (2001). Student and faculty perceptions of effective clinical instructors in ADN programs. *Journal of Nursing Education, 40*(8), 347–353.

Griffith, J. W., & Bakanauskas, A. J. (1983). Student–instructor relationships in nursing education. *Journal of Nursing Education, 22*(3), 104–107.

Jacobson, M. D. (1966). Effective and ineffective behavior of teachers of nursing as determined by their students. *Nursing Research, 15*(3), 218–224.

Karns, P. J., & Schwab, T. A. (1982). Therapeutic communication and clinical instruction. *Nursing Outlook, 30*(1), 39–43.

Kiker, M. (1973). Characteristics of the effective teacher. *Nursing Outlook, 21*(11), 721–723.

Knox, J. E., & Mogan, J. (1985). Important clinical teacher behaviours as perceived by university nursing faculty, students and graduates. *Journal of Advanced Nursing, 10,* 25–30.

Kotzabassaki, S., Panou, M., Dimou, F., Karabagli, A., Koutsoupoulou, B., & Ikonomou, U. (1997). Nursing students' and faculty's perceptions of the characteristics of "best" and "worst" clinical teachers: A replication study. *Journal of Advanced Nursing, 26,* 817–824.

Krichbaum, K. (1994). Clinical teaching effectiveness described in relation to learning outcomes of baccalaureate nursing students. *Journal of Nursing Education, 33*(7), 306–315.

Kruger, S. (1991). The patient educator role in nursing. *Applied Nursing Research, 4*(1), 19–24.

Li, M. K. (1997). Perceptions of effective clinical teaching behaviours in a hospital-based nurse training programme. *Journal of Advanced Nursing, 26,* 1252–1261.

Lowery, B. J., Keane, A. P., & Hyman, I. A. (1971). Nursing students' and faculty opinion on student evaluation of teachers. *Nursing Research, 20*(5), 436–439.

McKeachie, W. J. (1999). *Teaching tips* (10th ed.). Boston: Houghton Mifflin.

Mogan, J., & Knox, J. E. (1987). Characteristics of 'best' and 'worst' clinical teachers as perceived by university faculty and students. *Journal of Advanced Nursing, 12,* 331–337.

Nehring, V. (1990). Nursing clinical teacher effectiveness inventory: A replication study of the characteristics of "best" and "worst" clinical teachers as perceived by nursing faculty and students. *Journal of Advanced Nursing, 15,* 934–940.

O'Shea, H. S., & Parsons, M. K. (1979). Clinical instruction: Effective/and ineffective teacher behaviors. *Nursing Outlook, 27*(6), 411–415.

Parini, J. (1997, September 5). Cultivating a teaching persona. *The Chronicle of Higher Education,* p. A92.

Pascarella, E., Edison, M., Nora, A., Hagedorn, L. S., & Braxton, J. (1996). Effects of teacher organization/preparation and teacher skill/clarity on general cognitive skills in college. *Journal of College Student Development, 37*(1), 7–19.

Rodden, J. (2000). The teacher as hero. *The American Enterprise, 11*(6), 40–41.

Rodgers, A. T., Cross, D. S., Tanenbaum, B. G., & Tilson, E. R. (1997). Reflections on what makes a good teacher. *Radiologic Technology, 69*(2), 167–169.

Rogers, C. R. (1969). *Freedom to learn.* Columbus, OH: Charles E. Merrill.

Sufka, K. J., & George, M. D. (2000). Setting clear & mutual expectations. *Liberal Education, 86*(1), 48–53.

Tuckman, B. W., & Yates, D. (1980). Evaluating the student feedback strategy for changing teacher style. *Journal of Educational Research, 74*(2), 74–77.

Van Ort, S. R. (1983). Developing a system for documenting teaching effectiveness. *Journal of Nursing Education, 22*(8), 324–328.

Wong, S. (1978). Nurse-teacher behaviours in the clinical field: Apparent effect on nursing students' learning. *Journal of Advanced Nursing, 3*, 369–372.

Zimmerman, L., & Waltman, N. (1986). Effective clinical behaviors of faculty: A review of the literature. *Nurse Educator, 11*(1), 31–34.

Zimmerman, L., & Westfall, J. (1988). The development and validation of a scale measuring effective clinical teaching behaviors. *Journal of Nursing Education, 27*(6), 274–277.

2

Learning Theory

If you were to ask ten teachers on what learning theory they base their teaching, what kind of answers do you think you would get? Based on my own questioning of teachers, I found that they will rarely tell you they subscribe to a particular theory, but will rather talk about some propositions or concepts that are parts of different theories. For example, they may say, "I know that all children can learn if you spend the time to teach them how to think and solve problems," or "Adults learn best if what they are being taught is meaningful to them." I believe teachers develop a kind of personal philosophy of teaching based on segments of varied theories they have learned about that make sense to them based on their experience. There are other teachers who probably never give a thought to theory or philosophy of teaching, but who probably have developed an approach and style based on theories they learned sometime in the past.

In this chapter I will first explain the basics of the most commonly used learning theories and then describe the propositions on which many teachers base their teaching. Following the theories and propositions I will review types of learning, learning concepts, and learning styles that cross the varied schools of learning theory.

Learning Theories

Why do we need theories? Many students probably think we don't need them at all, but it is theories that tie together those concepts and propositions that teachers often repeat. Learning theories take concepts and *propositions* (statements of the relationships between concepts) and fit them together to explain why people learn and predict under what circumstances they will learn. The major learning theories that guide research and practice today are behaviorist theories, cognitive theories, and social learning theories.

Behaviorist Theories

The earliest formal theories of learning grew out of the behaviorist philosophy in the early twentieth century. Until then, psychologists had focused on studying thoughts and feelings.

John Watson broke with tradition when he began studying behavior because it was objective and practical (Hill, 1971). He defined behavior as muscle movement. He postulated that behavior is a result of a series of conditioned reflexes, and all emotion and thought is a result of behavior learned through conditioning. For example, fear of a hot stove is learned when a child's curiosity leads him to touch a stove (a stimulus followed by a response) and he feels pain (another stimulus and response). Because of an innate fear of pain, the child is now conditioned to avoid touching the stove even when it is cold. Even complex learning occurs through conditioning, according to Watson and his contemporary Guthrie. They believed (although many other experts do not) that even a skill like walking is learned through a series of conditioned responses. For example, shifting the body's weight to one foot, lifting the other foot and swinging it forward, etc. is learned because each muscular sensation becomes a stimulus for the next response, another muscle movement (Hill, 1971). Because Watson and Guthrie emphasized the contiguity of the stimulus and response, they are known as *contiguity theorists.*

Two other well-known behaviorists are Thorndike and Skinner. They are sometimes called *reinforcement theorists* (Hill, 1971). While Watson and Guthrie believed that stimuli and response bonds are strengthened simply because they occur together, Thorndike and Skinner proposed that stimulus–response bonds are strengthened by *reinforcements* like reward or punishment. The same example of the child touching the stove can be used for reinforcement theory. The child learns to avoid the stove because the pain was a negative reinforcer for the behavior. Skinner hypothesized that behavior that is rewarded is more likely to reoccur (Rosenstock, Strecher, & Becker, 1988).

Although the behaviorists could hardly deny the existence of thought processes, they believed them to be the result of stimulus–response activities, and they believed that the learning process was really very simple. Today, behaviorism is viewed as capable of explaining only simple behavior. Teachers who adhered to the behaviorist school extolled the value of drill and practice and memorization. They were wedded to behavioral objectives written in great detail. Newer thinking in the direction of cognitive theory emphasizes understanding and "meaningful learning" rather than rote learning (Glaser, 1984). Cognitive theorists believe higher order thinking to be the result of far more complex processing than just stimulus–response sequences, and research findings are providing support for cognitivism.

Cognitive Learning Theories

The field of cognitive psychology has been under development since the 1960s and is the predominant approach to psychology today. Cognitive science is the study of how our brains work in the process of perceiving, thinking, remembering, and learning (Breur, 1993). The term *information processing* is sometimes used to describe this field of study. Cognitive science has been a true paradigm shift from behaviorism. Instead of a focus on behavior, the focus is on mental processes that are responsible for behavior and its meaning. Learning, from a cognitive perspective, is an active process in which the learner constructs meaning based on prior knowledge and view of the world (Feden, 1994).

The earliest model of cognitive learning was developed by Ausubel in the 1960s and was called the Subsumption Theory of Meaningful Verbal Learning (Ausubel, 1963). Ausubel proposed that new information is subsumed into existing thought and memory structures. Meaningful learning is thought to occur only if existing cognitive structures are organized and differentiated. For example, in order to learn and remember information about aseptic technique, the person would first have to have some memory and understanding of germ theory and be able to differentiate helpful from harmful germs. Repetition of meaningful material and use in various contexts would enhance the retention of the material, according to Ausubel.

Rumelhart (1980) built a more comprehensive theory of cognitive learning, whose foundation was the concept of *schema* or *schemata* (plural). Schemata are knowledge structures that are stored in memory. According to Rumelhart, "all knowledge is packaged into units. These units are schemata" (p. 34). Examples of schemata are the processes of remembering the route to work and recognizing people (Cust, 1995). People don't just remember a series of street names or particular facial features. They remember patterns of facts or visual, auditory, or tactile cues—schemata, in fact. Rumelhart says that schemata function like theories; that is, they help us to comprehend events or situations and to make predictions about unobserved events. For instance, if you read a newspaper headline that says "West Nile Virus Found in Dead Crows, Ground Spraying to Follow," you would most likely understand the intent of the article because you already have schemata to help you. You probably have a schema related to viruses spread by insects, with birds as part of the infection chain. You would also have a schema related to ground spraying for insects and probably have a mental image of it. The variables and their relationships exist as a unit in your brain. So, you would understand that the ground spraying refers to mosquito spraying, not dead crow spraying. Schemata are not always accurate, and they can be modified. Anytime someone holds a misconception in memory, their schema is faulty. For example, someone may think incorrectly that West Nile virus is spread to people directly from crows. If that person is provided with correct information in a meaningful way, the schema can be altered.

In their theory, Rumelhart and Norman delineated three kinds of learning, all based on schema theory (Rumelhart, 1980; Shuell, 1986). The three different modes of learning are *accretion, tuning* (or *schema evolution*), and *restructuring* (or *schema creation*). *Accretion* is the learning of facts. New information is learned and added to existing schemata. No changes are made to existing knowledge. *Tuning* means that existing schemata evolve or are refined throughout the life span as new situations and issues are encountered. *Restructuring* is the development of new schemata by copying an old schema and adding new elements that are different enough to warrant a new schema.

There are other many narrow range theories and models of information processing such as Levels of Processing Theory, Parallel Distributing Processing Model, and the Connectionistic Model (Huitt, 2000). Levels of Processing Theory states that information is processed sequentially, from perception to attention to labeling and meaning. The processing sequence occurs in both memory storage and memory retrieval. The Parallel Distributing Model proposes that information is processed by different parts of the memory system simultaneously rather than being a sequential process. The Connectionistic Model says that information is stored in many places throughout the brain, forming a network of connections. The more connections that there are to an item in memory storage, the easier it is to retrieve it from memory. The Connectionistic Model has received significant research support.

Stage Theory of information processing also relates to memory activity. The core of this theory is that information is both processed and stored in three stages (Atkinson & Shiffrin, 1968). The first stage is *sensory memory*. Sensory memory is fleeting. Objects we see may last in sensory memory for only half a second. Things we hear remain in sensory memory for about three seconds. If these sensory items are not attended to in that time frame, they are usually forgotten. For them to be passed on to the next level of *short-term memory*, these sensations must be of some interest to the person or activate a known schema. Short-term memory consists of whatever we are thinking about or that which impinges on us from an external stimulus at any given time. This particular memory may last about 20 seconds unless we mentally or verbally repeat the item. We may retain the item indefinitely if it continues to be rehearsed or is especially meaningful to us. We have all had the experience of being introduced to a person and forgetting his or her name almost immediately. Indeed, you may forget it in three seconds if it is not important to you. If you want to remember it for the next hour, you would need to repeat or rehearse it to yourself. If you want to move it into *long-term memory*, you would have to firmly tie this name to an existing schema in the brain. Maybe you would use some mnemonic device, or relate the name to another similar name, face, or place or create a mental association picture. It would also help to practice the name periodically to fix it firmly in long-term memory. More information about memory will follow later in this chapter.

Educators who base their work on cognitive theories tend to focus on making learning meaningful and interesting and tying it to students' existing mental schemata. They focus on deep understanding of core material through active learning techniques. They use techniques such as *advance organizers*, which are statements made at the beginning of class to help students activate prior knowledge and relate it to the new material. They teach students how to learn through *elaboration* of concepts and ideas, applying them to various situations, drawing analogies, asking questions about them, and organizing and summarizing the information (Brandt, 1996; Feden, 1994).

Common Concepts of Cognitive Theories

There are several concepts that are central to cognitive psychology and appear in many of the cognitive learning theories. Following is a further exploration of some of those concepts that are of great interest to educators regardless of the particular theory. These concepts include *learning, metacognition, memory,* and *transfer.*

LEARNING

The definition of learning depends to some degree on the theoretical lens you use to look at it. The behaviorist lens sees learning as the acquisition of knowledge and skills that changes a person's behavior. The cognitive theorist's lens focuses more on the acquisition of knowledge than on the resulting behavior change. Cognitive psychologists are more concerned with what the knowledge means to a person than they are with whether the person's behavior will change as a result of it (Shuell, 1986).

Recent research has focused a great deal on the learning processes and knowledge of novices and experts. In fact, Breur (1993) actually defines learning as "the process whereby novices become more expert" (p. 45). This avenue of research has led to the belief that learning does not follow the same principles and path in every circumstance. In fact, the amount of knowledge and understanding you already possess on a subject will have a tremendous influence on what and how you learn (Feden, 1994). This discovery has led to the term *domain-specific learning.* That is, if you already possess a body of knowledge on a topic, it may be easier for you to learn more, because you have a schema in your brain already that helps you to make sense of new information and lodge it in memory. Experts have been shown to have better memory in their fields, but not in general. This fact helps dispel the myth that improving your learning ability or memory in one subject will build your mental muscles for learning other subjects (Breur, 1993).

METACOGNITION

The concept of *metacognition* has evolved from the study of information processing and is sometimes defined as thinking about one's thinking. It is a process learners use to gauge their thinking while reading, studying, trying to learn, or problem solving (Adams, DeYoung, & Just, 1997). This mental monitoring and control serves people well as they try to learn. Brown and Palinscar (1987) first recognized that some people are *intelligent novices*. They know what they know and what they don't know, and they plan to get the information and understanding they need.

The good news is that there is research to support the hypothesis that learners can improve their metacognitive abilities (Beitz, 1996). They can be taught how to reflect on what they are doing, to analyze their thinking, and to predict whether they know the answers to test questions. Such teaching strategies as journal writing, group dialogue, problem-based learning, and *think aloud* techniques when reviewing test questions with an instructor help students strengthen their metacognitive powers (Cust, 1995).

MEMORY

The Stage Theory of memory was discussed earlier, and sensory (or immediate) memory, short-term memory, and long-term memory differentiated. In addition to what has already been said, there is a *consolidation* function in the memory process (Gordon, 1995). It is through consolidation that items are stationed in memory. The more we connect new information to old, the more we ruminate over new information, and the more frequently we recall and think about it, the more long-lasting it will be. But theorists warn us that the more we recall and chew over memories, the more danger there is that we will actually change those memories (Bolles, 1998; Gordon, 1995). Haven't you noticed that other people's memories of certain events have changed over the years? Well, you may not realize it, but yours have too. Some theorists assert that it happens because we *construct* a memory rather than retrieve one fully formed (Bolles, 1998; Leamnson, 2000). We take different memory fragments and assemble them each time so that eventually the recalled memory may be quite different from the original.

Not every theorist believes in memory construction. Many believe in pure retrieval processes such as described in the Connectionistic Model discussed earlier. In this mode of thought, we simply retrieve information, events, or processes from memory if we have the right cues to prompt us and if the item was stored well in the first place.

This last item, the degree to which material is stored well in memory, is worthy of mention. Figure 2–1 shows a classic retention or forgetting curve. Examination of the graph reveals that in the case shown, less than two weeks after the material was "learned," about 90 percent of the information has been forgotten or cannot be retrieved from memory. Lest you become too despondent after realizing the implications of this curve, let me point out that this type of curve refers to the learning of meaningless lists of words or nonsense syllables. Little if any of this type of learning will be retained after a long interval because it has not

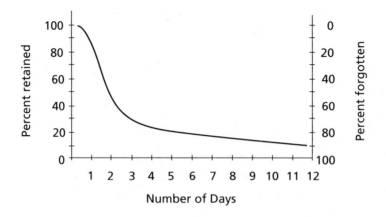

FIGURE 2-1 Typical Retention/Forgetting Curve

been attached to a schema in the mind. The learning of meaningful material presents another picture. Information that is meaningful to the person and that is studied may be retained very well. Meaningful material consists of information that is inherently meaningful (words, phrases, or ideas that make sense) and that is meaningful enough to the learner for him or her to want to retain it. It also consists of material that has been elaborated and consolidated during the learning process and then tied to an existing schema.

Just how much information a person can be expected to hold in short-term memory has been studied over many years (Bolles, 1988). Many studies have concluded that we can hold about seven items in short-term memory before immediate forgetting occurs. So, if you see a list of seven words and study them for a few minutes, you should be able to recite them from memory. To go beyond seven words, you would have to use some kind of mental strategy. Pure repetition doesn't help to extend beyond seven items, but serves only to increase the duration that they remain in short-term memory. A strategy that has been found to be very successful is *chunking* (Bruer, 1993). *Chunks* are formed when information is clustered into patterns. For example, a list of words may be grouped by some common element to form a chunk. If you were given the following list of 10 words and studied them for a minute, you could probably recite about seven of them from memory a few seconds later.

Tree	Battery
Closet	Lake
Food	Book
Road	Chicken
Boy	Chair

If you were to form chunks by grouping the words in some meaningful way, you could remember even more. For example, you could form chunks according to like elements such as:

Boy, Chicken, Tree (living things)
Closet, Chair (elements of a house)
Food, Book (things you desperately need)

Battery, Road, Lake (you need a battery in your car to ride
the road that takes you to the lake)

Using chunking you would probably have little difficulty remembering all 10 items or four chunks. Research into the differences between novice and expert chess players has revealed a great deal about the element of chunking. Novice chess players see the chessboard as a group of individual pieces and store the positions of only about six of them in short-term memory; they take the game one step at a time. Experts see several chess pieces together as a pattern or chunk and can store five to seven chunks in short-term memory. Thus, when they think about moving a piece, they also think about the implications of moving the chunk.

The flip side of the memory coin is forgetting. In addition to what has been said about remembering or forgetting, there are a few other hypotheses about why we forget things. Some researchers believe that memories are in our brains but we may not be able to retrieve them because the connections (networks) to the memory have been weakened. Weakening can happen with disuse over time, with disease, and with interference from new memories (Gordon, 1995; Leamnson, 2000). We know that axons and synapses degenerate if they are not used. We also know that new memories may interfere with old ones when there is some similarity between them. For example, you may find yourself forgetting your sixteenth birthday party if your eighteenth birthday party was somewhat similar and even more meaningful.

Other people have hypothesized that if you don't have the right stimulus or cue, you may not be able to remember something (White, 1997). For example, I have had many occasions when nursing students who have just graduated and taken the NCLEX examination call me to tell me they panicked because "half the test was on maternity nursing" (or some other aspect of nursing that they didn't expect). They felt they had forgotten all the information they learned about this specialty in nursing. In reality, what probably occurred was that a few maternity situations were described as sample cases, but the questions within the cases could have applied mental health principles or community health principles or principles of human sexuality. Nevertheless, the students panic because they see a cue or stimulus that throws them off track and makes the information seem unfamiliar. This phenomenon alerts us to the need to teach people information in varying contexts so they can relate to a variety of cues that will help them to retrieve information from memory.

Finally, some theorists have postulated that a person's *intent to learn* partly determines whether they will remember or forget something they have learned (White, 1997). If a person listens or reads or writes with the intent to learn the material and pays great attention to it because he or she knows the information will be used later, chances are greater that the material will not be forgotten. However, if the learner really was not interested in the first place or saw no future need for the information, that learner may have had no real intent to learn and therefore did not store any material in memory. In effect, it was forgotten almost as soon as it entered the brain.

TRANSFER

Some of the concepts and hypotheses related to remembering and forgetting are also related to *transfer of learning*. Transfer is the ability to take information learned in one situation and apply it to another. One could say that in nursing, transfer of learning is what teaching is all about. We don't teach learners about the principles of infection so they can apply them to just one particular patient situation. We teach them so they can apply the principles and adapt them to all clinical situations.

Successful transfer depends on several factors, including the following (Lauder, Reynolds & Angus, 1999; Voss, 1987):

1. The extent to which material was originally learned
2. The ability to retrieve information from memory
3. The way in which the material was taught and learned
4. The similarity of the new situation to the original

The first item seems to be common sense. You cannot transfer information if you have not learned it well in the first place. This is a fact that many young learners do not seem to understand. They think that if they read or practice something once, they have learned it sufficiently and that it will always be in their memory for future use. Unfortunately, it is not that simple. Retrieval from memory also emphasizes the need to learn, elaborate, and connect new information if it is to remain in long-term memory.

The second and third items focus on the responsibility of the educator. When teaching for transfer, the possibilities of transfer to various types of situations should be made explicit to the student. Emphasizing concepts and principles rather than facts prepares the learner for transfer. Teaching by means of simulations and problem-based learning will also help students to see the process of transfer. An example of the benefit of teaching for transfer is the staff development educator who demonstrates the use of a new infusion pump. She begins by referring to the basic principles of volume and rate control that were learned and used previously with the old equipment and then points out how these same principles underlie the use of the new equipment. The staff find the process of learning how to use the new pump to be quite simple because they can see the relationship of what they already know about pumps to this new situation. This example depicts a situation in which there is *positive transfer*. Positive transfer occurs when present learning is enhanced or accelerated by past learning. However, *negative transfer* can also occur, wherein past learning interferes with present learning. Negative transfer has occurred when a student, who has learned that unconscious patients should be in a side-lying position with the bed flat to facilitate drainage of secretions, places a head-injured unconscious patient in a similar position, not considering the danger of increased intracranial pressure.

Transfer of learning is a phenomenon that is acknowledged in all major theories of learning. In behaviorism it is seen as stimulus–response generalization or interference. In cognitive learning theory it is related to schema restructuring. In social learning theories, to be discussed next, transfer is seen in the modeling process.

Social Learning Theory (Social Cognitive Theory)

The person best known for his Social Learning Theory is Albert Bandura (1977). In later work he renamed his theory Social Cognitive Theory (Rosenstock, Strecher & Becker, 1988), but this new designation has not really caught on. Social Learning Theory takes a very different view of learning from those already discussed. There are several key components of this theory. First, people learn as they are in constant interaction with their environment. Most learning occurs as a result of observing other people's behavior and its consequences (Bandura calls this *modeling*). Second, *attentional processes* determine which modeled behaviors will be learned. People perceive and attend to only a certain number of modeled behaviors. Characteristics of the individual, the modeled activities themselves, and the social interactions in which the learner engages determine which behaviors are attended to. Third, *retention processes* refer to the ability to retain modeled behaviors in permanent memory. For retention to occur, people must retain a mental image of the modeled behavior (e.g., picturing a skill being carried out) or a verbal symbol that is easily recalled (an example is remembering a numbered list of activities involved in a skill). These mental images or verbal symbols are types of schemata. Rehearsal is seen as a significant way of committing learned material to memory. Bandura (1977) emphasizes that although observation starts the learning process, expertise is developed through practice with external and internal (self-regulatory) feedback.

According to Social Learning (Social Cognitive) Theory, motivation for learning will determine which modeled behaviors are enacted. A person is motivated when he or she sees the possibility of valued outcomes as opposed to unrewarding or punishing outcomes. Perceived reward, therefore, is a good motivator and helps people attend to modeled behavior and enact it. An example of a valued outcome as a motivator is a situation in which a student always hands assignments in early because each time he or she receives praise from the teacher for doing so.

A Model of Adult Learning

Malcolm Knowles (1984) is by no means the only scholar to theorize or write about adult learning concepts, but he may be the best known. In the 1970s he began to crusade for a model of education for adults that was different from the education of children. He adopted the term *andragogy* to differentiate the teaching of adults from *pedagogy*, the teaching of children. Table 2–1 displays the concepts that Knowles (1984) used to differentiate andragogy from pedagogy. His model of adult learning can be summarized by saying first that adults are motivated to learn information for which they understand the purpose and see practical applications. Second, they want to take some control of their learning process and be self-directed. Third, they want their life experience to be considered in the learning situation and also want to learn from others' experiences.

TABLE 2-1   Comparison of Pedagogy to Andragogy According to Knowles

	Pedagogy	Andragogy
Need to know	Learn what the teacher wants them to learn	Need to know why they need to learn something
Self-concept	Perception of being dependent on the teacher for learning	Feel responsible for their own learning
Role of experience	The teacher's experience, not the children's is what counts	Adults learn from each other's experience
Readiness to learn	Must be ready when the teacher says they must or they will not be promoted	Ready to learn when they feel the need to know
Orientation to learning	Subject-centered orientation	Life-centered or task-centered orientation
Motivation	Externally motivated	Primarily internally motivated, with some external motivation

Brookfield (1995) states that although much has been written about adult learning and several models have been developed, we are far from developing a general theory of adult learning. He believes the roadblocks to theory development are the widely held myths about adult learning that many educators hold dear. They include the ideas that adult learning is by nature joyful, that adult learners are inherently self-directed, and that adult learning is totally and uniquely different from learning in children.

Any of us who have spent time teaching adults know very well that all adult learning is not joyful. In fact, it can be painful, and adult students are the first to tell you so. Some adult learners are not self-directed at all but want to be led each step of the way. Finally, as Brookfield says, "a strong case can be made that . . . variables of culture, ethnicity, personality and political ethos assume far greater significance in explaining how learning occurs and is experienced than does the variable of chronological age" (p. 1). So, theorists seemingly have a long way to go in developing a realistic and explanatory theory of andragogy.

From what most people do agree on, we can state that the teacher who takes an adult learning model into consideration when teaching will be less of a disseminator of information and director of the learning process and more of a facilitator. He or she will take on the roles of guide, coach, mentor, role model, challenger, and motivator (Galbraith, 1991). This teacher should have confidence in most adult learners' abilities to self-plan learning experiences and should see him- or herself as taking part in a dialogue among equals.

Learning Propositions with Which Most Psychologists Will Agree

To synthesize the commonalities of the theories that have been discussed, I will present the following list of some of the propositions about learning identified by Watson in his classic 1960 article and by Knowles, Holton, and Swanson (1998) in their book on andragogy. These are propositions on which most psychologists from varied schools of thought (behaviorist, cognitivist, and adult learning) would agree. Following the proposition is an application to nursing education.

1. "Behaviors which are rewarded (reinforced) are more likely to occur" (Watson, p. 254). Positive feedback, or reward, is a powerful tool in the hands of a teacher. If a learner performs well in the clinical setting, and the teacher gives praise or a positive written evaluation, the learner's desirable behavior is more likely to be repeated than if the teacher had said or written nothing. In fact, absence of feedback is usually interpreted as negative feedback.

2. "Sheer repetition without indications of improvement or any kind of reinforcement is a poor way to attempt to learn" (Watson, p. 254). Most nurse educators have had experience with learners who spend a great deal of time practicing skills on their own and yet perform them incorrectly when being observed or evaluated. That usually occurs because the learners have been practicing without any external feedback or reinforcement and develop poor habits, or at least fail to improve on each repetition. Thus, to be useful, practice must include feedback.

3. "Threat and punishment have variable and uncertain effects upon learning; they may make the punished response more likely or less likely to recur; they may set up avoidance tendencies which prevent further learning" (Watson, p. 254). Threats to learners are sometimes used in nursing, unfortunately. A new nurse may make a medication error during orientation and be informed that he will be let go if he makes any more errors. While such ultimatums may sometimes be necessary, the effect on learning is unpredictable and may actually increase the likelihood of more errors. It is usually more effective to stress the positive aspects of improvement of performance.

4. "Reward (reinforcement) to be most effective in learning, must follow almost immediately after the desired behavior and be clearly connected with that behavior in the mind of the learner" (Watson, p. 254). The student who gives a good answer to a question raised in the classroom should be given an immediate "Good" or "Right" rather than be told after class that it was a good answer. A learner in the clinical area should be given positive feedback at the time something is done well; the instructor shouldn't wait until the end of the course to give the reward on the final evaluation. The success of computer-assisted instruction can be attributed in part to the immediate feedback given to students. Immediate knowledge of success encourages students to proceed and learn even more material.

5. "Learners progress in any area of learning only as far as they need to in order to achieve their purposes. Often they do only well enough to 'get by'; with increased motivation they improve" (Watson, p. 254). "Adults are motivated to learn to the extent that they perceive that learning will help them perform tasks or deal with problems that they confront in their life situations" (Knowles, Holton, & Swanson, p. 67). Some learners have intrinsic motivation that helps them to excel. Intrinsic motives include wanting to be the best at whatever job one undertakes and wanting to learn because learning brings its own satisfaction. Teachers can also use extrinsic motivation to help learners rise above mediocrity. Curiosity is a great motivator. The educator who can arouse the learners' curiosity and help set them on a path to discovering the things they are curious about, can help them want to do more than the minimum. Teachers can help nursing students see the concrete rewards of providing quality nursing care: patients returned to a higher level of health than they would have achieved without help, patients who look to one as a caring and reliable professional, and colleagues who value one's judgment and expertise. Nurse educators can help patients see how learning certain information can improve their quality of life.

6. "Forgetting proceeds rapidly at first—then more and more slowly; recall shortly after learning reduces the amount forgotten" (Watson, p. 254). Even when the material to be learned is meaningful, we forget much too quickly to make any of us happy. However, we can reduce the amount of forgetting by manipulating the information and applying it soon after the time of initial learning. For example, learners should be encouraged to study each night the class material learned that day. There is probably no better way to help fix it in memory.

7. "Learning from reading is facilitated more by time spent recalling what has been read than by rereading" (Watson, p. 255). Simply rereading is a passive endeavor. However, recalling information forces us to construct a memory and makes us use the information in an active way.

8. "The best way to help pupils form a general concept is to present the concept in numerous ways and varied situations, contrasting experiences with and without the concept, then to encourage precise formulations of the general idea and its application in situations different from those in which the concept was learned" (Watson, p. 255). We teach many concepts in nursing education. Take the concept of *priority setting*. For the newly licensed nurse, setting priorities can be difficult. During orientation, it may help to give examples of a typical day of setting priorities from the standpoint of a staff nurse, a unit manager, and a patient. Demonstrate how priorities differ in these varied situations and discuss how things can turn out wrong if priorities are not set carefully.

9. "When children or adults experience too much frustration, their behavior ceases to be integrated, purposeful, and rational. Blindly they act out their rage, discouragement or withdrawal. The threshold of what is 'too much' varies; it is lowered by previous failures" (Watson, p. 255). Have you ever tried to teach a patient colostomy care and have a number of things go wrong? Maybe the patient had trouble viewing the stoma or keeping the colostomy bag in place, or a full bag empties onto his lap. These kinds of mishaps on top of previous frustrations in the postoperative period can be "too much" for some people. They say they are giving up, or they become angry or start to cry. Understanding and compassionate guidance can make all the difference in the learning outcome.

10. "No school subjects are markedly superior to others for 'strengthening mental powers.' General improvement as a result of study in any subject depends on instruction designed to build up generalizations about principles, concept formation, and improvements of techniques of study, thinking, and communication" (Watson, p. 256). Requiring nursing students to take chemistry or calculus out of the belief that it will help them think more scientifically or will increase their memory abilities will not work. If science or math teachers spend time teaching students how to solve problems or analyze situations or how to apply learned principles in new situations, then "mental powers" may be strengthened. The same is true, however, for nursing courses. Although nursing content, like other course content, will not in itself improve mental skills, nurse educators may help students learn more effectively by helping them with study and memory techniques and with practice in problem-solving and logical thinking.

11. "What is learned is most likely to be available for use if it is learned in a situation much like that in which it is to be used and immediately preceding the time when it is needed" (Watson, p. 256). The proposition that people should learn subject matter in a situation much like that in which it will be used lends support to the teaching method of simulation. Written or laboratory simulations place the content in a clinical context that, although not as complex as the real world, helps learners see how the information actually can be applied.

12. "Children (and adults even more) . . . remember new information which confirms their previous attitudes better than they remember new information which runs counter to their previous attitudes" (Watson, p. 256). Nursing students or nursing aides enter nursing with values and attitudes that may contradict the values of the profession or the nurse educator. Those entering the field may not accept the values they are being taught, and they may resist learning information that doesn't fit with their existing schema. For instance, some students or aides may have little interest in or concern for the elderly. Lecture material about the needs and problems of the elderly may have little effect on this person unless he or she can first be brought to feel empathy for the elderly and interest in them as a group. Changing attitudes is not an easy task, but it is possible to do so with techniques such as providing positive clinical experiences with the elderly or assigning groups of learners to work together on interesting assignments to uncover the problems or interests of the elderly. The following chapters will provide some insight into teaching strategies that are helpful in changing attitudes.

13. "Adults need to know why they need to learn something before undertaking to learn it" (Knowles, Holton, & Swanson, p. 64). In nursing, this proposition presents little problem. Nurses and patients can easily be led to see how the material they are being asked to learn will apply to their professional or personal lives. It is a good idea to begin a class by helping learners to see how the information will fit into a real-life setting.

Application of these 13 propositions of learning along with the unique viewpoints of the various schools of educational psychology will enable the nurse educator to be effective in achieving the goals of instruction. They can aid in understanding not only how people learn, but also why they sometimes act the way they do and why certain teaching strategies work in a particular situation while other strategies do not.

Types of Learning

There is yet another classic work that will provide insight into learning processes. This classic work is Gagne's *Conditions of Learning* (1970). Gagne delineated a hierarchy of eight types of learning. I will quickly describe all eight types and then focus in more depth on the most complex type—problem solving.

Signal Learning

The first type of learning is *signal learning*, or the conditioned response. On this simplest level of learning, the person develops a general diffuse reaction to a stimulus. For example, a nursing aide student may feel fear every time the term *skill test* is mentioned because he or she has felt fear whenever taking an actual skill test. Because of the association, just the term *skill test* is enough to evoke fear. The words have become the signal that elicits the response.

Stimulus–Response Learning

Stimulus–response learning involves developing a voluntary response to a specific stimulus or combination of stimuli. An example of stimulus–response learning is the nursing student learning to monitor an intravenous infusion. Initially, the instructor may tell the learner, "If you see that an intravenous infusion is not dripping, first open the clamp farther." Eventually, the learner responds automatically to an intravenous line that is not running by opening the clamp before doing anything else. This behavior can also occur at a higher conscious level of learning, but the simple, almost automatic muscular reaction of reaching out and opening the clamp can be a simple stimulus–response sequence.

Chaining

Chaining is the acquisition of a series of related conditioned responses or stimulus–response connections. After learning to open the clamp farther if an intravenous line is not dripping, the nursing student is taught that if opening the clamp is not successful, checking the line for a return blood flow is in order. This second step becomes another automatic response in a chain of responses.

Verbal Association

Verbal association is really a type of chaining and is easily recognized in the process of learning medical terminology. A nurse's aide already knows that the word *thermal* refers to temperature. The instructor introduces the word hyperthermia and its definition. The aide recognizes that the syllable *therm,* connects the two words, and thus finds it easier to learn the new term because of a previous association.

Discrimination Learning

A great deal can be learned through forming large numbers of stimulus–response or verbal chains. However, the more new chains that are learned, the easier it is to forget previous chains. To learn and retain large numbers of chains, the person has to be able to discriminate among them. This process is called *discrimination learning.* For instance, a nurse practitioner student tries to learn a long list of drugs and their actions. Halfway down the list, the learning of new chains interferes with the memory for old ones. If the student can find a means of discriminating between the drugs, maybe finding something unique or noteworthy about each, retention will be increased.

Concept Learning

Concept learning is learning how to classify stimuli into groups represented by a common concept. People learn many concepts as they go through life. They learn concepts ranging from *up* and *down* to *near* and *far* to *justice* and *democracy.* When they encounter the health care field, they learn new concepts. A patient with a chronic wound infection who has to learn to empty a drain and change a dressing has to learn about the concepts of *infection* and *inflammation* and the concept of *asepsis.* This person learns to see symptoms like redness, swelling, and yellow drainage as being stimuli that are grouped together under the concept of infection.

Rule Learning

A *rule* can be considered a chain of concepts or a relationship between concepts. If you were a home care nurse teaching a wife to prevent decubitus ulcers in her post-stroke husband, you would have to teach the rule that expresses the relationship between pressure and ulceration. Rules are generally expressed as "If . . . then" relationships. So, you would teach the wife that "If you leave your husband in one position too long, the pressure on a body part can cause ulceration." She might also need to learn the rule that "If your husband does not eat a balanced diet, he will be more prone to ulceration." Rule learning is a fairly sophisticated level of learning. Some people do fine at the lower levels up through discrimination and concept learning, but they have more difficulty learning and applying rules. If a learner does not learn and truly comprehend a lot of rules in a particular area of study, she or he will have difficulty with the highest level of learning called *problem solving.*

Problem Solving

To solve problems, the learner must have a clear idea of the problem or goal being sought and must be able to recall and apply previously learned rules that relate to the situation. If you were teaching a nurse refresher course for RNs and wanted to explore the problem of noso-comial urinary infections in patients with indwelling catheters, you might ask the nurses to recall any rules they know that apply to this type of situation. They would probably be able to recall rules like "a break in aseptic technique can lead to infection"; "a break in a closed ster-ile system can lead to the entry of pathogens"; and "raising a catheter above the level of the bladder can cause backflow of urine and therefore infection." By combining these rules, the nurses could develop a higher-order rule like "a break in a closed sterile system with break in aseptic technique, or backflow of urine into the bladder can lead to infection." This new higher-order rule would now be available for use in similar situations in the future, without having to start over with basic problem solving each time the situation is encountered.

Another way of viewing problem solving is as a process of formulating and testing hypotheses. A learner, confronted with a problem, begins to formulate hypotheses, a process analogous to combining recalled rules to form a higher-order rule. The hypotheses are then mentally tested and accepted, rejected, or modified.

An educator can teach and model the problem-solving process. An example of how a nursing student might use problem solving might be helpful at this point. Suppose the stu-dent is planning care for a patient who has been stabilized after an extensive myocardial infarction but is still on bedrest. As the instructor, you ask the learner how he or she is going to prevent muscle weakness in this patient yet also prevent strain on the heart. The problem has now been identified. The student will recall rules that relate to exercise, muscle tone, and strength and will remember that passive isotonic exercise puts the least demands on the cir-culatory system, making it relatively safe for the stabilized myocardial infarction patient to maintain some muscle strength. The student will then test the solution in actual practice. He or she has now learned a solution to this exact problem and related problems and will prob-ably be able to recall the solution in future situations. If the learner had simply been told the solution, problem solving would not have taken place; the learner might not have truly understood the concepts involved and might not have retained the information.

You, as the nurse educator, play an important role in problem-solving learning. First, you can help the student to define the problem and the goal. You may simply state the prob-lem or help the student put it into words by verbal coaching. You should be fairly certain at this point that the student has already learned the concepts and rules that will be needed to solve the problem. In the second step, you help the student recall the necessary rules by means of questions, suggestions, or demonstration.

Returning to the problem of the cardiac patient on bedrest, let me illustrate how the teacher could help the learner through the problem-solving process, allowing the learner to reach the solution:

Teacher: What is Mr. X's activity order?
Learner: He's on bedrest, but he can bathe and feed himself.
Teacher: Why is he on bedrest?
Learner: Because the doctor ordered it.
Teacher: I meant, why did the physician write that order?
Learner: I guess so that Mr. X's heart can rest.
Teacher: Good. There shouldn't be any strain on his heart muscle. But while his myocardium is resting, what is happening to the rest of the muscles of his body?

Learner: They're resting too—getting weak.

Teacher: Yes. Is there anything we can do to prevent the skeletal muscles from getting any weaker, yet not put strain on his heart muscle?

Learner: Maybe he could do isometric exercise—that doesn't cause much movement.

Teacher: It doesn't cause much movement because the muscle fibers don't shorten, but it does cause other physiologic effects.

Learner: I remember now. Isometric exercise raises blood pressure.

Teacher: Right! It not only raises blood pressure, it also increases cardiac output.

Learner: Well, we can't do that. (Pause) Could he do range-of-motion exercise?

Teacher: What kind of exercise is range of motion—what classification?

Learner: It's isotonic exercise. The muscles move and the fibers shorten.

Teacher: Yes, they move, but they actually require less oxygen than isometric exercise.

Learner: I guess Mr. X could do active range of motion of his arms because he is allowed to wash and feed himself. What about his legs?

Teacher: You can check with the physician about how much leg exercise Mr. X should do.

In this example, the teacher led the learner through the problem-solving process, aiding in the recall of principles and rules, helping the student think clearly and to arrive at a goal. Students who can recall principles and rules independently do not need this much guidance from the instructor in arriving at a solution. Individual differences among students affect their ability to learn through problem solving (Gagne, 1970). A student who has learned a large repertoire of rules is more likely to have access to some rules that will apply to the situation at hand. But students also vary in their ability to recall those rules. Gagne also notes differences in *concept distinctiveness* among students; that is, some students are more able to select useful and relevant concepts that will help to define and solve the problem. Students may also differ in their ability to combine rules into hypotheses and to apply specific solutions to a general class of problems. These intellectual and creativity factors account for why some students do so well at problem solving while others find it a struggle.

Learning Styles

Research into learning styles or cognitive styles has been conducted for decades. The topic is of interest to the fields of psychology and education because we observe that people learn in uniquely different ways. Some of us are global thinkers and some are analytic; some prefer to learn from auditory sources and some from visual sources; some process information actively and some reflectively; some like to learn independently and some in groups (Anderson, 2001). These kinds of preferences make us wonder if there is indeed a formula for learning in the brains of children and adults. In the 1970s and 1980s, when research into learning styles became popular, the term *cognitive style* was most frequently used. Newer theorists tend to use the term *learning style* because they believe more is involved than just cognitive style; learning style includes physiologic, affective, and cognitive styles (Thompson & Crutchlow, 1993). Today, the terms *cognitive style* and *learning style* are often used synonymously. There are as many definitions of learning style (or cognitive style) as there are articles written on the subject. For our purposes, I will define learning style as the habitual manner in which learners receive and perceive information, process it, understand it, value it, store it, and recall it.

Why should researchers bother to study learning styles; how can this knowledge benefit us? Because we hope that if we understand the way individuals learn, we can intervene when they are having difficulty, or we can enhance effective learning to make it even better. Many schools today test students' learning styles and base their remediation programs on those styles. For example, a student is having difficulty in learning a body of knowledge or a skill while in a classroom setting. Testing reveals that the student deals with information in a very concrete and analytical way, yet the class material is very abstract and the teacher is teaching it with a broad conceptual approach. Remediation will attempt to help this student make this abstract material more concrete in his own mind, perhaps with diagrams, examples or stories. If students become aware of their own learning styles, they can be helped to learn how to learn (Flannery, 1993).

Learning Style Models

There are dozens of learning style models and instruments to measure them. I will discuss three of the most commonly used, especially in nursing. First, though, I will elaborate on the basic concepts of cognitive style that cross the boundaries of many of the models. These concepts include wholistic versus analytic thinking, and verbal versus visual representation.

Holistic (or global) thinkers want to get the whole picture quickly, or get the gist of things. They want to see broad categories before they look at details. They process information simultaneously rather than in a step-by-step manner, and they need to see how new information connects to what they already know and value. They retain an overall or global view of information. Analytic thinkers, on the other hand, process the details of a picture, outlining the component parts in a logical progression. They perceive information in an objective manner and do not need to connect it to their personal values or experiences (Flannery, 1993).

People who have a habitual verbal approach to learning represent, in their brains, information they read, see, or hear in terms of words or verbal associations. Those with a visual approach experience information they read, see, or hear in terms of mental pictures or images (Sadler-Smith & Riding, 1999).

It is important to understand that these concepts are not dichotomies but rather continuums. No one is a purely holistic learner and not at all analytic and vice versa, and no one is a totally verbal learner and not visual and vice versa. These concepts weave together, along with other factors, as we see in the following models.

Kolb's Theory of Experiential Learning

Kolb's model depicts learning as a four-stage cycle beginning with an *immediate concrete experience* during which the person makes *observations* and *reflections*. Then the person develops an *abstract theory* from which he or she develops ideas on how to proceed. Finally, the person *actively experiments* with actions to test them out. Kolb then hypothesized that learners need four abilities in order to be effective:

1. Concrete experience (CE) abilities: Learning from actual experience
2. Reflective observation (RO) abilities: Learning by observing others
3. Abstract conceptualization (AC) abilities: Creating theories to explain what is seen
4. Active experimentation (AE) abilities: Using theories to solve problems

He states that these four abilities or modes of learning occur on two continuums—the abstract conceptualization to concrete experience continuum (or thinking versus feeling) and the active experimentation to reflective observation (external versus internal) continuum (Truluck & Courtenay, 1999). Most people tend toward a pattern of preference of one bipolar opposite over the other, resulting in their unique learning style. Kolb identified four possible learning styles based on the above concepts (see Figure 2–2):

1. *Converger:* A person who learns by abstract conceptualization (AC) and active experimentation (AE). This person is good at decision making and problem solving and likes dealing with technical work rather than interpersonal relationships.
2. *Diverger:* A person who stresses concrete experience (CE) and reflective observation (RO). This person excels in imagination and awareness of meaning. He or she is feeling oriented and people oriented and likes working in groups.
3. *Accommodator:* A person who relies heavily on concrete experience (CE) and active experimentation (AE). He or she likes to actively accomplish things, often using trial-and-error methods to solve problems. This person may be impatient with other people. He or she acts on intuition and is a risk taker.
4. *Assimilator:* A person who emphasizes abstract conceptualization (AC) and reflective observation (RO). The strengths of this person are in inductive reasoning, creating theoretical models, and integrating ideas. He or she prefers playing with ideas

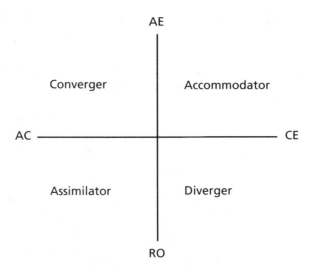

FIGURE 2-2 Kolb's Learning Styles

to actively applying them. This person is more concerned with ideas than people (Linares, 1999).

Kolb developed a Learning Style Inventory (LSI), which was originally a 9-item questionnaire, and is now a 12-item tool with sentence completion items. This inventory is the one that has been used most frequently in measuring learning styles of nursing students (DeCoux, 1990).

Gregorc Cognitive Styles Model

Gregorc hypothesized that the mind has the mediation abilities of *perception* and *ordering;* that is, the perception and ordering of knowledge affects how the person learns. Perception ability, or the way you grasp incoming stimuli, is on a continuum ranging from *abstractness* to *concreteness*. Ordering ability, or the way you arrange and systematize incoming stimuli, is on a continuum from *sequence* to *randomness* (Seidel & England, 1999). Gregorc states that everyone processes information in all four of the dimensions, but they have a preference for one end or the other on the perception and ordering continuums. The preferences fall into what he called the four mediation channels (see Figure 2–3):

1. Concrete sequential (CS)
2. Concrete random (CR)
3. Abstract sequential (AS)
4. Abstract random (AR)

Concrete sequential learners like highly structured, quiet learning environments and do not like being interrupted. They often focus on details, they like concrete learning materials, especially those that are visual, and they may interpret words literally. *Concrete random* learn-

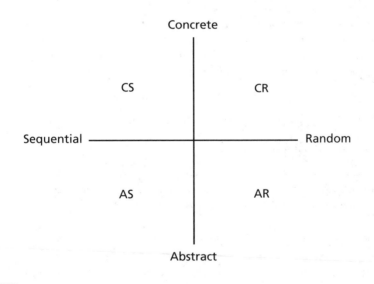

FIGURE 2-3 Gregorc's Cognitive Styles Model

ers are intuitive, use trial-and-error methods, and look for alternatives. They tend to order new information mentally into a three-dimensional pattern. *Abstract sequential* learners are holistic thinkers who seek understanding of incoming information. They need consistency in the learning environment and do not like interruptions. They have good verbal skills and are logical and rational. *Abstract random* learners think holistically and benefit greatly from visual stimuli. They like busy, unstructured learning environments and are often focused on personal relationships (Wells & Higgs, 1990).

Gregorc developed the Gregorc Style Delineator, a self-report inventory. There are 10 columns on the inventory and each contains four words. The subject chooses the word that best describes him or her. After completing the selection of words, the scores are added to get a subscore for each of the four learning styles. The highest score indicates the preferred learning style.

Field Independence/Dependence Model

This cognitive style model is associated primarily with Herman Witkin, who conducted a large body of research into these concepts. Witkin identified a continuum of perception that ranges from a *field-independent* style in which items are perceived relatively independently of their surrounding field, and a *field-dependent* style in which a person has difficulty perceiving items aside from their surrounding field (Witkin, 1976). The field-dependent style is more global (seeing the whole more than the parts) while the field-independent style is more analytical (seeing the parts more than the whole). Witkin found that this learning style is fairly stable over the years and that women and girls in Western cultures tend to be more field dependent than men and boys. Table 2–2 highlights the learning style differences between people on two ends of the continuum (Cleverly, 1994; Witkin, 1976). It must be kept in mind, however, that few people fall at the far ends of the continuum.

Several tests have been developed to measure field independence/field dependence. The easiest to use in an educational setting is the Embedded Figures Test. In this test, the person looks simultaneously at a simple figure and a complex figure in which the simple figure is embedded. The person is asked to find the simple figure within the complex figure. For field-independent people, the simple figure seems to jump out of the complex figure. Field-dependent people have difficulty finding the embedded simple figure.

TABLE 2–2 Differences Between Field-Independent and Field-Dependent Learning Styles

Field Independent	Field Dependent
1. Mathematical reasoning may be strong	1. More difficulty with mathematical reasoning
2. Analyzes the elements of a situation	2. Analyzes the whole picture; less able to analyze the elements
3. Recognizes and recalls details	3. Does not perceive details
4. More task oriented	4. More people oriented
5. Forms attitudes independently	5. Attitudes guided by authority figures or peer group
6. More pronounced self-identity	6. See themselves as others see them

Matching Learning Styles to Instruction

Research results are inconclusive about the effectiveness of matching teaching style to learning styles. Some studies have shown increased levels of student *achievement* when the learner's style was matched with a similar teaching style; some have not. Some studies have shown more student *satisfaction* when the teacher matches the student's learning style, but some have not (Cleverly, 1994; Cranston, 1985; Seidel & England, 1999; Thompson & Crutchlow, 1993).

There are obvious feasibility and even ethical issues that come into play in this discussion. How can a classroom teacher match the learning style of every student in the class? How many teachers are testing their students to even know what the learning styles are? Is it good for students to settle into one learning style and not be encouraged to expand their repertoire? Should matching be done only in remedial learning settings?

Many experts support the position that although students have preferred learning styles, they can be helped to work on developing other learning styles (Cleverly, 1994; Flannery, 1993; Grasha & Yangarber-Hicks, 2000; Reynolds, 1997). Helping students to diversify their learning styles will serve them well over time as they encounter a variety of learning environments. At the same time, teachers should be encouraged to use a variety of teaching strategies so that various students' learning needs may be addressed.

How Useful Is Learning Style Theory?

Many professionals are skeptical about the usefulness of learning style theory at this point in its development. There is neither a clear agreed-upon definition of learning styles nor a unifying theory behind learning style research (Thompson & Crutchlow, 1993; Truluck & Courtenay, 1999). As one author states, "different researchers pursue their own pet distinctions in cheerful disregard of one another" (Thompson & Crutchlow, 1993, p. 36). The lack of clarity and commonality makes it difficult to extricate principles or draw any generalizations. There are over 100 instruments to measure learning styles, 20 of which are generally well known (James & Blank, 1993; Reynolds, 1997), but none of which seem to unify all aspects of the concepts in the literature. Also, repeated research done using the same instruments seems to yield inconsistent results.

What conclusion can be drawn then? Should we forget about learning styles? Most educators and psychologists would probably say that we should continue to investigate this field, because there seems to be a nugget of truth in there somewhere. Further studies may find it.

CASE STUDY

A nursing student has been earning low grades on her examinations in a Parent–Child Nursing course. She tells you, the instructor, that she studies "all the time," but it doesn't seem to help.

1. What factors would you assess in this situation?
2. What questions would you ask her?
3. Would it help to test her learning style?
4. Based on your assessment, what initial steps might you suggest that would help her?

CRITICAL THINKING EXERCISES

A young diabetic patient is having difficulty maintaining a controlled blood sugar if he has any changes from his daily routine. For example, if he is nauseated and cannot eat usual meals, he doesn't compensate with "sick-day diets." If he exercises more than usual on the weekend, he has trouble keeping his blood sugar stable.

1. How can you determine if the cause of the problem is lack of motivation, lack of knowledge, or lack of adaptive abilities?
2. Since part of the difficulty seems to be lack of problem solving, which of the following might be a root cause?
   a. He doesn't know enough rules to apply to the situation.
   b. He cannot formulate and test hypotheses.
   c. He cannot transfer information he was taught.
3. How would you help this young man think through the handling of those days when he has problems and assist him to do a better job of problem solving?

IDEAS FOR FURTHER RESEARCH

1. Conduct a qualitative study of how nursing students learn might yield valuable information. Interview students and ask them how they approach learning situations. What do they find helpful to maximize their learning? Do they sense preferences in themselves for the way they begin to learn something?
2. Evaluate a curriculum. On what learning theories does the curriculum seem to be built? What types of learning are supposed to take place? Do the learning activities mesh with the anticipated types of learning?
3. Research the extent to which transfer of learning takes place in an orientation program for new staff. What concepts or activities included in the didactic portion of the orientation program are observed being carried out in the clinical portion? If they are not being transferred, why does the orientee think he or she is not doing so?

REFERENCES

Adams, E., DeYoung, S., & Just, G. (1997). Metacognitive strategies used by nursing students who are good and poor readers. *Journal of Nursing Science, 2*(3–4), 73–82.

Anderson, J. (2001). Tailoring assessment to student learning styles. *AAHE Bulletin, 53*(7), 3–7.

Atkinson, R. C., & Shiffrin, R. M. (1968). Human memory: A proposed system and its control processes. In K. W. Spence & J. T. Spence (Eds.), *The psychology of learning and motivation* (pp. 89–195). New York: Academic Press.

Ausubel, D. P. (1963). Cognitive structure and the facilitation of meaningful verbal learning. *Journal of Teacher Education, 14,* 217–221.

Bandura, A. (1977). *Social learning theory.* Englewood Cliffs, NJ: Prentice Hall.

Beitz, J. M. (1996). Metacognition: State-of-the-art learning theory implications for clinical nursing education. *Holistic Nursing Practice, 10*(3), 23–32.

Bolles, E. B. (1988). *Remembering and forgetting: An inquiry into the nature of memory.* New York: Walker and Company.

Brandt, B. L. (1996). Cognitive learning theory and continuing health professions education. *The Journal of Continuing Education in the Health Professions, 16,* 197–202.

Breur, J. (1993). The mind's journey from novice to expert. *American Educator, 17,* 6–15, 38–46.

Brookfield, S. (1995). Adult learning: An overview. Retrieved November 5, 2001, from the World Wide Web, *http://nlu.nl.edu/ace/Resources/Documents/AdultLearning.html.*

Brown, A. L., & Palinscar, A. S. (1987). Reciprocal teaching of comprehension strategies: A natural history of one program for enhancing learning. In J. D. Day & J. G. Borkowski (Eds.), *Intelligence and exceptionality: New directions for theory, assessment, and instructional practices* (pp. 81–132). Norwood, NJ: Ablex.

Cleverly, K. (1994). Learning styles of students: Development of an eclectic model. *International Journal of Nursing Studies, 31*(5), 437–450.

Cranston, C. M., & McCort, B. (1985). A learner analysis experiment: Cognitive style versus learning style in undergraduate nursing education. *Journal of Nursing Education, 24*(4), 136–138.

Cust, J. (1995). Recent cognitive perspectives on learning—implications for nursing education. *Nurse Education Today, 15,* 280–290.

DeCoux, V. M. (1990). Kolb's learning style inventory: A review of its applications in nursing research. *Journal of Nursing Education, 29*(5), 202–207.

Feden, P. D. (1994). About instruction: Powerful new strategies worth knowing. *Educational Horizons, 73,* 18–24.

Flannery, D. D. (1993). Global and analytical ways of processing information. In D. D. Flannery (Ed.), *Applying cognitive learning theory to adult learning.* San Fransisco: Jossey-Bass.

Gagne, R. M (1970). *Conditions of learning.* New York: Holt, Rinehart and Winston.

Galbraith, M. W. (1991). *Facilitating adult learning.* Malabar, FL: Krieger Publishing.

Glaser, R. (1984). Education and thinking: The role of knowledge. *American Psychologist, 39*(2), 93–104.

Gordon, B. (1995). *Memory: Remembering and forgetting in everyday life.* New York: Mastermedia Limited.

Grasha, A. F., & Yangarber-Hicks, N. (2000). Integrating teaching styles and learning styles with instructional technology. *College Teaching, 48*(1), 2–10.

Hill, W. F. (1971). *Learning: A survey of psychological interpretations.* Scranton: Chandler Publishing Co.

Huitt, W. (2000). The information processing approach. Retrieved November 5, 2001, from the World Wide Web, *http://chiron.valdosta.edu/whuitt/col/cogsys/infoproc.html.*

James, W. B., & Blank, W. E. (1993). Review and critique of available learning-style instruments for adults. In D. D. Flannery (Ed.), *Applying cognitive learning theory to adult learning.* San Fransisco: Jossey-Bass.

Knowles, M. (1984). *The adult learner: A neglected species.* Houston: Gulf Publishing.

Knowles, M., Holton, E. F., & Swanson, R. A. (1998). *The adult learner* (5th ed.). Woburn, MA: Butterworth-Heinemann.

Lauder, W., Reynolds, W., & Angus, N. (1999). Transfer of knowledge and skills: Some implications for nursing and nursing education. *Nurse Education Today, 19*(6), 480–487.

Leamnson, R. (2000). Learning as a biological brain change. *Change, 32*(6), 34–40.

Linares, A. Z. (1999). Learning styles of students and faculty in selected health care professions. *Journal of Nursing Education, 38*(9), 407–414.

Reynolds, M. (1997). Learning styles: A critique. *Management Learning, 28*(2), 115–133.

Rosenstock, I. M., Strecher, V. J., & Becker, M. H. (1988). Social learning theory and the health belief model. *Health Education Quarterly, 15*(2), 175–183.

Rumelhart, D. E. (1980). Schemata: The building blocks of cognition. In R. J. Spiro, B. C. Bruce, & W. F. Brewer (Eds.), *Theoretical issues in reading comprehension: Perspectives from cognitive psychology, linguistics, artificial intelligence, and education* (pp. 33–58). Hillsdale, NJ: Lawrence Erlbaum Associates.

Sadler-Smith, E., & Riding, R. (1999). Cognitive style and instructional preferences. *Instructional Science, 27*(5), 355–371.

Seidel. L. E., & England, E. M. (1999). Gregorc's cognitive styles: College students' preferences for teaching methods and testing techniques. *Perceptual and Motor Skills, 88*, 859–875.

Shuell, T. J. (1986). Cognitive conceptions of learning. *Review of Educational Research, 56*(4), 411–436.

Thompson, C., & Crutchlow, E. (1993). Learning style research: A critical review of the literature and implications for nursing education. *Journal of Professional Nursing, 9*(1), 34–40.

Truluck, J. E., & Courtenay, B. C. (1999). Learning style preferences among older adults. *Educational Gerontology, 25*(3), 221–236.

Voss, J. F. (1987). Learning and transfer in subject-matter learning: A problem solving model. *International Journal of Educational Research, 11*, p. 607–622.

Watson, G. (1960). What psychology can we feel sure about? *Teachers College Record, 61*(5), 253–257.

Wells, D., & Higgs, Z. R. (1990). Learning styles and learning preferences of first and fourth semester baccalaureate degree nursing students. *Journal of Nursing Education, 29*(9), 385–390.

White, W. F. (1997). Why students can't remember: The problem of forgetting. *Journal of Instructional Psychology, 24*(2), 140–143.

Witkin, H. A. (1976). Cognitive style in academic performance and in teacher–student relations. In S. Messick (Ed.), *Individuality in learning* (pp. 38–72). San Francisco: Jossey-Bass.

3

Planning and Conducting Classes

The most formidable task a new teacher may face is the planning of classes. Even with a well-developed curriculum in place, the novice instructor must decide:

> What should I include in each class and what should I leave out?
> What methods should I use in the classroom?
> How do I know how long it will take to teach this amount of material?
> How can I keep learners interested and make sure they learn?

It is not only new teachers who face such questions; all teachers have to deal with planning classes in such a way that they help meet curricular objectives and individual student learning needs, while keeping intellectually stimulated, even if you have taught the same information many times over. In this chapter I propose some helpful hints for both planning and conducting classes, based on research findings and on my own experience. Much of the material in this chapter applies to patient education (especially groups of patients), staff development, and academic teaching. Some of the material, especially the information on planning assignments and choosing textbooks, applies mainly to academic settings, and application to those settings will be made clear in the following pages.

The Planning Sequence

Before you enter a classroom, you must do a tremendous amount of planning. You need to formulate objectives, select and organize content, choose teaching methods, and design assignments. You also have to decide how you are going to evaluate learning. Ideally, you will complete all these steps before beginning to teach the first class. In reality, time constraints may force you to continue with class preparation even after the course has begun. For your own sanity and the sake of the learners, stay at least a few steps ahead of the learners. However, even if your class preparation is ongoing, your planning of objectives, content, and evaluation methods should be completed before the course begins.

Developing a Course Outline or Syllabus

Whether you are teaching in an academic, inservice, or patient education setting, a course outline or syllabus should always accompany a course. The information included in the outline may vary by setting and institution. As a general guideline, the course outline should include the name of the course, the name of the instructor, a one-paragraph course description, and a list of course objectives. You may also wish to include a topical outline, the teaching methods to be used, the textbook or other readings, and the methods of evaluation, if appropriate. A course outline helps learners to gauge just what is to be learned and what is expected of them.

A course outline or syllabus is considered a contract between teacher and learners. Whatever you say you are going to do in the outline, follow through with it. If you say you are going to cover four objectives, do it. If you list three methods of evaluating learning, use them. To protect yourself legally, you may also include a statement at the end of the outline that states changes in course material or evaluation may be necessary at times, but that the learners will be notified in writing of any changes.

Formulating Objectives

You will need to write the course objectives for the course outline or syllabus, and you will need objectives for each class. All nurses are familiar with objectives and goals in relation to patient care, and probably all have received reams of objectives written by professors in college courses. However, not all objectives are readable and useful. Some seem much too broad and some too specific. You should try to write objectives that have meaning not just for you but also for the learners. They should reflect what the learner is supposed to do with what is taught (Holmes, 1990).

THE VALUE OF OBJECTIVES

Why do you need objectives? First, you need them to guide your selection and handling of course materials. If your assignment is to teach a class on mental defense mechanisms, decide what you want the students to learn about such mechanisms before you outline your content. Once you have settled on your objectives, the content should flow naturally and easily from them.

Second, you need objectives to help you determine whether people in the class have learned what you have tried to teach. You may have several vague ideas about what you would like the learners to know about defense mechanisms, but unless you have specific objectives, your teaching and your evaluation of their learning may miss the mark. Your objectives should be specific enough that they enable you to know what the learners will say, do, or think if they have learned this material. Because of the focus on the expected behaviors at the end of the class or course, educational objectives are sometimes called learning outcomes (Houlden & Collier, 1999).

Third, objectives are essential from the learners' perspective. They need to know more about a course than they can get from a course description or a list of course content. They must receive objectives that communicate clearly what they will be expected to know and do with the course material. If tests are given in a course, the objectives should guide the students in their studying. For example, in a course on psychological reactions to stress and illness, a session might be devoted to mental defense mechanisms. If the students have only a list of class topics, they will be unprepared for studying specifics about defense mechanisms. They will not know what material they will be held responsible for unless the teacher spends a lot of time before each test explaining just that. Suppose, however, that the learners are provided with objectives such as these:

1. Explain the rationale for people's use of defense mechanisms.
2. Analyze in a given situation which defense mechanisms are being used by an individual.

In this case, the students will know more specifically what types of knowledge and skills are expected of them.

Objectives for a course are naturally broader than class objectives. The number of course objectives usually varies from 5 to 15. In addition to appearing in the course outline or syllabus, they should be discussed in the first class session so learners are immediately clear about what they will be expected to learn.

Course objectives should be designed to be achievable by most or all learners in the class; they may be viewed as minimal competencies. It is the instructor's duty to plan learning experiences that will enable learners to meet the objectives. If the objectives are unrealistic, either because the teacher's expectations are too high or because the needed learning experiences are inaccessible, they are worthless.

TAXONOMY OF OBJECTIVES

Bloom (1984) developed a taxonomy of educational objectives. He identified three learning domains: cognitive (knowing), psychomotor (doing), and affective (feeling, valuing). One of the challenges of writing good course objectives is making the objectives in each domain measurable. It is relatively easy to write objectives and measure learning in the cognitive and psychomotor domains. In the cognitive domain you can measure knowledge, comprehension, application, analysis, synthesis, and evaluation (categories in Bloom's Taxonomy) by using written or oral tests. For example, you might say the learner will "decide how much insulin to take (or give) depending on the number of carbohydrates consumed." This objective could be measured by presenting the learner with a written case about a diabetic who is using carbohydrate counting as a method of determining insulin doses and ask the learner to calculate the insulin dose based on the situation.

In the psychomotor domain you can observe what learners are actually doing when they perform a skill. Learners can demonstrate what they have learned and you can rate their performance. An objective in the psychomotor domain may state that the learner will "correctly mix two types of insulin in one syringe." The teacher can observe the person drawing up the insulin to see if the performance meets the stated criteria.

Objectives in the affective domain are not so easy to write and measure. Many educators avoid writing objectives related to beliefs, attitudes, and values. The reasons given are that it is very difficult to write test questions that measure the affective domain, and that you cannot readily observe whether students, nurses, or patients have accepted the beliefs and values inherent in the health care professions, and even if you could, the process is rather subjective. Yet, the danger is that if we don't write and attempt to measure such objectives, we may forget about teaching the beliefs and values that are so important in nursing, especially those in the American Nurses Association's (ANA's) Code for Nurses and ANA Social Policy Statement. Maier-Lorentz (1999) suggests that educators can infer attitudes or feelings from what is observed. For example, if a student is reluctant to share with her classmates something a patient has told her, the educator could infer that the student understands the principle of confidentiality. Objectives can be written in the affective domain for both classroom and clinical settings. An example of an affective objective that can be measured by a written assignment is "defends in writing the refusal of a nurse to divulge confidential information given by a patient." An example of an affective objective that can be measured in a clinical setting is "accepts responsibility for identifying one's own learning needs" (Andrusyszyn, 1989). Although it may be difficult to capture the full flavor of the affective domain in a behavioral objective, it is better to try than to abandon the effort.

WORDING OF OBJECTIVES

Course objectives (as opposed to class objectives) may be fairly broad in order to keep the list a manageable length. For example, consider the objective "Recognizes the parameters of effective hemodialysis." This course objective is quite broad and not directly measurable; the implication is that this objective could be measured, however, either by a written or an oral test or in clinical practice. Some educators with a behaviorist philosophy believe that an objective is incomplete unless it contains the intended learner, the behavior to be performed, the conditions under which it is to be performed, and the expected degree of attainment of specific standards (Cummings, 1994; Ferguson, 1998). An example of this type of detailed objective is "The nurse will list and explain, with 95 percent accuracy, the parameters by which effective hemodialysis is measured." Many educators believe this degree of structure and detail is not necessary in course objectives, but may use detailed objectives like this for each class within a course. Note the action verbs *list* and *explain* in the last objective. See Table 3–1 for a partial listing of behavioral verbs that can be used in writing objectives.

Individual class session objectives are usually few—only three to five per class session. They may be written and distributed to the learners on a weekly basis, or they may be presented verbally or on an overhead transparency at the beginning of a session. Class objectives are invaluable in helping the teacher to evaluate learning and in helping learners to focus their attention on what the outcomes of their studying should be.

TABLE 3–1 Behavioral Verbs Useful for Writing Objectives

Cognitive Domain	
Knowledge:	Define, delineate, describe, identify, list, name, state
Comprehension:	Classify, discuss, estimate, explain, rephrase, summarize
Application:	Adjust, apply, compute, demonstrate, generate, prove
Analysis:	Analyze, compare, contrast, critique, defend, differentiate
Synthesis:	Create, develop, propose, suggest, write
Evaluation:	Assess, choose, conclude, defend, evaluate, judge
Psychomotor Domain	Arrange, assemble, calibrate, combine, copy, correct, create, demonstrate, execute, handle, manipulate, operate, organize, position, produce, remove, revise, show, solve
Affective Domain	Accept, agree, choose, comply, commit, defend, explain, influence, integrate, recommend, resolve, volunteer

Selecting Content

The general guidelines for course content are usually prescribed by the curriculum of the school, health agency or proprietary agency for which the educator works. Sometimes the only direction the educator is given is the course description, but more often someone's files contain previous course outlines or course objectives to guide the instructor in deciding what to teach. It is generally left to the instructor's discretion to determine exactly what to include on a particular topic and what can safely be skipped over.

Let's imagine that you are responsible for teaching a physical assessment course. You are handed a course description and a list of course objectives indicating that the learners will perform and write a nursing history and complete a physical assessment of each body system. You want to start developing objectives and a content outline for your first class session. The topic is going to be "The value of a good nursing assessment." After you jot down that heading, your pen may come to a stop. How much information should you include, and into how much detail should you go? Several factors can guide your decisions. The first consideration is how much time you can devote to the topic. The content you select will vary greatly if you have 30 minutes or 60 minutes. The second factor is the kind of background the students have. If you are teaching undergraduate students, your approach may be quite different than if you are teaching a refresher course for RNs. Third, if a textbook has already been selected for the course, its depth of content can give you some hints as to what you need to include.

Cramming too much information into a class session is one of the pitfalls some teachers, especially new ones, fall into. Give yourself time to discuss the meaningfulness of the subject and cover important points without getting bogged down in details that the learners will never remember or need a month later. Obviously, some details are necessary, but details such as dates and places when nurses first began performing physical assessments are something learners could probably well do without. It is better to spend your time discussing broad related issues and concepts and have the learners apply the information in some active way in class.

The best way to determine how long it will take you to teach the content is to plan it out and then rehearse it orally (preferably in front of a mirror). Build in time for questions and any active learning techniques you plan to use. You will generally find that the first time you teach a class it will take less time than you planned because you keep up a fast pace to "get it all in." In subsequent classes you are more relaxed, and it may take longer to teach the same material.

Organizing Content

The way in which class content is organized can make all the difference between sessions that are enjoyable and smooth running and those in which students are irritated and grumbling. Lectures, especially, need to be organized. Sharing class objectives with the group sets the stage for an organized lecture. You can indicate, in the progress of your lecture, the headings and subheadings under which you are discussing the subject of the day. Nothing is more distressing than trying to take notes from a lecturer who skips all over a topic with no apparent rhyme or reason. I still retain a vivid memory of a professor who taught one of my research courses. In the space of a two-hour class, this teacher would flit from random sampling to reliability and validity to correlation theory and back to sampling again, apparently unaware that the students were bewildered. We clung to the textbook as a lifeline for the whole semester in order to keep our heads above water and make sense of the research process. If you are in any doubt about the organization of your classes, you can have a colleague sit in on a class and critique that aspect of it, or you can tape the class and attempt to take notes on the content while playing it back. The results should be enlightening.

There are several ways to structure content so that it follows a logical sequence. You can move from generalizations to specifics or vice versa. For example, you may start a preop class for patients by talking about effects of general anesthesia and then mention a few specific anesthetic effects that the patients may experience. Some classes lend themselves to a time sequence structure. An example of this could be the history of nursing research over the past few centuries. You can form a class around problems and solutions or concepts and their applications (McKeachie, 1999).

It is not only lectures that need to be organized. Discussions, role-playing, computer applications, and problem-based learning as well as other strategies also require structure and organization if learning is to proceed smoothly. In a research class I taught, one class involved the use of a statistical computer program. The class began in the regular classroom, then moved to a nearby computer lab, and finally returned to the original classroom. The moving alone necessitated planning and organization. The content also required strict organization lest the class disintegrate into a session of computer games. I began by giving objectives for the day, then reviewed the particular statistical tests we were going to use, and handed out some raw data (in simulation format) that the students would run on the computer. When we went to the computer lab, the challenge was to achieve a balance between allowing students to work at their own pace (in small groups) and maintaining organization by helping each group run the program and understand what they were doing. On the return to the classroom, students had many questions. I attempted to organize my responses by fielding questions pertaining to one aspect of the process at a time. I finished with a summary of how to interpret the printouts. So you see, organization is important to any class session, regardless of methods used.

Selecting Teaching Methods

Deciding which teaching method to use, given the wide assortment available, is not easy. Which method is the best for teaching a certain body of information or learning process? Weston and Cranton (1986) believe that selection of teaching methods is one of the most complex parts of teaching, yet it receives the least attention in instructional planning. It may receive little attention because educators, unless taught otherwise, assume that the way they were taught is the best way to do it. They select strategies with which they are familiar and comfortable, without much thought as to whether those strategies are the most appropriate way to teach the material. For educators who are aware of the many teaching methods available to them, and who wonder which is the best, there are several factors they should consider.

Factors Affecting Choice of Method

First, the selection of method depends on the objectives and type of learning you are trying to achieve. If you want to present facts and rules, a lecture with handouts or a computer tutorial may be appropriate. If you want to mold attitudes, case studies, discussion, or role-playing may work the best. If your goal is to motivate the learners, gaming would be a good choice. If you want to encourage creativity and problem-solving skills, your best approach might be problem-based learning or individual projects. Different teaching strategies yield different outcomes; you have to be clear about your goals for learning if you are to choose an appropriate method.

Course content also dictates methodology to some extent. A class on isolation technique may be effectively taught by demonstration, computer simulation, or hands-on practice, but would be poorly taught by means of Socratic questioning. The ethical aspects of euthanasia could be handled nicely with a discussion or with audiovisuals, but would not be taught as effectively by a computer tutorial. Because nursing is a practice discipline, a lot of the learning should be active learning; that is, the learner should be an active participant in the learning process. The teaching methods selected should therefore emphasize student activity: discussion, case studies and simulations, role-playing, cooperative learning, computer use, and so on. Overdependence on lecture is indefensible in teaching material for a practice profession.

Choice of teaching strategy also depends on the abilities and interests of the teacher. As you begin to use various methods, you will find that you feel comfortable with some and not others. Every educator should capitalize on personal strengths and use those methods that are compatible with his or her personality and teaching style. At the same time, the teacher should keep an open mind about new methodologies and have the courage to try and persevere with new techniques.

Compatibility between teachers and teaching methods is important, but so is compatibility between learners and teaching methods. You have to know the capabilities and background knowledge level of your students. You might choose different strategies, for example, for a group of people in a new parents class who have less than a high school education compared to those who have a college education. Or educational background may not be as important as life experience they have had. Different groups of learners may also have different motivation levels that might influence the methods you choose. Consideration should be given to student learning styles that were discussed in Chapter 2. Using a variety of teaching strategies in one class or course can help to meet varied learning styles.

Another factor that influences the selection of teaching methods is the number of people in the class. Having a single learner versus 30 learners will obviously affect the way you teach. Teaching individuals can be done best through modules, computer programs, or handouts with explanations. With small groups, discussions, role-playing, or cooperative learning can be effective. Large groups lend themselves to lectures, audiovisuals, and maybe case studies.

Finally, an educator's instructional options are limited to the resources of the institution. Classroom size, furniture, lighting, availability of technology, and availability of other instructional equipment and supplies all determine which strategies may be used.

Effectiveness of Teaching Methods

A great deal of research has been conducted in which comparisons are made about the effectiveness of two teaching methods. The findings depend on the outcome criterion (dependent variable) used in the various studies. When the outcome is the acquisition of knowledge, performance is about the same for all methods (Gage, 1976; Weston & Cranton,

1986). When the outcome being measured is problem-solving ability, time saved in learning, or transfer of learning abilities, some methods prove to be better than others, as will be seen in subsequent chapters. So, it would be inappropriate to claim that any one method is superior to another without asking, "Superior in which regard?"

Most methodology research has compared some "newer" methods to "traditional" methods such as the lecture method. Comparing gaming to lectures is an example. But the very fact that a "new" or experimental method is being used can confound the study results. The educator who is teaching the new method may have a sense of excitement about it that is conveyed to students. Students who know they are part of the study may respond differently, causing the *Hawthorne effect* (i.e., acting differently just because you know you are part of a study).

Another extraneous variable that can affect the research outcomes is the fact that it is often the same teacher who uses both teaching methods. That is, the instructor using gaming with the experimental group may be the same person lecturing to the control group. The problem in this case is that the personality, style, and approach of the teacher can play a significant role in the success of a particular teaching method. Some personality styles work well with some methods but not others. Therefore, as with any research, the results must be weighed carefully in light of the design and procedures. Full confidence should be placed only in results that have been replicated and confirmed.

Choosing a Textbook

Educators who use a textbook in a course should not underestimate the importance of either the textbook or its selection process. Courses are often built around the content and approach of a textbook. Texts provide a stable and uniform source of information for students to use in their individual study, and teachers expect students to use the book extensively (Besser, Stone, & Nan, 1999). In some academic settings, individual teachers select their own course textbooks; however, in others, the text must be reviewed by not only the individual teachers, but by a textbook review committee.

To begin the process of textbook selection, talk to publishers' representatives or call publishers for review copies of likely texts so you can examine them in some detail in order to make the right decision. Try to put yourself in the students' place and decide whether students would see the book as interesting, appealing, well organized, and well written. A unique study was conducted by Besser, Stone, and Nan (1999) in which they asked over 1,000 college students to report the value of the textbooks they bought. Students overwhelmingly reported that it was the quality of writing in a book that determined how helpful it would be to their learning. The aspects of writing they said was most helpful were examples given in the text and easy-to-read, clear writing. The next most frequently reported elements of quality were how the book was organized and the graphics that were included. Students liked introductions to chapters that give an overview of content; key words that appear in boldface; end-of-chapter summaries; study questions; and charts, tables, and pictures. Interestingly, they were not impressed with sidebars.

Many considerations should guide you when choosing a textbook. Sicola and Chesley (1999) suggest evaluating the content scope and quality; credibility of authorship; format (table of contents, index, organization, length, graphics); and issues like cost, permanency, quality of print, and the like. They developed a valid and reliable tool that can be used to rate any nursing text (see Figure 3–1). I suggest beginning with the preface to the book. The preface is the author's description of what the book is all about, its general objectives, the types of people who can use it, and its intended use. If a preface is done well, you can tell immediately if the book's approach is appropriate to your needs. Then look at the table of contents to see how closely the content mirrors the content of your course. You may not always find an exact fit, but you should be able to find at least one text that comes pretty close. You can supplement the text with outside readings, if you wish.

The next step is to examine some of the chapters. Spend time with a few chapters that cover content in which you are most expert. Evaluate the accuracy, currency, and breadth and depth of content. If all of the vital information is acceptable, read the chapter for clarity and style. Will the material be understandable for the level of reader intended? Will it hold the reader's interest?

Next, examine the book's appearance. Is the print easy to read, and are the diagrams or charts easy to follow? Do the graphics add interest to the content rather than distracting from the content? Is the page layout attractive, cluttered, or boring? Is more than one color used? Is the paper heavy enough that print does not show through the pages? Parsons and O'Shea state that "an attractive, easily understood, accurate textbook can be a servant in the finest sense" (1986, p. 344). The converse is also true, however. An unattractive, overly difficult, or inaccurate text serves little purpose except to make teaching and learning more difficult.

Another important factor to consider before selecting a textbook is the way in which the book will be used. Some instructors prefer a comprehensive, in-depth text from which they will choose topics for discussion or application. The student will not only use the text to prepare for class but will presumably use the book as an ongoing reference. Other teachers prefer books that cover broad topics in less detail. Their class presentations are then built around adding depth and detail to those topics. The success of the chosen book and of the method used often depends on the abilities of the learners. Novices and nonprofessionals such as nurses' aides and clients might do better with a more simplistic text, for example.

The cost of textbooks is a practical issue that should be considered. Instructors should be conservative with learners' money and should find out the cost of books under consideration. If two books are nearly equal in all other respects, why not select the less expensive one? Cost should also be kept in mind when considering the value of supplementary books such as workbooks and study guides. Will they really be used? That factor should be paramount when deciding whether to require them.

Using a Textbook

The degree to which teachers use the textbook ranges from ignoring it and letting students use it if or how they will, to having the learners bring the book to class and using it as an integral tool for the learning session. If you believe that a textbook is a valuable learning tool, it seems logical to build its use into the course. The teacher's goal should be to ensure that students indeed do the reading and understand the information they have read.

Instructors can take several approaches toward reading assignments. A common approach is to assign pages for homework, assume the students have read and understood

Name of Textbook _____ Author:_____

Publisher: _____

Textbook Evaluation Scale　　　Directions: Circle your rating for each item.
3 = Excellent　　2 = Average　　1 = Poor　　0 = Non Applicable for this Text

Topic		Rating	Topic		Rating
Topic I:	*Nursing Specialty Content*		**Topic III:**	*Content Quality*	
1	Appropriate Standards of Practice	3 2 1 0	1	Comparable (with other books)	3 2 1 0
2	Broad Based Knowledge	3 2 1 0	2	Content Areas Related	3 2 1 0
3	Cites Clinical Research	3 2 1 0	3	Up to Date Bibliography	3 2 1 0
4	Content Easily Located	3 2 1 0	4	Current Content	3 2 1 0
5	Grounded in Research	3 2 1 0	5	Current Medical Vocabulary with Definitions	3 2 1 0
6	Keypoints Highlighted	3 2 1 0	6	Illustrations Match Content	3 2 1 0
7	Nursing Orientation	3 2 1 0	7	Organization of Content	3 2 1 0
8	Rationale for Procedures Present	3 2 1 0	8	Photographs (appropriate)	3 2 1 0
9	Uniqueness of Content	3 2 1 0	9	Readability	3 2 1 0
10	Useful Information	3 2 1 0	10	Reading Level	3 2 1 0
Total Score		Total No. Rated	11	References [From Nursing Literature]	3 2 1 0
			12	Theoretical Appropriateness	3 2 1 0
			Total Score		Total No. Rated
Topic II:	*Credibility*		**Topic IV:**	*General Content*	
1	Print Date/Reprint Date	3 2 1 0	1	Appropriate Standards of Practice	3 2 1 0
2	Content Written by Authorities	3 2 1 0	2	Broad Based Knowledge	3 2 1 0
3	Credentials of Authors	3 2 1 0	3	Cites Clinical Research	3 2 1 0
4	Publishing Company's Attention to Errors after First Printing	3 2 1 0	4	Content Easily Located	3 2 1 0
5	Update Every Four Years	3 2 1 0	5	Grounded in Research	3 2 1 0
Total Score		Total No. Rated	6	Nursing Orientation	3 2 1 0
			7	Uniqueness of Content	3 2 1 0
			8	Useful Information	3 2 1 0
			Total Score		Total No. Rated

FIGURE 3-1 Texas Textbook Evaluation Tool

Permission granted by *Nurse Educator*.

Total		Rating		Topic		Rating
Topic V:	*Format*		Topic VI:	*Tangible Issues*		
1	Content [Close to Table/Unit]	3 2 1 0	1	Availability in Paperback and Hardcover		3 2 1 0
2	Errors are Minimal	3 2 1 0	2	Cost of Text		3 2 1 0
3	Headings	3 2 1 0	3	Permanency of Print		3 2 1 0
4	Index	3 2 1 0	4	Quality of Binding		3 2 1 0
5	Length	3 2 1 0	5	Quality of Paper		3 2 1 0
6	Organization	3 2 1 0	6	Readability/Quality of Print		3 2 1 0
7	Purpose/Objectives	3 2 1 0	7	Type Size		3 2 1 0
8	Quality of Photographs	3 2 1 0	8	Typesetting/Spacing		3 2 1 0
9	Summary/Conclusions [At End of Chapter Unit]	3 2 1 0	Total Score		Total No. Rated	
10	Table of Contents	3 2 1 0				
11	Table/Graphs	3 2 1 0				
12	Appendices	3 2 1 0				
Total Score		Total No. Rated				

Directions for Scoring:
Add the ratings for each item to obtain Total Score of Topic. To obtain the Average Score for each topic divide the Total Score by the Total Number rated under the topic. Exclude the non-applicable items.

Rating-Score Sheet

Rating
3 = Excellent   2 = Average   1 = Poor

Topic	Total Score	÷	Total No. Rated	=	Rating	Percentage Score	Conversion Scale			
							Overall Rating	Percentage Score	Overall Rating	Percentage Score
Topic I		÷		=			3.00	100	1.9	63
Topic II		÷		=			2.9	97	1.8	60
Topic III		÷		=			2.8	93	1.7	57
Topic IV		÷		=			2.7	90	1.6	53
Topic V		÷		=			2.6	87	1.5	50
							2.5	83	1.4	47
Topic VI		÷		=			2.4	80	1.3	43
							2.3	77	1.2	40
					Overall		2.2	73	1.1	37
					T-Test Rating	Percentage Score	2.1	70	1.0	33
							2.0	67		
Sum of Topic I to Topic VI		÷		=						

+ Exclude non applicable items from calculations.

FIGURE 3-1   Texas Textbook Evaluation Tool *(continued)*

the material, and carry on the next class as if the students have all the information mentally digested, catalogued, and stored for future use. Other instructors assume that few people in the class have read or understood the assigned reading, so they rehash it all in class, which simply serves to reinforce the nonreading behavior. A third approach is to use the information from assigned reading as a basis for classroom discussion, making sure that everyone participates in the discussion at one time or another. Finally, some instructors do the assigned reading themselves, make some notes about what to have the learners focus on, and explain to them in advance how they should read the material and how it will be used in class. Gallo and Gallo (1974) refer to this last approach as *guided reading.*

Guided reading, Gallo and Gallo contend, will help keep students from underlining everything in the book, trying to memorize all the facts, or getting so bogged down in the mass of information that they just give up and close the book. Students should read the assignment knowing what they should be focusing on, what they should get out of the assignment, and how the information will blend with class material. For example, an instructor may assign 15 pages of reading related to myocardial infarction. He or she tells the students to pay special attention to risk factors, because a preventative teaching plan will be formulated in class the next time. They are to come prepared with any questions about the pathophysiologic process, which will be briefly outlined in class. This kind of direction will help many students to learn from the reading assignment.

Pestel (1997) uses another way, called *discovery questions,* to help students get the most out of their reading. Students are assigned short passages to read before class. In class, this author distributes questions that help students to understand and evaluate the material in the text. Students work in groups at the beginning of class to answer the questions, and the questions and answers then guide the rest of the day's discussion.

I have used a variation of the above methods. A week or two ahead of time I distribute Reading/Discussion Guides for material that lends itself to this format and for which students may have difficulty extracting important information from the text. Students write their answers on the Guide, and that information becomes the basis for in-class discussion on the topic. Table 3–2 shows an example of a Guide for the material in the beginning of this chapter.

There are any number of ways a textbook can be used in teaching. Creative and effective use of a textbook is one of the challenges of teaching. Teachers may expand their creativity in using a text if they purchase an accompanying Instructor's Manual and a student Study Guide. There are many exercises and active learning techniques built into these supplemental materials.

Planning Assignments

Planning learning assignments is challenging work. Some courses may require only reading assignments; others have objectives that can be met only by other means. In academic settings, one of the favorite teaching devices is the term paper, sometimes disguised as the topic paper, research paper, or position paper. Such papers frequently are assigned in introductory nursing courses, current issue courses, or professional theory courses. The standard term paper, usually 10 to 15 pages long, in which a student must research a topic and write it up in "scholarly form," is rarely appropriate or necessary. What does a teacher expect the student to learn from such an assignment: how to write a scholarly paper? How to organize one's thoughts? How to think analytically? How to find answers to questions and solutions to prob-

TABLE 3-2 Reading/Discussion Guide for Chapter 3

1. Explain why course objectives are also called learning outcomes.
2. What is the difference between goals and objectives?
3. Is it important to write objectives in behavioral terms? Why or why not?
4. Write three class objectives that pertain to this chapter.
5. If this chapter were turned into a lecture, could it be organized differently? How?
6. If you were teaching a class on the material in this chapter, what teaching methods would you use?
7. What are the advantages and disadvantages of using a textbook versus a collection of periodicals?
8. Rate this textbook using the Texas Textbook Evaluation Tool.

lems? Few of these goals are actually met by term-paper writing in a nursing course. What actually occurs is that students learn a great deal about one topic (which may or may not have later usefulness). They may learn something about how to write and edit a paper, but probably learn little else that contributes to meeting the learning outcomes of the course.

If you want to see whether students can think analytically, assign a short essay in which they have to analyze a particular patient problem or issue related to the course. This kind of assignment forces students to use their own analytical powers and not just rephrase someone else's ideas from the literature. If you want to test students' ability to use resources to answer specific questions, ask them the questions, let them investigate the answers, and have them write up the answers in a short paper. You might even ask students to write lists of pertinent questions that need answers.

There are other types of creative and worthy assignments. Students could be asked to devise assessment forms or patient teaching materials. They could solve a problem in the real world of nursing and report on the solution. They could do personal interviews, formulate ideas for research, or keep logs and journals. They could do a concept map of physiologic processes involved in certain medical conditions. Countless types of assignments are available that would help achieve objectives and yet not involve a lot of busywork and repetition.

Nursing care plans of some type are an indispensable part of the nursing instructor's assignments. Care plans need to be written for most clinical courses, but they are sometimes misused. The objectives for preparing care plans should be clear in the instructor's mind. Will students be writing them as a means of learning the nursing process? Planning care for an assigned patient? Learning about typical nursing diagnoses and related nursing care? All three objectives can be met by writing care plans, but the type and size of the care plans may vary.

Beginning students who are learning the nursing process need to write simple, short care plans on simulated or real patient situations. They can learn the process without writing comprehensive, lengthy plans. If the student's goal is to write a plan of care for a particular patient, it will vary in length and comprehensiveness. For example, a "working" care plan that has to be devised every week in order to provide safe care should be as short as possible, maybe in card form. Occasionally, a teacher may be justified in asking students to enlarge these working care plans to include scientific rationale and documentation.

Once students have a basic grasp of the nursing process, it may be best for them to start their planning with a standardized care plan or care map and learn to individualize it for the patient. There is no need for students to keep writing the basics once they have mastered them. They need to move on to higher-level learning.

Care plans that become term-paper length are really case studies. Objectives for a case study should be different from objectives for a care plan, and the teacher should be clear about the intent. Case studies may be useful if they are written on common recurring cases that students will encounter frequently, and if the essence of the case is shared with class members.

Conducting the Class

The planning is done. You are prepared to enter the classroom the first day of a course. What is the best way to proceed so the class gets off to a good start, with an optimal atmosphere for learning? Let's explore some of the ways you can make each class as positive and productive an experience as possible, for both you and the learners.

The First Class

The way you approach the first session often sets the tone for the whole course. Unless you already know every learner in the class, begin by introducing yourself. If you have a preference for a form of address, first name or last name, or title, make it known at the outset. At some point in the first session, tell the class a little about yourself (professional or personal, whichever information is pertinent and you feel comfortable sharing). You can establish a pleasant atmosphere by welcoming the class, reading names and getting correct pronunciations, making sure that everyone gets the handouts, and commiserating about the early or late hour, the weather, or parking. A little humor is helpful on the first day if it flows naturally.

The first session is the best time to communicate your expectations for the course. Review the course syllabus or outline (do not read it aloud word for word) and take time to answer questions about content, methods, and assignments. Give the class a general idea of the workload and your expectations in terms of preparation for class and in terms of learning outcomes.

Besides content expectations, you should cover general classroom rules. If you have rules or policies about attendance, lateness, eating in class, and bathroom breaks, let everyone know right away. It is poor practice to let the class think they can do what they like in terms of these things while you continue to get more and more annoyed about behavior that doesn't meet your expectations.

A positive way to end this introductory portion of the course it to try to whet the learners' appetites for what is to come. Try to place the course or class in a larger perspective of their professional or personal lives. Talk about why they should learn this information, how it will help them, how they will be able to apply it to their lives, and what they will like about it. If you can communicate your enthusiasm for the subject by the end of the first class, you may have given the group something to look forward to for the rest of the course.

Subsequent Classes

In each following class, it is important to begin by gaining and controlling the attention of the learners. You can easily get the attention of some groups with just a look; others practically need a police whistle. But you must gain their attention before you start to teach. If you begin talking while the group is still moving around or conversing, not only will they miss what you say, but also you will establish an impression of lack of control. It sometimes helps to walk around the periphery of the room instead of standing behind the desk or lectern. Your close proximity may help establish your presence and authority. When you are close to the learners, it is also easier for them to hear you as you ask them to settle down. Many educators have also found they can relax the atmosphere if they move about the room periodically throughout the class time and sometimes stand in front of the teacher's desk rather than behind it.

As you begin the work of the course, you will need to assess the learners to determine their backgrounds and how much they already know about the content of the course. This assessment can be done formally by giving pretests or short questionnaires or more informally by asking questions during class. It is equally as harmful to assume that the learners already know a lot about the subject as to assume that they know nothing. If they indeed know little about the subject, you will cause great confusion by beginning to teach above the introductory level. If they already know the material you are covering, boredom may set in.

A course that has been well planned and that starts out well on the first session is already on the way to success. If you follow the planning sequences suggested in this chapter and continue to refine your approach to teaching, you will be rewarded with rich and memorable teaching experiences. The process is hard work, but the outcome is well worth the effort.

CASE STUDY

You are a community educator for a large health care system. You are preparing a series of two classes on smoking cessation that will be followed by a support group for people who want to quit smoking.

1. What resources might you use to help you with content for the classes?
2. Write objectives for the course in all three learning domains. Indicate how you plan to measure each of them.
3. Write objectives for the first class, with one at each of the six levels of the cognitive domain.
4. What teaching methods would you use in these classes? What resources would you need for these methods?

CRITICAL THINKING EXERCISES

1. You are responsible for selecting a medication computation workbook for an RN refresher course you are going to teach. A friend has recommended a book to you, but you want to be sure that it is the best book for your course. Which of the following factors might make this book appropriate or inappropriate for your course, and why?

    a. It reviews basic math like addition, multiplication, and working with fractions.

    b. Conversions between metric and apothecary systems are included.

    c. Intravenous rate calculations are included.

    d. Dimensional analysis is used as an approach instead of the desired/have method.

    e. Formulas are given for titrating drugs used in critical care units.

    f. A computer disk with tutorials and sample quizzes is included with each book.

2. An experienced teacher once said that it can be good if learners feel a little confused during class. How can it be a good thing? If there is some merit to that thought, why should we work hard at organizing our content delivery in order to avoid confusion?

3. How could you design an experiment to test the effectiveness of a new teaching method that would minimize some of the pitfalls of educational research identified on page 46?

IDEAS FOR FURTHER RESEARCH

1. Survey educators to see how many learning objectives in their courses cover the affective domain. Ask them about their experience in measuring affective objectives.

2. Replicate the study of textbooks by Besser, Stone, and Nan (1999) referred to in the chapter.

3. Conduct an experiment to measure learning that occurs with guided reading versus student self-reading of a textbook.

4. Interview experienced and novice educators to discover how they decide which teaching strategies to use in their classes. Do the two groups differ? Do patterns emerge?

REFERENCES

Andrusyszyn, M. A. (1989). Clinical evaluation of the affective domain. *Nurse Education Today, 9*(2), 75–81.

Besser, D., Stone, G., & Nan, L. (1999). Textbooks and teaching: A lesson from students. *Journalism & Mass Communication Educator, 53*(4), 4–17.

Bloom, B. S. (1984). *Taxonomy of educational objectives.* New York: Longman.

Cummings, C. (1994). Tips for writing behavioral objectives. *Nursing Staff Development Insider, 3*(4), 6, 8.

Ferguson, L. M. (1998). Writing learning objectives. *Journal of Nursing Staff Development, 14*(2), 87–94.

Gage, N. L. (Ed.). (1976). *The psychology of teaching methods.* Chicago: University of Chicago Press.

Gallo, B. M., & Gallo, D. R. (1974). Guided reading: A strategy to enhance learning. *Journal of Nursing Education, 13*(1), 21–25.

Holmes, S. A. (1990). Getting started: Writing behavioral objectives. *Journal of Nursing Staff Development, 6*(1), 40–44.

Houlden, R. L., & Collier, C. P. (1999). Learning outcome objectives: A critical tool in learner-centered education. *The Journal of Continuing Education in the Health Professions, 19*(4), 208–213.

Maier-Lorentz, M. M. (1999). Writing objectives and evaluating learning in the affective domain. *Journal for Nurses in Staff Development, 15*(4), 167–171.

McKeachie, W. J. (1999). *Teaching tips* (10th ed.). Boston: Houghton Mifflin.

Parsons, M., & O'Shea, H. S. (1986). Textbook selection: Perils and pointers. *Journal of Nursing Education, 25*(8), 343–345.

Pestel, B. C. (1997). Facilitating the reading/discussion connection in the interactive classroom. *Journal of College Science Teaching, 27*(1), 44–46.

Sicola, V., & Chesley, D. A. (1999). Development of the Texas Textbook Evaluation Tool. *Nurse Educator, 24*(2), 23–28.

Weston, C., & Cranton, P. A. (1986). Selecting instructional strategies. *Journal of Higher Education, 57*(3), 259–288.

Part II

The Learner

4

Motivation and Behavior Change

Teaching is part of nursing practice. For education to be effective, the nurse must not only be knowledgeable about the subject matter being taught, but also about the teaching/learning process. This chapter applies primarily to patient or client teaching, but some applications to other learners are apparent.

Learning is a multifactorial activity that is often taken for granted, since we all learn all the time. However, in a medical or nursing situation, there are many variables that play into the patient's or client's ability to learn that must be taken into account. There are theories that, when used by the nurse to guide the development of educational interventions, can improve the likelihood of effectiveness.

Teaching a client new information and having him or her use it are two different things. An effective health education intervention encompasses more than just the giving of new information, for information alone does not always result in behavior change, compliance, or improved health status.

Successful educational interventions increase compliance with medical regimens and improve health outcomes. They are based on learner characteristics, his or her educational needs, theory, and a sound educational plan.

Learner Characteristics

There are many factors that influence a client's ability, motivation, and desire to learn. Addressing these factors when planning educational interventions is essential, because the effectiveness of the intervention can be at stake. Learner characteristics include, among others, culture/ethnicity, literacy, age, health status, education level, and socioeconomic status.

Culture

Culture is defined as invisible patterns that form the normal ways of acting, feeling, judging, perceiving, and organizing the world (Shade, Kelly, & Oberg, 1997). In a country where the population is relatively homogenous, culture is not an issue. All of the people function from a common set of acceptable behaviors. This is not so in a diverse population as the one we have in the United States. Even with the different geographic regions of the United States, there are variations of diversity. The population mix in the New York metropolitan area is quite different from that which is found in the Los Angeles area, which is different from that found in the Miami area.

Culture affects health behaviors and the teaching/learning process in many ways. Culture influences gender roles, sexual behavior, diet, personal hygiene, body image (i.e., obesity, slimness, etc.), drug use (alcohol, hallucinogens, coffee, tea), exercise, and communication, among others (Nakamura, 1999). For example, in Hispanic or Latino populations, the decision to follow medical orders might involve other family members or the head of the household. The decision may be based on what these individuals feel is best for the family (Huff & Kline, 1999). Knowing this, it may be best to include the entire family in an educational session, rather than just the client.

In the many diverse Native American and Alaska Native tribal groups, traditional healers and herbal medicines are still very important components of caring for the sick (Huff & Kline, 1999). Thus, questions about the use of herbs might be asked to prevent untoward drug interactions with medically prescribed treatment, which will result in noncompliance.

In Asian cultures that follow the traditions of Buddhism, Taoism, or Confucian ideology, there can be aversion to public admission of mental or physical illness or of personal weakness. This, coupled with the need to achieve harmony with nature or freedom from symptoms (Huff & Kline, 1999), may affect the likelihood of an accurate assessment of the patient's condition or with compliance with our Western approach to treating illness and evaluating treatment effectiveness.

In Pacific Island populations, there is the belief that certain illnesses must be treated with traditional remedies, and certain others that are considered "Western" illnesses that can be treated with Western medicine (Huff & Kline, 1999). This belief may greatly impact compliance, especially if the treatment and illness (traditional versus Western) are incompatible with each other. For further discussion on the impact of culture on learning, see Chapter 5.

Literacy

The client's ability to read and understand what is being read is an essential component of learning. Establishing the reading level and using materials that are consistent with the client's ability is paramount. Materials at too high a level will be useless, as they will not be understood. Materials at too low a level, while of some value, may be too simplistic and may even be seen as insulting.

For those who are illiterate, written communication obviously cannot be used. What is not obvious is who is illiterate. Illiteracy is often embarrassing and is not readily disclosed. However, it can have a profound affect on compliance, learning, and health. Chapter 6, Literacy and Readability, discusses this issue in more depth and suggests ways to address it in the clinical setting.

Age

As more of our population live longer, it is increasingly the aged who are our clients. Teaching the older adult presents some challenges, although none are insurmountable. The older adult usually needs more time to learn. Educational sessions either need to be for a longer period of time or broken down into more sessions for a shorter time covering less information. Regardless of how the time factor is addressed, bear in mind that older adults tend to learn best when the information is relevant to them and has a practical application.

As with all clients, emotional or mental status should be acknowledged and taken into account when planning an educational intervention for this population. Depression, denial, fear, and anxiety can all have an impact on the effectiveness of teaching. These issues may need to be addressed before teaching and learning can progress.

Older adults often enjoy learning in a group. If possible, plan group sessions with time allotted for socialization. This may improve the outcome of the educational intervention.

Be cognizant of possible hearing and visual deficits. Deficits can be addressed by making sure always to face the client while speaking clearly, slowly, and loudly if necessary, while avoiding shouting. To address visual impairments, use large-print materials or print in larger letters if using a flip chart or chalkboard. For those whose eyesight is such that reading is not possible, make a tape recording of pertinent instructions.

Education Level and Health Status

A client's education level may have an impact on learning. It has been well documented that education level is significantly associated with health status (i.e., the more educated the healthier). This does not presuppose that only the less educated become ill. What it may mean for the nurse is that the more educated client is the one who seeks treatment earlier in the disease process, and the less educated client is sicker.

When teaching, it is important to establish the client's level of knowledge or depth of understanding of his or her condition. This will enable you to provide information at an appropriate level—basic or in great medical detail.

Using medical terminology, anatomical labels for body parts, abbreviations for medical procedures, or just "big words" may hinder the learning process for some. In contrast, using more simple language and lay terminology may be insulting for others and not provide the degree of information they want or need.

Socioeconomic Level

The impact of socioeconomic level on learning has more to do with being able to use the information being taught rather than the process of learning. Simply, the resources needed to comply with the medical regimen may not be available. Changes in diet, for example, may include increasing the intake of fresh fruits and vegetables. Fresh produce is expensive, does not keep well, and may not be available to some at a neighborhood store. While the information is learned, the behavior cannot be changed because of factors beyond the client's control, income, transportation, and local availability.

Socioeconomic level may dictate where a client lives. Although this may not seem to be related to learning or changing behavior, it is. For example, if part of a cardiac rehabilitation program is to walk several times a week and the client lives in a high crime area, then even though the value of walking is understood, it will not be carried out.

In teaching patients and clients, it is important to identify as many variables as possible that may affect learning or ultimately on complying with health care. The more the nurse knows about the person, the better able he or she will be to develop an educational intervention that will be successful.

Planning for Learning

Learning is a complex process. Having people learn new information and skills and change their behavior can be daunting. Approaching this with a plan that incorporates factors that increase the likelihood of learning, and based on a theory that explains why people behave the way they do, increases the chances that learning will take place, change will occur, compliance will improve, and education will be effective.

To increase the likelihood of compliance, it is helpful to understand the basics of how people learn or those factors that impact on learning. Approaching the educational process from a theoretical basis enables the nurse educator to identify methods most likely to produce the best results.

Learning Principles

There are a number of factors that affect the learning process. Some we have control over, such as the learning environment or the rate at which information is taught or presented. Others we don't have control over, such as the client's innate ability to learn, interest in the information, or desire to learn.

The following learning principles (Breckon, Harvey, & Lancaster, 1998; Moss, 1994) are helpful in motivating people to learn and in planning for the most effective educational experience possible (see Table 4–1).

1. *Use several senses.*

   People retain 10 percent of what they read, 20 percent of what they hear, 30 percent of what they see, 50 percent of what they hear and see, 70 percent of what they say, and 90 percent of what they say and do. Based on this principle, learning is more likely to occur if clients are allowed to practice what they are being taught. This prin-

TABLE 4-1 Learning Principles to Use in Motivating Learners

1. Use several senses.
2. Actively involve the patients or clients in the learning process.
3. Provide an environment conducive to learning.
4. Assess the extent to which the learner is ready to learn.
5. Determine the perceived relevance of the information.
6. Repeat information.
7. Generalize information.
8. Make learning a pleasant experience.
9. Begin with what is known; move toward what is unknown.
10. Present information at an appropriate rate.

ciple is used regularly when teaching new diabetics how to administer insulin. Practicing how to draw up insulin into a syringe and injecting it is an integral component of this educational process. In this situation, compliance is crucial. Compliance will certainly be enhanced if the skill of injecting has been mastered.

In any educational situation in which it is appropriate, time should be planned for practicing what is being taught. Obviously, this principle is most effective when a new psychomotor skill must be learned. In situations in which psychomotor skill development is not the educational aim, reading out loud while clients follow along increases learning much more than simply distributing printed information for them to read at home.

2. *Actively involve the patients or clients in the learning process.*

This principle relates to the teaching methods used, whether they are passive or active. Passive methods include lecture, videos, and print materials. While these do allow for learning, learning is much enhanced if more active methods are used.

The more interactive the educational experience, the greater the likelihood of success. Use methods that engage the participants, such as discussion, role-playing, small group discussion, and question and answer, rather than lecture. Ask clients to assist in the demonstration of the skill being taught, or to share personal experiences related to the information being presented. If appropriate, use case studies or scenarios from which discussion questions can be generated or problem-solving techniques can be practiced.

3. *Provide an environment conducive to learning.*

Do you remember trying to learn in a classroom that was freezing cold, or sweltering hot? One that was too noisy, or in which the seats were uncomfortable, or too close to the person next to you? All of these environmental factors can make a huge difference in the outcome or success of an educational intervention. Learning takes place best when people are comfortable and extraneous interference is kept to a minimum.

Ideally, the room should have good lighting and temperature control and comfortable seating with enough space between seats. It should be free of unpleasant odors (mold, mildew, cigarette smoke, heavy perfume) and signs of deterioration (falling ceiling tiles, peeling paint, graffiti, dirty carpeting). It should have adequate acoustics, that is, no echo, and if it is a large space, a sound system.

While attention to these factors may seem trivial, they can make the difference between a successful education program and an unsuccessful one. "Creature features" do count.

4. *Assess the extent to which the learner is ready to learn.*

In general, people learn only if they are emotionally and physically ready. Client or patient readiness, unfortunately, is not often—if ever—in your control. An adolescent who is in denial about a diabetes diagnosis may not be ready (able) to learn how to inject insulin or follow a prescribed diet. Anxiety, fear, and depression can all hinder the learning process. Physical readiness to learn can be hampered by pain, the effects of anesthesia, visual or auditory impairment, language barriers, and lack of privacy.

The first step in the educational process is to assess client readiness for learning. Assessment data can be obtained directly from the clients or families (primary data), or it can be gathered from a variety of other sources such as charts or reports (secondary data). Primary data have an advantage over data from other sources in that the sources can directly answer questions about the needs of the specific client or group for whom the educational intervention is being planned (McKenzie & Smeltzer, 2001).

Keep in mind that readiness assessment aims to provide information about what clients want to know and want to learn (or perhaps do not want to learn), their beliefs, family dynamics, housing situation, skills, educational level, fears or concerns about their condition, or the effect of their condition on others.

Further information can be obtained from talking with families. What do family members feel the client should know or learn? What is the support system like at home? What are the family dynamics, from the family's perspective, that might affect compliance with the medical regimen?

In situations in which the patient or family members are not ready, the educational process may need to be tailored to fit what they are ready for. This may mean the learning process will take longer. However, extra time is worth it if the educational goal is met and the likelihood of compliance is increased.

5. *Determine the perceived relevance of the information.*

People generally are willing to learn what they perceive as being important. Sometimes, this is not consistent with what we think is important. The easiest way to determine what is important and what is not is to simply ask. Keep in mind that this may vary from person to person, depending on how ready they are to learn.

6. *Repeat information.*

Repetition enhances learning. When new information is presented, it should be presented several times, in a variety of ways. Reword the information, discuss a practical application of the information, and have the person provide a situation in which the information could be used. Repetition is particularly important when the information is complex or completely new. Information can also be repeated throughout the educational session by referring back to material that was previously discussed.

7. *Generalize information.*

Information is more readily learned if it is applied to more than one situation. Using a variety of examples and applying the information to specific situations in the client's life promotes learning and contributes to a better chance of compliance.

8. *Make learning a pleasant experience.*

Learning is enhanced if the learning experience is pleasant. This can be accomplished through frequent encouragement and positive feedback. People usually enjoy learning, and learning is enhanced when obvious progress is being made. Frequent recognition of accomplishment, even for seemingly small successes, can go a long way toward a successful education intervention.

9. *Begin with what is known; move toward what is unknown.*

Information should be presented in an organized fashion. It should begin with the basics or general information that is known and move toward new information, or that which is unknown. Using this approach will also contribute to a pleasant learning experience. Starting with information that people generally have knowledge of and building on that increases the likelihood of a pleasant, but most importantly a successful, learning experience.

10. *Present information at an appropriate rate.*

Nothing is more frustrating for learners than to have new information presented at such a rapid pace that they cannot keep up. The rate at which information is taught must be tailored to the client. Depending on the client's knowledge level, a faster or slower pace may be necessary.

The pace of presentation may be affected by physical limitations of the client. For example, a client who has difficulty hearing may need to lip read, and consequently may need the information to be presented at a slower rate. A client with a long history of dealing with the particular disease entity being taught may be well versed and not need the basic information. For this person, a somewhat faster pace would be appropriate.

Motivation and Behavior Change Theories

Theories are used by the nurse educator to plan and implement the most effective educational intervention possible. A theory is "a set of interrelated concepts, definitions, and propositions that presents a systematic view of events or situations by specifying relations among variables in order to explain and predict the events of the situation" (Glanz, Lewis, & Rimer, 1997). More simply put, a theory is a set of ideas that help to explain the relationship among factors or predict the outcome of their interrelation. Theories help us to understand why people do or don't do certain things in a given situation.

In general, the purpose of most educational interventions is to change behavior. Behavior change is often at the root of increasing compliance with treatment regimens or preventing complications or further illness. To accomplish behavior change, it is important to understand why people do what they do in a given situation and to use the best possible approach to initiate the targeted change, for change does not come easy to most people.

Using theory as the basis for an educational intervention does not guarantee success, but it increases the likelihood of success that change will occur. There are no right or wrong theories. Each situation, each client, each behavior change may be influenced by many different variables, as discussed earlier in this chapter. The following are among the most commonly used theories for health education interventions, but again, these are but a sampling of the many theories that may be used to initiate change. Table 4-2 summarizes the essentials of these theories.

Health Belief Model

The *Health Belief Model* explains behavior or predicts whether behavior change will occur based on a set of beliefs or perceptions, which include perceived seriousness, susceptibility, benefits, and barriers. These perceptions are modified by cues to action (Elder, Ayala, & Harris, 1999; Glanz et al., 1997).

TABLE 4-2 Essential Components of Motivation and Behavior Change Theories

Theory	Components
Health Belief Model	Based on perceptions of seriousness or severity of the health problem; personal belief of susceptibility to or risk of the illness; benefits of adopting the new behavior or changing the old behavior; barriers to changing or adopting the behavior. Change is triggered by cues to action and supported or hindered by modifying variables.
Transtheoretical or Stages of Change Model	These are five stages people go through in the process of change: Precontemplation—before they even begin to think about the change Contemplation—when they weigh the pros and cons of changing the behavior Preparation—when they decide on how they will undertake the change, what they will do Action—when they start the change, they put the plan into motion Maintenance—keeping the new behavior and resisting the old Termination—when the behavior becomes a habit
Theory of Reasoned Action	This is based on a person's intention to do something. Intention to change behavior is the result of: A person's attitude toward the behavior—whether it is positive or negative Subjective norms—significant others' reaction to the behavior Behavioral control—how easy or difficult the person believes the new behavior is
Social Cognitive Theory	This is based on reciprocal determinism, that behavior is the result of an interaction between the behavior, the person or personal factors, and the environment. If one is changed, all are changed. This uses self-efficacy, modeling, reinforcement, locus of control.
Self-Efficacy Theory	This is based on the idea that people will do only what they think they can do. Four variables determine the strength of a person's belief in ability: performance accomplishments, vicarious experience, verbal persuasion, and physiological state. The most important determinant of behavior change is learning a new behavior by doing it.
Behavior Modification Theory	The underlying basis is the idea of rewards and punishment. If the person does what is wanted, then the person is given something pleasant—a reward. If the person does not do what is wanted, then something unpleasant is given or something is taken way—a punishment. Although both rewards and punishment will change behavior, using rewards is more likely to be effective.

The beliefs or perceptions are the individual's beliefs about the seriousness of an illness, either the one he or she has just been diagnosed with, is at risk for, or that needs to be prevented, as in the case of complications from failure to follow medical treatment.

The belief that an illness is not serious can significantly alter an individual's desire to change behavior relative to that illness. For example, if the belief is that hypertension is not serious, because after all, the person feels fine, has no pain or discomfort, and is not restricted or incapacitated by it, then compliance with medical treatment is less likely to occur.

However, if the perception is that hypertension is a serious illness, then the likelihood of compliance, behavior change, is increased.

Perceived susceptibility is the belief of personal risk or threat of a particular health problem. If the perception is that there is great risk of developing or contracting a particular disease, then the likelihood of changing behavior to avoid or prevent this disease from occurring is increased.

Using HIV as the example, if the perception is that the risk of contracting the virus is minimal, then the likelihood of safer sex behaviors being adopted is also minimal. However, the perception of risk may be based on misinformation or lack of information, and if corrected, the perception may be altered, and safer sex behaviors adopted.

The perception of benefit is that which could be derived from following the prescribed course of action (i.e., is the behavior change worth it). The benefit of changing behavior is impacted by the extent to which the health problem is perceived as being serious and the extent to which the person believes he or she is at risk.

The change must be perceived as being beneficial or advantageous for the new behavior to be adopted. In the case of cigarette smoking, for example, a smoker may perceive lung cancer as a very serious health problem, and may perceive him- or herself as being at risk for this disease. If the perceived benefit of quitting smoking is a significant reduction in the risk of developing this serious condition, the person is more likely to quit smoking.

Conversely, if a smoker perceives lung cancer as serious, and believes he or she is at greater risk for lung cancer, but does not believe that quitting will alter the risk of developing it, then the benefit of quitting is not a strong enough motivating factor and the likelihood of quitting is minimal. However, there may be other benefits from quitting smoking that are perceived as being greater incentives than increased health status. For instance, it may be saving money, elimination of tobacco smoke smell on clothing, whiter teeth, or pleasing a significant other, all of which are nonhealth benefits. Whether the outcome of quitting is a benefit is determined by the individual's perception, not the perception of the educator. Thus, behavior change may be perceived as having both health benefits and nonhealth benefits. Regardless, adoption of the new behavior is not likely to take place unless the person believes that the change will be effective (Glanz et al., 1997).

Barriers to behavior change are those factors that prevent the adoption of a new behavior. Barriers might include the perception that a treatment is expensive, painful, not effective, embarrassing, or inconvenient. These beliefs may stem from misconceptions, lack of information, previous experience, or hearsay. In order for a behavior to be adopted, the barriers must be addressed and removed.

Educational interventions based on the Health Belief Model depend on the combined perception of severity and susceptibility as the force that leads one to act. The perceived benefits of the proposed behavior, minus the barriers, leads to the course of action (Rosenstock, 1974).

Social Cognitive Theory

Social Cognitive Theory (originally introduced as *Social Learning Theory*) explains that behavior is the result of an interaction among the person (characteristics, personality, etc.), the environment (physical, social, etc.), and the behavior itself (Baranowski, Perry, & Parcel, 1997). A change in one of these factors changes all of them, a phenomenon called *reciprocal determinism*.

Using this theory to elicit behavior change requires that one or more of the person, environment, or behavior factors be modified. Factors that affect behavior include the anticipated outcomes of engaging in the behavior, learning by observing others, self-efficacy, and self-control (Bandura, 1986).

By providing opportunities for the client to watch others perform the targeted behavior and mimic or copy it, the personal factor may change and result in the adoption of the new behavior. Similarly, addressing the concept of self-efficacy, that is, the person's belief in his or her ability to perform the new behavior, may also lead to behavior change. If a person does not believe he or she can do something, then most likely it won't be done. By providing opportunities for clients to increase their perception of ability, perhaps through skill-building exercises, practice sessions, support group interactions, or by learning the new behavior in small parts over time, a stronger sense of self-efficacy can occur and perhaps a greater likelihood of changing behavior. (Self-efficacy is discussed later in this chapter.)

Attitude toward the expected outcomes of the behavior is a personal factor that also plays a role in determining whether a new behavior is adopted. Outcome expectations may be influenced by past experiences in similar situations, through observation of others in similar situations, and through word of mouth or hearing about others in similar situations. These expectations may be realistic or based on misinformation or lack of information. Consequently, what the client expects to happen as a result of adopting the new behavior (i.e., being compliant with a medical regimen) may need to be modified in order for the educational intervention to be successful.

In addition to outcome expectations, the value a person places on these outcomes also influences compliance with or adoption of a new behavior. This value placed on outcomes is termed *expectancies,* or *incentives.* The extent to which the new behavior is seen as a positive thing—that is, the behavior is valued—affects the likelihood that it will be adopted. Positive expectancies are a motivating force and an incentive to adopt the behavior (Baranowksi et al., 1997).

Characteristics of the behavior also affect whether it will be adopted. The extent to which the client has control over the behavior, that is, self-control, may be an important factor in its adoption and ultimately in improved compliance. Allowing the client to set his or her own goals may be the most important determinant. For example, instead of asking a client to cut down on certain foods, the client might be more likely to comply with a new diet if he or she is able to choose a specific limited amount of food instead. This allows for a sense of control over the situation, provides parameters against which success can be measured, and improves the likelihood of a successful educational intervention (Baranowski et al., 1997).

The environment in which the behavior takes place is also important. Environment encompasses more than the physical surroundings, the classroom, clinic, physician's office, or worksite. It also entails the social environment, including the family, friends, peers, and colleagues (Baranowski et al., 1997). An example of the role environment plays in determining compliance with behavior change can be seen in the adoption of more healthy behaviors when smoking restrictions in the workplace are put into effect (Biener, Abrams, Follick, & Dean, 1989) or when healthy foods replace junk foods in vending machines.

Using Social Cognitive Theory to change behavior, to increase compliance with medical treatment, or to improve the likelihood of success of an educational intervention means that the nurse educator needs to learn as much as possible about the client. Understanding the importance of the interrelationship among the client's beliefs, attitudes, and environment will go a long way in enabling the desired change in behavior to occur.

Self-Efficacy Theory

Self-efficacy is a very powerful determinant of health behavior, as is seen from its use in the Social Cognitive Theory. However, self-efficacy on its own has been presented as a means by which behavior can be predicted or explained. Self-efficacy is a determinant of motivation. The stronger someone's belief in his or her ability to accomplish something, the more effort will be exerted and the longer he or she will persevere (Bandura, 1989).

The *Theory of Self-Efficacy* proposes that behavior change occurs because of the expectations or expected result of the new behavior and one's belief about his or her ability to perform a specific behavior in a specific situation (Strecher, DeVillis, Becker, & Rosenstock, 1986). There are four sources from which a person's degree of self-efficacy arises: performance accomplishments, vicarious experience, verbal persuasion, and physiological state. *Performance accomplishment* refers to learning that occurs through personal mastery of a particular skill or task. Accomplishments attained through personal mastery are the most powerful sources of efficacy expectations (Bandura, 1977). Simply stated, the most important determinant of behavior change is when people learn (master) a new behavior by doing it. Knowing this, the nurse educator needs to be aware of or provide for experiences whereby the clients can learn by doing.

People also increase their belief in their own ability to perform a specific behavior when they watch someone else perform the behavior. This is *vicarious experience,* or learning through observation. The people or events being observed are called models (Strecher et al., 1986). Modeling enables people to learn by watching, through demonstration. For example, in teaching a child how to use an inhaler with a spacer, having another child of similar age demonstrate its use and explain the difficulties he or she had and how they were overcome increases one's belief in the ability to also master the behavior. *Verbal persuasion* involves acting as the coach and providing encouragement. Patients may need to be prompted to continue trying to master the targeted behavior.

Transtheoretical Model/Stages of Change Theory

The *Transtheoretical Model* or *Stages of Change Theory* is useful when the targeted behavior change is the discontinuation of an unhealthy behavior. It is often used for smoking cessation and weight management interventions.

This theory postulates that people go through stages before a change in behavior occurs. These stages include precontemplation, contemplation, preparation, action, maintenance, and termination (Prochaska, Redding, & Evers, 1997).

During the *precontemplation stage,* there is no serious thought being given to changing the behavior in the next six months. This could be because the person is unaware that the behavior is unhealthy or he or she is uninvolved, meaning that the person knows that the behavior needs to be changed but does not see it as being very important. It could also be because the person is undecided in thinking about the positives and negatives of changing the behavior (Weinstein, Rothman, & Sutton, 1998). The time frame of six months is used because that seems to be about as far into the future as people plan for behavior change

(Prochaska, Redding, Harlow, Rossi, & Velicer, 1994). Educational interventions targeting individuals in this stage should be focused on increasing awareness, increasing the perception of seriousness of the unhealthy behavior, and highlighting the benefits of adopting the new behavior.

People in the *contemplation stage* are at least aware of the need to change their behavior and are thinking about making a change in the next six months. They are weighing the pros and cons of the new behavior. This stage can last for long periods, and when it does it is termed *behavioral procrastination* (Prochaska et al., 1997).

People progress from the precontemplation stage to the contemplation stage when the perceived benefits of change (the pros) increase. The pros represent the perceived advantages and act as facilitators of change. The cons are the disadvantages and act as barriers to change (Prochaska et al., 1994). Thus, is it more likely that people will move from precontemplation to contemplation when they perceive the advantages as being greater than the disadvantages. This idea of decisional balance (Prochaska et al., 1997), weighing the pros and cons, can be useful when planning a health education intervention.

To enable people to move from precontemplation to contemplation, the focus of education needs to be on the positive aspects or benefits of the new behavior rather than the negative aspects. For example, quitting smoking will make it easier to breathe, to walk, and to climb stairs and will save money. Focusing on these positive factors is more effective than focusing on the negative aspects of quitting, such as dealing with the withdrawal and weight gain.

Once the decision to change has been made, people move into the *preparation* or *planning stage.* During this time, people are planning to make the behavior change in the immediate future, often within the next month (Prochaska et al., 1997). The plan of action or means by which they will implement the change has been identified. For instance, continuing with the smoking example, the person may have already planned to use a nicotine patch and made an appointment with his or her health care provider.

People in this stage are the most receptive to health education interventions that are action oriented. These are the individuals who will attend a smoking cessation program, will keep appointments for blood pressure monitoring, or will make an appointment for counseling. These clients are ready to change. Many people in the preparation stage have already begun trying the new behavior. The smoker may have begun delaying that first morning cigarette (Prochaska et al., 1994), or the hypertensive may have already started to experiment with condiments other than salt.

During the *action stage,* the person is actively involved in the behavior change or adopting the new behavior. For the smoker, this means that he or she has quit smoking; for the hypertensive, it means that a low-salt diet is being carefully followed. Action is necessary for behavior to change, but changing behavior and keeping it changed are two different things. Ask any smoker how easy it is to quit. Most have quit many times. Maintaining the changed behavior is much more difficult a task than is making the change in the first place.

Thus, *maintenance* is the next stage of change. It begins after six months of adherence to the new behavior. It is a period of constant attention to the new behavior to prevent relapse, although relapse is less likely to occur in this stage than in the previous one. Sustaining the new behavior can be difficult, especially when there are cues in the environment that can trigger the old behavior (Prochaska et al., 1994).

People are in the maintenance phase for as long as there is temptation to revert to the problem behavior in certain situations. Behavior change has been completed and maintenance comes to an end when temptation in problematic situations no longer is a threat and the ability to resist relapse has developed (Basler, 1995). Individuals have reached the *termination stage* when the new behavior has become a habit, and they require no further intervention.

Theory of Reasoned Action

The *Theory of Reasoned Action* proposes that adoption of a new behavior results from individual intention to engage in the behavior. Behavioral intention is determined by attitude toward the behavior and the associated subjective norm (Montano, Kasprzyk, & Taplin, 1997).

Attitude toward the behavior is determined by beliefs about the outcome or attributes of the behavior. If it is believed that the behavior will result in a positive outcome, the attitude toward the behavior will be positive and there is a greater likelihood of adopting the new behavior. Conversely, if the attitude toward the behavior is negative, the likelihood of adopting the new behavior is diminished.

The subjective norm is determined by normative beliefs, or whether important others approve or disapprove of the targeted behavior (Montano et al., 1997). Important others may be family members or significant others. It is important to determine who the "important others" are for each individual client if this theory is to be used.

So, behavior change will result if a person plans to (intends to) change. If the behavior is seen as being good, and if the significant others believe the behavior is good, then the likelihood of adopting the behavior is increased. If the person does not plan to change his or her behavior, and if the behavior is not believed to be good and the significant others do not see the behavior as being good, then the likelihood of behavior change is decreased.

The key to using this theory effectively is to address the variables needed to ensure behavioral intention. This may mean changing the attitude toward the behavior or changing the subjective norm through including those significant others in the education process.

Behavior Modification Theory

Behavior Modification Theory, first proposed by B. F. Skinner in 1938, is based on the premise that behavior occurs because of its consequences (i.e., reinforcements or rewards). Changing the consequences, reinforcements or rewards (Skinner, 1938, 1953), then, can change behavior.

The consequences of a behavior can be a positive reinforcer, giving something that is wanted, or punishment, giving something that is not wanted or taking away something that is wanted (Hergehahn, 1994). Parents commonly use this approach, albeit they may not know they are using Skinner's theory. In potty training, a child is rewarded whenever he or she uses the toilet. The reward might be a favorite food, or snack, or a small toy. The child learns that if he or she uses the toilet, the reward will be given; hence, toilet use is continued.

Conversely, if a child is being taught not to run into the street, the consequence of running into the street would be a punishment rather than a reward. Hence, the child learns to avoid the street and avoid the negative consequence.

Although both positive reinforcers and punishment will shape behavior, Skinner believed that positive rewards should be used. Positive rewards strengthen behavior, but punishment does not necessarily eliminate it (Hergehahn, 1994). This is most profoundly demonstrated by our penal system. Imprisoning as a means of punishment for illegal behavior does not necessarily stop the person from ever engaging in the offensive behavior again.

Not only does the type of reinforcement shape behavior, but the rapidity with which it is given does also. Reinforcement given immediately after the target behavior is more powerful than one that is delayed. When the reinforcement is positive, even a small reward given right away is more effective than a large one that is delayed (Abrams, Emmons, & Linnan, 1997).

Behavior, according to this theory, does not entail reasoning, thought, or knowledge, but only external immediate rewards. As a result, the challenge to the nurse educator is to replace positive rewards associated with behaviors that hinder health with positive rewards for behaviors that enhance health (Butler, 1997).

Because behavior modification does not provide clients with information and skills or reasons so that they may change behavior themselves, there is the risk that these types of interventions are directly manipulating behavior. To address this concern, obtain informed consent from the client prior to the intervention (Kothari, 1999). By doing so, the client is making the decision to engage in an intervention designed to change his or her behavior. In addition, because the strength of the reward is such a powerful determinant of behavior, having the client choose the reward (or punishment) also diminishes the risk of behavior manipulation (Kothari, 1999).

Effectiveness of Health Education

Educational interventions, even if perfectly planned and implemented, will fail if the patient or client does not follow through or continue with the behavior changes. After all is said and done, changing behavior is a voluntary activity. Clients can be taught what to do, but it is up to them to do it. This aspect of education is often frustrating and can make teaching seem futile. It is not!

Health education interventions do work, and they work well. Hathaway's (1986) meta-analysis of 68 studies on the effects of preoperative education on postoperative outcomes revealed that 67 percent of clients who received preoperative instruction had more favorable surgical outcomes.

In a meta-analysis conducted by Devine (1992), 191 studies were examined for the effects of education on surgical recovery. This investigation found education to have beneficial effects on recovery, pain, and psychological distress.

Education programs have resulted in the reduction of physician office visits for stress-related palpitations, gastrointestinal problems, sleep disorders, chronic pain, physical symptoms of premenstrual syndrome, upper respiratory infections, and osteo- and rheumatoid arthritis (Grandinetti, 1996); reduction in hospitalizations for diabetes and emergency room visits for asthma (Barlett, 1995); and increased pregnancy rates for infertile couples and a reduction in preterm births (Barlett, 1995; Grandinetti, 1996). Education decreases anxiety, increases participation in self-care, and increases feelings of control over one's life (Wilson-Barnett & Osborne, 1983).

Teaching is an integral component of nursing practice. To teach effectively means that the educational experience has to be planned. Planning must take into account the client's unique characteristics, be based on the most appropriate theory for the given situation, and be presented in the most likely manner to attain success. The goal of any intervention is to meet the educational needs of the client, increase the likelihood of compliance, and, ultimately, improve health status.

CASE STUDY

Mr. R, 69 years old, comes to the cardiology physician practice where you work and is told he needs open heart surgery. You are responsible for his preliminary preoperative teaching.

1. What questions would you ask Mr. R to elicit his readiness to learn?
2. You know from experience that although many patients want as much information as you can give them, others do not want to be told too many details. How can you find out which group Mr. R is in?
3. How can you discover if Mr. R has any cultural beliefs that may affect the teaching/learning process?
4. You want to send Mr. R home with some pamphlets that give more information about his upcoming surgery. Assuming you have a wide variety of pamphlets, what types would you want to give Mr. R to reinforce your teaching?

CRITICAL THINKING EXERCISES

1. You are preparing to teach a young woman recently diagnosed with lupus how best to manage her illness. How would your approach differ if you base your teaching on the Health Belief Model versus Self-Efficacy Theory?
2. If you are a clinical preceptor in a health care agency, how could Social Cognitive Theory assist you in teaching your preceptee?
3. What data would you need in order to determine what stage of change a person is in according to the Transtheoretical Model?
4. What ethical principle(s) might be violated if you use Behavior Modification as a way of trying to change health-related behaviors, without the informed consent of the client?

IDEAS FOR FURTHER RESEARCH

1. We read a lot of statistics about what percentage of information is retained when we *hear* it versus *read* it versus *say* it, and so on. However, there is not much research data to support the figures we read. Design an experiment to test the amount of retention given these various sensory inputs.

2. Interview patients who have had open heart surgery or joint replacement surgery to determine their remembered and perceived readiness to learn preoperatively. Ask them what health care professionals could have done to enhance their readiness and better prepare them for surgery.

3. Conduct a longitudinal study of smokers. Study whether the Health Belief Model helps explain their smoking behavior over time.

4. Survey women who have yearly mammograms done versus women who don't. Ask questions designed to elicit their beliefs about outcomes of the mammogram and what are the beliefs of their significant others. Determine whether the Theory of Reasoned Action explains their behavior.

REFERENCES

Abrams, D. B., Emmons, K. M., & Linnan, L. A. (1997). Health behavior and health education: The past, present and future. In K. Glanz, F. Lewis, & B. Rimer (Eds.), *Health behavior and health education: Theory, research and practice* (2nd ed.) (pp. 453–478). San Francisco: Jossey-Bass.

Bandura, A. (1977). *A social learning theory.* Upper Saddle River, NJ: Prentice Hall.

Bandura, A. (1986). *Social foundations of thought and actions: A social cognitive theory.* Upper Saddle River, NJ: Prentice Hall.

Bandura, A. (1989). Human agency in social cognitive theory. *American Psychologist, 44*(9), 1175–1184.

Baranowski, T., Perry, C. L., & Parcel, G. S. (1997). How individuals, environments and health behavior interact. In K. Glanz, F. Lewis, & B. Rimer (Eds.), *Health behavior and health education: Theory, research and practice* (2nd ed.) (pp. 153–178), San Francisco: Jossey-Bass.

Bartlett, E. E. (1995). Cost–benefit analysis of patient education. *Health Education and Counseling, 26,* 87–91.

Basler, H. D. (1995). Patient education with reference to the process of behavioral change. *Patient Education and Counseling, 26,* 91–98.

Biener, L., Abrams, D. B., Follick, M. J., & Dean, L. (1989). A comparative evaluation of a restrictive smoking policy in a general hospital. *American Journal of Public Health, 79,* 192–195.

Breckon, D. J., Harvey, J. R., & Lancaster, R. B. (1998). *Community health education.* Gaithersburg, MD: Aspen.

Butler, J. T. (1997). *Principles of health education & health promotion.* Englewood, CO: Morton.

Devine, E. C. (1992). Effects of psychoeducational care for adult surgical patients: A meta-analysis of 191 studies. *Patient Education and Counseling, 19,* 129–142.

Elder, J. P., Ayala, G. X., & Harris, S. (1999). Theories and intervention approaches to health behavior change in primary care. *American Journal of Preventive Medicine, 17*(4), 275–284.

Glanz, K., Lewis, F., & Rimer, B. (Eds.). (1997). *Health behavior and health education: Theory, research and practice* (2nd ed). San Francisco: Jossey-Bass.

Grandinetti, D. (1996, November 25). Teaching patients to take care of themselves. *Medical Economics,* 83–92.

Hathaway, D. (1986). Effect of preoperative instruction on postoperative outcomes: A meta-analysis. *Nursing Research, 35*(5), 269–281.

Hergehahn, B. R. (1994). An introduction to theories of personality. Upper Saddle River, NJ: Prentice Hall.

Huff, R. M., & Kline, M. V. (1999). *Promoting health in multicultural populations.* Thousand Oaks, CA: Sage.

Kothari, S. (1999). The ethics of behavior modification. *Topics in Stroke Rehabilitation, 5*(4), 66–69.

McKenzie, J. F., & Smeltzer, J. L. (2001). *Planning, implementing and evaluating health promotion programs* (3rd ed.). Needham Heights, MA: Allyn & Bacon.

Montano, D. E., Kasprzyk, D., & Taplin, S. H. (1997). The theory of reasoned action and the theory of planned behavior. In K. Glanz, F. Lewis, & B. Rimer (Eds.), *Health behavior and health education: Theory, research and practice* (2nd ed.) (pp. 85–112). San Francisco: Jossey-Bass.

Moss, V. A. (1994). Assessing learning abilities, readiness for education. *Seminars in Perioperative Nursing, 3*(3), 113–120.

Nakamaura, R. M. (1999). *Health in America: A multicultural perspective.* Boston: Allyn & Bacon.

Prochaska, J. O., Redding, C. A., & Evers, K. E. (1997). The transtheoretical model and stages of change. In K. Glanz, F. Lewis, & B. Rimer (Eds.): *Health behavior and health education: Theory, research and practice* (2nd ed.) (pp. 60–84). San Francisco: Jossey-Bass.

Prochaska, J. P., Redding, C. A., Harlow, L. L., Rossi, J. S., & Velicer, W. F. (1994). The transtheoretical model of change and HIV prevention: A review. *Health Education Quarterly, 21*(4), 471–486.

Rosenstock, I. M. (1974). Historical origins of the Health Belief Model. *Health Education Monograph, 2,* 328–335.

Shade, B., Kelly, C., & Oberg, M. (1997). Creating culturally responsive classrooms. Washington, DC: American Psychological Association.

Skinner, B. F. (1938). *The behavior of organisms.* East Norwalk, CT: Appleton & Lange.

Skinner, B. F. (1953). *Science and human behavior.* New York: Macmillan.

Strecher, V. J., DeVillis, B. M., Becker, M. H., & Rosenstock, I. M. (1986). The role of self-efficacy in achieving health behavior change. *Health Education Quarterly, 13*(1), 73–92.

Weinstein, N. D., Rothman, A. J., & Sutton, S. R. (1998). Stages of change theories of health behavior: Conceptual and methodological issues. *Health Psychology, 17,* 1–10.

Wilson-Barnett, J., & Osborne, J. (1983). Studies evaluating patient teaching: Implications for practice. *International Journal of Nursing Studies, 20*(1), 33–44.

5

Multicultural Aspects
of Learning

The focus of this chapter is instructing learners from diverse cultural backgrounds. The learners may be nursing students, nurses, or patients and clients from a culture that is different from the teacher's. Topics include the examination of the concepts of culture and cultural competence; assessment of the learner; use of explanatory models; effective teaching strategies; and communicating with people for whom English is a second language. Finally, gender issues will be discussed.

Nurse educators are seeing more learners from various cultures in the classroom due to the dramatic increases in ethnic minorities in the United States. It is predicted that by the year 2010, the U.S. population will increase by 42 million and this includes increases in the number of Hispanics (37 percent), African Americans (22 percent), Asians (18 percent), and European Americans (13 percent) (Davidhizar, Dowd, & Giger, 1998).

Nurse educators in clinical settings recognize the importance of culture in interacting with clients and colleagues. As the U.S. population continues to become more diverse, the ability to recognize different cultural values and practices and to address these factors in interventions are likely to lead to more successful treatment outcomes (Bonder, Martin, & Miracle, 2001). Eliason and Raheim (2000) contend that in dealing with culture, there are two major roles for nurse educators: (1) creating specific multicultural curricular content and (2) providing a learning environment for learners from all backgrounds.

A major problem confronting nurse educators is how to present content on cultural diversity without stereotyping. Classifying all cultural and ethnic groups as having the same characteristics and attributes negates the uniqueness of the individual. There are great cultural variations between cultural and ethnic groups, and it is important to consider each student, registered nurse, and client as an individual. Teaching learners cultural competence skills is beyond the scope of this chapter and has been addressed by several authors (AAN Expert Panel Report, 1992; Abrums & Leppa, 2001; Sommer, 2001).

Learning About Culture

Cultural diversity has been defined broadly (Eliason & Raheim, 2000). Characteristics of culture include gender, race, and ethnicity, sexuality identity, age, physical ability, social circumstances, and religion. With cultural diversity come identifiable differences in language, communication, dress, behavior, and socialization among groups.

Bonder, Martin, and Miracle (2001, p. 36) offer the following points about culture:

1. Culture is learned and transmitted from one generation to another.
2. Culture is localized and is created through specific interactions with specific individuals.
3. Culture is patterned. These patterns emerge from the repetition of specific behaviors.
4. Culture is evaluative. Values are the central components of culture and are reflected in individual behaviors. Values also reflect shared beliefs that facilitate the social interaction with others.
5. Culture has continuity, with change. In general, cultural identity is stable but one's cultural knowledge changes over the life course as one encounters new objects, situations, and ideas in the environment.

Promoting Cultural Knowledge

There are three main approaches to promoting cultural knowledge and competency for health care providers and nurse educators. First is the fact-centered approach, which provides information about the health beliefs and behaviors of specific ethnic groups. The advantage of this approach is that it is a starting place for interactions with one individual. Factual knowledge of an ethnic group is vital to effective cross-cultural interactions. Keep in mind, however, that African Americans, Hispanics, Native Americans, and Asian groups are not single cultures but consist of many diverse groups.

The second approach to culture is attitude centered, emphasizing the importance of valuing and respecting all cultures. The advantage of this approach is the acknowledgment of culture and fostering of positive attitudes. The focus on cultural sensitivity is an example of this approach.

A third method is an ethnographic approach to cultural competence. This approach offers a practical strategy of "learning how to ask." The focus of this approach is on inquiry, reflection, and analysis as a means of getting to know an individual. This approach will further be clarified in the discussion on explanatory models.

A Cultural Competence Model

Cultural competence is the ability to work effectively in a cross-cultural situation. Nurse educators in both clinical and academic settings need to develop cultural competence themselves before they can help students and nurses become more culturally competent.

One model of cultural competence, proposed by a nurse, presents an understanding of the processes involved in becoming culturally competent. Campinha-Bacote (1998) defines cultural competence in the delivery of health care services as "the process in which the healthcare provider continuously strives to achieve the ability to effectively work within the cultural context of a client, individual, family or community" (p. 6). This model allows nurses to see themselves as *becoming* culturally competent, rather than *being* culturally competent. This model involves the five interrelated aspects of cultural competence seen in Table 5–1 and explained below.

CULTURAL AWARENESS

Cultural awareness is the process whereby the nurse becomes respectful, appreciative, and sensitive to the values, beliefs, practices, and problem-solving strategies of a client's culture. It involves self-examination of one's own prejudice and bias about other cultures, in addition to an in-depth exploration of one's own cultural background. Cultural awareness is viewed along a continuum that ranges from ethnocentrism to ethnorelativism.

Ethnocentrism is a behavior in which a person is totally unaware of others' cultural beliefs and values. The ethnocentric individual assumes that his or her values, beliefs, and practices are the only correct perceptions. Leininger (1978) emphasized that if you are not aware of the influence your own cultural values, there is a risk that you may engage in *cultural imposition,* which is the tendency to impose your own beliefs, values, practices, and patterns of behavior on another. Cultural imposition also may lead to noncompliance with health care regimens. Campinha-Bacote (1998) reports that noncompliance is not a client problem, but rather may be the nurse's failure to provide culturally responsive care that incorporates the client's cultural beliefs and values.

In contrast, *ethnorelativism* reflects an attitude of nurses who value, respect, and integrate cultural differences into their practice. They are aware of their cultural backgrounds, along with prejudices and biases about other cultures. This awareness alone does not ensure culturally responsive interventions. Nurses must develop other needed components of cultural competence.

CULTURAL KNOWLEDGE

Cultural knowledge involves the process of seeking and obtaining factual information about different cultures. Campinha-Bacote (1998) describes four stages of obtaining cultural knowledge:

1. *Unconscious incompetence* is identified as an individual's being unaware that he or she lacks cultural knowledge.

TABLE 5-1 **Aspects of Cultural Competence**

Cultural awareness: Becoming respectful and appreciative of another's culture

Cultural knowledge: Obtaining factual knowledge about different cultures

Cultural encounters: Engaging in cross-cultural encounters with people from other cultures

Cultural skill: Collecting relevant cultural data about a client's health history and accurately performing culturally specific physical assessment

Cultural desire: Wanting to engage in learning cultural competence

Source: Campinha-Bacote, J. (1998). *The process of cultural competence in the delivery of health care services* (3rd ed.). Cincinnati, OH: Transcultural CARE Associates Press.

2. *Conscious incompetence* is the awareness that he or she lacks knowledge about another culture and is willing to seek and obtain the knowledge.
3. *Conscious competence* is the act of learning about a client's culture, verifying generalization, and providing culturally responsive nursing interventions.
4. *Unconscious competence* is the ability to automatically apply knowledge and culturally congruent care to clients from diverse cultural backgrounds. The nurse who has unconscious competence interacts naturally and easily with clients from diverse cultures.

CULTURAL ENCOUNTERS

A *cultural encounter* is the process whereby a nurse engages directly in cross-cultural interactions with clients from culturally diverse backgrounds. One of the purposes of this encounter is to refine or modify one's belief about those groups to prevent possible stereotyping.

CULTURAL SKILL

Cultural skill is the ability to collect relevant cultural data about a client's health history and health problems, as well as to accurately perform culturally specific physical assessment. Leininger (1978) defined a cultural assessment as a "systematic appraisal or examination of individuals, groups and communities as to their cultural beliefs, values, and practices to determine explicit needs and intervention practices within the context of the people be evaluated" (pp. 85–86). The literature offers several assessment tools that nurses can use when conducting a cultural assessment (Giger & Davidhizar, 1999; Purnell, 2000).

CULTURAL DESIRE

Cultural desire is the nurse's motivation to engage in the process of cultural competence. Nurses need to want to work toward cultural competence as they provide individualized and safe care to clients.

Nurse educators who work in academic settings also face the challenges of becoming culturally competent themselves and teaching their students about culturally appropriate care. Eliason and Raheim (2000) reported that a majority of nursing students still come from the Western dominant culture and are raised within families and educational systems with inherent racial biases and other prejudices. It is important for nurse educators to be aware of potential areas of bias in beginning nursing students, so that these biases are addressed directly before students encounter clients from diverse backgrounds. Research conducted by Eliason and Raheim measured the relationship of prenursing students' exposure to 14 culturally diverse groups. The study took place in a major Midwestern university. One hundred ninety-six white undergraduate students in a nursing prerequisite course volunteered for the study. Participation included completing an open-ended questionnaire designed to examine comfort levels with people from 14 groups. Four major themes emerged from the data.

1. Discomfort caused by lack of knowledge, skills, or exposure to group members
2. Discomfort caused by disapproval or negative attitudes toward group members
3. Discomfort as a result of feeling threatened by group members
4. Discomfort caused by feelings of guilt, sympathy, or pity toward group members

In order to provide a learning environment conducive for all learners, nurse educators need to understand learners' cultural attitudes and perceptions of others and of authority figures.

Higher-education programs need to prepare teachers who can effectively provide instruction to students of diverse backgrounds and cultures (Pettus & Allain, 1999). Studies have shown that "a high correlation exists among educators' sensitivity (attitudes, beliefs, and behaviors toward students of other cultures) knowledge and application of cultural awareness information, and multicultural students' successful academic performance" (Larke, 1990, p. 24).

The Culture of Teachers and Learners

In addition to the characteristics of nurse educators described in the other chapters of this book, there are specific characteristics of effective teachers related to working with multicultural students.

Many, if not most, nurse educators are from the dominant culture and have never examined their own culture. Some educators have stated that they don't have a "culture" since their families have been in the United States for three generations or more. They may respond to different values and behaviors exhibited by multicultural students with confusion, uncertainty, and possibly bias.

Faculty in institutions of higher learning tend to be homogenous with 93 percent of professors from Caucasian backgrounds, while 70 percent are male and 42 to 54 years old (McKenna, 1989). In nursing, the majority of faculty are from Caucasian European backgrounds.

There is a need for increased numbers of ethnic minority nurse educators who have been successful in the Western educational system to serve as role models for multicultural students. Some authors reported that differences in interactions between teachers and students are attributable to race, ethnicity, or gender, and the differences are reflected in student performance (Brophy & Good, 1984; Fennema & Peterson, 1986).

Variables found to promote successful student learning and achievement include faculty commitment and advisement, prompt and individualized attention to students, and satisfying relationships with faculty, staff, and peers (Courage & Godbey, 1992). Nurse educators who work with multicultural students should consider the following:

1. Become self-aware of your own cultural values, norms, and beliefs and the influence they have on your view of life, family, and relationships.
2. Develop and maintain an attitude of respect for the broad range of cultural differences and their importance to individuals. Identify and value the strengths in different cultural values and beliefs rather than becoming critical of them.
3. Develop a strategy for continuing education about predominant cultures in a given community or institution.
4. Explore the possibility of integrating the appropriate use of teaching strategies and communications.
5. Consider the use of other professionals and members of the community from other cultures to learn more about the culture.

Assessing the Culturally Diverse Learner

Educating culturally diverse learners presents a challenge to nurse educators. We must be aware of the fact there are varying cultural behaviors and that these behaviors are the result of past educational experiences, cultural beliefs, and cultural heritage. Cultural differences may have a significant impact on the way learners think and learn. Therefore, learners from different cultures vary in the manner in which they receive information, process information, and apply information.

Davidhizar, Dowd, and Giger (1998) propose one model for assessing differences between people in cultural groups. Learners may vary according to six factors: communication, space, time, social organization, environmental control, and biological variations. Understanding these interrelated factors provides a first step toward appreciating the diversity that exists between people from varied backgrounds as applied to an educational setting.

COMMUNICATION

Communication is the means by which culture is transmitted and preserved through the generations. Cultural patterns consisting of verbal and nonverbal expression of each cultural group affect the way the group expresses ideas and feelings, the way they make decisions, and the way they communicate. Certain communication patterns may be culture specific. For example, Native Americans may value nonverbal and passive approaches to communication, while European Americans may value more verbal and active approaches. However, educators must be cautious about assuming that a certain communication pattern can be generalized to all persons in a designated cultural group, because communication patterns are often unique and variable.

Nurse educators need to be aware of the complexity in communication, especially in learners whose primary language is other than English. Misunderstandings are not necessarily due to problems in translation. This topic will be further addressed later in this chapter.

SPACE

An individual's level of comfort is related to personal space or distance, and discomfort is experienced when one's personal space is invaded. Personal space is an individual matter and varies with the situation. The proximity of the comfort zone also varies from culture to culture. For example, Puerto Ricans and African Americans may communicate with others in closer proximity than do Americans from European backgrounds. A distance of three feet is usually acceptable with individuals in the United States while a distance of one to two feet may be accepted in other cultures. Davidhizar, Dowd, and Giger (1998) note that the educator must be aware that students may have differing spatial needs when conversing with others, conducting group work, or concentrating when taking a test.

SOCIAL ORGANIZATION

Cultural behavior, or how one acts in certain situations, is socially acquired and learned. These patterns of cultural behavior are important to the teacher because they provide explanations for people's behavior. Individuals are not generally conscious of their cultural behavior.

A recent study examined the differences between two groups of nursing students. Pacquiao (1996) reported that European American nursing students identified with core values of individualism, honesty, truthfulness, straightforwardness, self-assuredness, self-confidence, and self-motivation. In contrast, ethnically diverse students reported values related to mutual interdependence and group centeredness. These attributes involve sensitivity, respect, loyalty, generosity, sense of belonging, cooperation, tolerance, and accommodation of others.

Values such as those held by students in Pacquiao's study affect learning and the learning environment. One useful method of recognizing differences in beliefs and values is to ask students to share their views, based on their culture, with the class or with the instructor.

TIME

Temporal orientation refers to how time is viewed. It includes the ordering of past, present, and future in terms of behavior and outlook. In education, getting assignments done in a specific time frame is more important for a learner who is present or future oriented. If the cultural value is "let it go until tomorrow," a student may have difficulty meeting deadlines for term papers and being on time for classes. Assisting all students to focus on beginning tasks on time and sticking to a deadline to achieve a goal may be an important cultural adjustment for someone with a future time orientation. Assisting students to identify their own values in relationship to time is helpful.

ENVIRONMENTAL CONTROL

Environmental control refers to a person's ability to plan activities that control nature. It also refers to the person's perception of his or her ability to direct factors in the environment.

Dominant North American values tend to stress the ability to use, control, and master the environment. Americans want to examine and explain environmental phenomena in a rational and critical manner. On the other hand, cultures that view nature as greater than human beings tend to be fatalistic. People from cultures that tend to accept the status quo do not require rational explanations for uncommon phenomena. Rather, they emphasize providing harmonious relations with nature. In an educational setting that values independent problem solving and initiative to achieve rational explanations, a person oriented to accepting things as they are and striving for integration rather than control may be at a disadvantage. An example of how a teacher might intervene to aid such students is when the teacher helps them to see that poor grades or failure on an exam are not destined as fate but rather something that can be influenced or changed.

BIOLOGICAL VARIATIONS

Last, educators should know that learners from different backgrounds have genetic biological differences that may affect their classroom performance. One such difference may be susceptibility to disease.

Using Explanatory Models

An *explanatory model* is a tool that helps a culturally different patient or client to explain his or her viewpoint or perspective on health and illness. Explanatory models have relevance for assessing clients, planning care, and teaching clinicians to deliver culturally appropriate care. In order to individualize care planning, it is essential to have an understanding of the client's interpretation of a specific illness event and cultural views of health. Eliciting a client's explanatory model, as one aspect of a routine nursing history, provides the following information: (a) similarities and differences between the client's explanatory model and that of Western biomedicine; (b) potential points of differences that may inhibit planning of care;

and (c) history of the client's self-care actions and use of resources (McSweeney, 1993). Nurse educators are encouraged to use explanatory models in teaching nurses and nursing students to further their understanding of a client's experience with illness.

Kleinman (1980) reported that explanatory models contain any one or all five parts of an illness:

- Etiology
- Time of onset of symptoms
- Pathophysiology
- Course of sickness
- Treatment

Kleinman demonstrated that culturally based knowledge and beliefs concerning health and illness could be elicited by exploring eight questions. The questions listed in Table 5–2 can be added to any health assessment.

Explanatory models tend to change over time and are influenced by social environment, ethnicity, subjective interpretation of past experiences, and tacit knowledge. Because explanatory models can change, an ongoing illness experience, new knowledge, or a significant health event may modify them. Nurses can influence explanatory models by health teaching, or family members and peers may influence them by modeling health behaviors (McSweeney, 1993).

Blumhagen (1982) suggests that explanatory models provide a substantive link between a person's beliefs and accepted treatments, and several research studies have supported this link (Luyas, 1991; McSweeney, 1993). Therefore, justification to comply, modify, or ignore advice may flow from personal explanatory models.

Exploring a client's explanatory model can lead to culturally appropriate treatment plans addressing lifestyles, illness concerns, and priorities in the context of their daily lives. In nursing research and practice, the concept of explanatory models has relevance. The concept provides one way to understand phenomena relevant to health needs of multicultural populations. Specifically, researchers and clinicians can use explanatory models to explore health and illness beliefs, linkages between beliefs and actions, help-seeking behaviors, and nurse-to-client communication (McSweeney, Allan, & Mayo, 1997).

TABLE 5-2 Questions That May Be Asked in Eliciting an Explanatory Model

1. What do you call your problem? What name does it have?
2. What do you think has caused your problem? (Etiology)
3. Why do you think it started when it did? (Time of onset)
4. What does your sickness do to you? How does it work? (Pathophysiology)
5. How severe is it? Will it have a short or long course? (Course of sickness)
6. What do you fear most about your sickness?
7. What are the chief problems your sickness has cause for you? (Personally, in your family, and at work.)
8. What kind of treatment do you think you should receive? What are the most important results you hope to receive from the current treatment?

Source: Kleinman, A. (1980). *Patients and healers in the context of culture.* Berkeley, CA: University of California Press.

Teaching Strategies

Nurse educators should use their knowledge of cultural diversity to adapt teaching strategies for multicultural groups.

Learning Styles

Several researchers address the concept of learning style in respect to teaching multicultural learners. Learning style has been defined as "characteristic cognitive, affective, and physiological behaviors that serve as relatively stable indicators of how learners perceive, interact with, and respond to the learning environment" (Keane, 1993, p. 215). Generally, it is agreed that learning styles do not imply intelligence but rather a way by which individuals process stimuli (Even, as cited in Pacquiao, 1996).

In an early study, Messick (1976) reported that research does not support definitive links between learning style and race, culture, and gender, yet there are consistent findings that suggest a correlation exists. Ethnic groups, independent of socioeconomic differences, demonstrate characteristic patterns of abilities that are different from one another. Lesser (1976) reported that students of similar ethnic background have similar patterns of mental capabilities that significantly differ from other cultural groups. Pacquiao (1996) reported that nursing faculty working with a sample of ethnic minority students had concerns that these learners preferred rote learning and memorization. The faculty reported that students' cognitive style was concrete and visual. These learning patterns are attributed to past learning experiences in the family and in schools.

Keane (1993) noted that correct identification of students' learning preferences and instructional methods appropriate to their learning preferences positively affected their academic achievement. In addition, helping students to achieve understanding of their own learning style and how they learn assisted them in their ability to process information.

Sullivan (1993) noted that although some people may learn without using their learning style preferences, many students achieve significantly better when they capitalize on their preferences. No single instructional method works for all students. Some teaching approaches may help students perform well, while other teaching approaches enable the student to perform only marginally, and others may contribute to poor performance (Dunn & Griggs, 1995).

Based on the research literature identified by Dunn and Griggs (1995, pp. 41–67), and Yurkovich (2001), the following are findings of learning style characteristics of major cultural groups.

Native Americans
- Use imagery, symbolism, mediation, and relaxation.
- Use reflective learning, taking time before responding; being quiet in a group setting.
- Respond to learning by using advance organizers, making connections between the content and real life problems.
- Prefer activities that create cooperation rather than competition.
- Prefer listening, observing, and doing.

Hispanics

- Hispanics are a highly diverse group and include very distinct subcultures that differ significantly as to customs, values, and education orientation.
- First-generation Hispanic students usually communicate more freely in Spanish.
- Prefer formal settings, conformity (especially for first generation), peer-oriented learning (dependent on socioeconomic status and geographic region), kinesthetic instructional resources, and a high degree of structure.

African Americans

- Tendency to prefer global learning.
- Prefer bright light warm temperatures and informal design while learning.
- Require collegial support and presence of authority while learning.
- Visual kinesthetic learners who reject the auditory modality.

Asian Americans

- Environmental preferences for formal design.
- Emotional requirements for a high degree of structure.
- Some are strongly visual but a majority appear to prefer kinesthetic and tactual.
- Analytic field independent cognitive style.

See Chapter 2 for more information on learning styles.

Teaching/Learning Process

The teaching/learning process begins with assessment. Assessment provides the nurse educator with information about the knowledge and skills needed as well as the learner's characteristics within the context of ethnic and cultural considerations. An understanding of the learner's verbal and nonverbal cues, language, level of understanding, and preferred learning styles are important assessment information in this phase.

The second step is development of a teaching plan. The teaching plan is a carefully organized written presentation of what the learner needs to learn and how the nurse educator is going to provide the teaching. The teaching plan needs to include culturally relevant skills for the learner. The learning goals can be negotiated with the learner in the educational and clinical settings. A culturally congruent teaching strategies plan should include visual, auditory, and psychomotor strategies or a combination of two or more strategies, as well as the appropriate reading levels for the learner. The focus of every lesson or class session should include multiple strategies when teaching multicultural learners. The nurse educator can select from a variety of multimedia formats, presentations, group work, and assigned readings, as well as access activities through the Internet.

Following assessment and planning comes implementation and application of the teaching plan. The implementation should consider the learner's previous understanding, knowledge, and readiness in the learning situation.

Other teaching approaches have been found to be effective with culturally and ethnically diverse learners:

- Negotiation of learning goals (mentioned previously)
- Providing for immediate application and learning to help reinforce newly learned content
- Creating opportunities for learners to test their own ideas, take risks, and be creative. These activities enhance self-esteem.

Cross-Cultural Issues in Computer-Based Learning

Morgan (2000) reports, ". . . cross-cultural considerations can be a major influence in the successful understanding of educational and instructional concepts" (p. 491). Therefore, interactive computer/learning designers need to address cross-cultural considerations in software development. Nurse educators in designing or using computers as a teaching/learning strategy should consider the importance of using symbols and methods that users can recognize from their own cultural background and experience.

- *Symbols:* Care should be taken with the use of symbols or icons in the presentation of simulations. Some symbols, which appear quite innocent to the Western eye, can be of great religious significance. For instance, the symbol for the human or animal eye can be disturbing to many cultures as a symbol of evil.
- *Sounds:* The use of sound within a system adds life and interest to the learning situation. However, many innocent sounds may have a meaning other than the one intended to someone from another culture. For instance, the cries of some animals can denote evil to some cultures.
- *Directional flow:* The designer should be aware of the national directional flow that language takes in the users' cultures. The Western written flow is from left to right. In some Asian countries, the directional flow of writing is from right to left.
- *Selection of words and phrases:* The tone and use of language has a major impact on the effect of communication and on the interactive learning environment. Many words or phrases that are in common use within the computing industry can be highly offensive to many groups of users. For example, the words *kill* and *abort* are highly emotive words and can be replaced with descriptive words *end* and *cancel.*
- *Words, sounds, and mistranslation:* Caution should be used when making direct translations of words and to the meanings of the sounds of words used within a system.
- *Selection of human voices:* An increasing number of simulations include the use of human voices to add impact and realism to the interactive learning environment. However, care should be taken with the selection of these voices. In some cultures, a female voice giving instruction would not be as effective as a male voice because females are considered to have a lower social status. In many cultures, it has been found that female voices get more attention and are less irritating, so the solution for the simulation designer might to be include both female and male voices and allow users to select the voice they prefer.
- *Behavior stereotyping:* One of the most frequently cited criticisms with regard to the computer-based portrayal of people is behavior stereotyping. This phenomenon is one in which individuals of certain gender, age, occupation, religion, or ethnic backgrounds are shown consistently behaving or dressing in a particular way.

- *Colors:* Certain colors can be associated with death and disease based on one's culture. This may not be obvious from a typical Western viewpoint. For example, white is considered a color of death in some Asian countries.
- *Gestures:* Similar problems can arise from the use of animated gestures. In some cultures, a nod can be taken as a sign of a negative response. The soles of the feet can be highly offensive in some Middle Eastern countries.
- *Handedness:* In some cultures, passing or touching items with the left hand can be highly offensive.

Educational programs should consider developing a committee or panel to review instructional modules, including interactive simulations, for culturally appropriate materials. Ideally, the composition of the committee should include members from diverse cultural backgrounds.

Communication Issues

In this section, issues surrounding communication with a learner for whom English is not the primary language, patient education, and literacy will be discussed.

Cross-Cultural Communication with Nursing Students

There have been great efforts to recruit and retain students from underrepresented groups into nursing. Underrepresented groups include U.S.-born ethnically diverse students and immigrant English as a Second Language (ESL) students. Because of numerous cultural and language challenges, the rates of successful completion of the NCLEX-RN of ESL nursing students have been lower than those students who speak English as a first language (Johnston, 1989).

ESL students are learners who speak a native, first, home, or primary language other than standard English and are not fluent in standard English (Malu & Figlear, 1998). These students include many of the ethnic and cultural groups in the United States, immigrant students who come to the United States to either reside for an extended or indefinite period of time, or international students who usually come to study and return to their country when their studies are completed.

Villarruel, Canales, and Torres (2001) reported that Hispanic nursing students who had accents and for whom English was a second language experienced difficulties in school. Specifically, the students reported that faculty believed they were not capable of succeeding in the program.

Communicating and writing effectively in a second language has been identified as a major challenge facing ESL nursing students. Strategies identified to assist them include assessment of language proficiency, language assistance throughout the program, and measures taken by faculty to decrease test bias and facilitate test taking.

In one nursing program, prospective students are given the SPEAK test (Speaking Proficiency English Assessment Kit). This test is available from the Educational Testing

Service, Princeton, New Jersey. The test provides a valid and reliable assessment of the English speaking proficiency of people who are not native speakers of the language. Students who do not pass the SPEAK test on the first attempt are offered one-to-one tutoring. The goal of tutoring is to improve English comprehension, speaking, and writing. Tutoring is also available in accent reduction, pronunciation, and fluency of speech (Klisch, 2000).

ESL nursing students are not necessarily remedial students but need to be perceived and taught as foreign-born language students who have not quite mastered English. Keane (1993) identified several strategies to help these students:

- Use collaborative projects.
- Conduct small groups.
- Have students summarize main points from lectures.
- Read assignments and/or vignettes.
- Teach anxiety-reduction techniques.
- Teach group process as a study skill.

According to Malu and Figlear (1998), there are several problems with nursing's language, which cause difficulties for ESL students. One problem is that words are used interchangeably. Terms such as *nursing measure, intervention, order, approach,* and *implementation* are just a few examples of how confusing our vocabulary can be. Another problem is that some words have dual meanings, such as *tablet.* The non-ESL student would be able to discern the word *tablet* from the context in the sentence, whereas the ESL student would not be able to do so. Words do not always translate literally, such as *pouring* in other cultures. Another concern is words that look similar but have different meanings such as *internal* versus *interval.* These words can cause difficulty for ESL and non-ESL students.

Nurse educators need to help their students explore and build nursing terminology. Malu and Figlear (1998) suggest nurse educators begin by preparing a handout or outline of examples of problem words or categories of problem words. Nurse educators can require students to keep a vocabulary notebook in which students write the word, its definition or translation in English, its synonyms, and any personal connections they can make with the word. The vocabulary words in the notebooks can also be transferred to note cards and used as flash cards when reviewing exams. The authors further suggest that students can use these cards to build a concept map, categorize words, and connect interrelated concepts.

ESL nursing students may require assistance during examinations. Klisch (2000) recommends that beginning students be allowed to bring bilingual dictionaries and have additional time to complete examinations. Nurse educators could provide synonyms on exams for everyday words that ESL nursing students do not understand. However, a nursing content word such as *asepsis,* a word that students should know, should not be clarified. These suggested practices regarding use of dictionaries, time for examinations, and language clarification need to change as students progress through the curriculum as they become more proficient with English and the academic content of nursing courses.

Nurse educators need to encourage ESL students to immerse themselves in English. Immersion activities include participation in study and class discussion groups, attendance at extracurricular activities sponsored by the school, involvement in a nursing organization, participation in English language church services, or shopping in a predominantly English-speaking mall (Malu & Figlear, 1998). Improving the academic success of ESL students is a collaborative process between the nurse educator and student that begins early in the nursing program.

Cross-Cultural Communication and In-Service Education

Nurse educators in clinical settings who are responsible for orienting new nurses need to be aware of strategies that promote transition for ESL nurses. Sep and Jezewski (2000) reported five areas of concern when recruiting and hiring international nurses:

1. Relieving psychological stress
2. Overcoming the language barrier
3. Accepting U.S. nursing practice
4. Incorporating the styles of U.S. problem-solving strategies
5. Implementing the styles of U.S. interpersonal relationships

International nurses preparing for the NCLEX exam or going through new staff orientation need many of the same interventions explained in the previous paragraphs in reference to nursing students.

Cross-Cultural Communication with Patients and Clients

Nurses must use cross-cultural communication skills when teaching patients (Petaschnick, 2001). The nurse educator must know when and how to present material that respects cultural values. The nurse educator must also learn how to mediate cultural differences and how to promote modifications when necessary (Chachkes & Christ, 1996).

It is important to assess the various patterns of communication among nurses and clients. There are differences in verbal expressiveness and affective behaviors. In some cultures, highly expressive modes of communication are valued, while in others, more subdued modes are preferred. For example, Asians place a high value on polite, restrained behavior and will approach professionals in a nonconfrontational manner. Hispanics value more emotive expressions while European Americans value directness and openness in communication.

Nonverbal communication styles also vary. In some groups, physical touching is acceptable, while in others, it is considered taboo. For instance, Orthodox Jewish men will not shake hands with women. A woman never touches a man other than her husband, even to shake hands. In many Asian groups, touching the head, eye-to-eye contact, waving arms with palms upward, and pointing at things with one's feet are considered rude and disrespectful. Native Americans may value nonverbal and more passive approaches to communication than European Americans, and responses to questions may be short and offered only when requested. Understanding cultural patterns will help in the development of educational strategies that are more acceptable to clients from diverse cultures.

When the client is from a culture that differs from that of the care provider, it is important to be alert to cultural barriers to effective client education. Initial assessment is necessary to determine whether the client understands the language being spoken (Davidhizar & Brownson, 1999). If the client cannot understand instructions given, an in-person interpreter or telephone interpreter should be obtained. When an agency interpreter is not available, a family member may be used. Recruiting a child to serve as an interpreter can be problematic since a child does not necessarily understand or adequately explain information.

In addition to language, it is important to assess other elements of communication when a client from another culture is being treated. These include dialect, style (language and social situations), volume (silence), use of touch, context of speech (emotional tone), and kinetics (gesture, stance, and eye behavior). Note that each of these factors varies within the same cultural group and between cultural groups. For example, in certain cultures, individuals may appear loud while talking, while in other cultures, people tend to speak in a soft voice. As a result, a nurse can erroneously correlate loudness with anger, and softness of voice with timidity, indecisiveness, lack of assertiveness, and incompetence.

Another barrier to communicating with a client from another culture may be the client's view of the family. Gender roles significantly influence attitudes about health and health education. For instance, Amish, Hispanic, and many Asian American families are male dominated. In the Amish society, taboos related to sexual behavior have special significance for client education. In Hispanic and Arab cultures, gender role differences are pronounced. Women are expected to be modest and submissive.

LITERACY

In 1996, the Joint Commission on Accreditation of Healthcare Organizations (JCAHO) identified client and family education as an important function necessary to client care. Not only was education required, but all members of the interdisciplinary treatment team were required to provide education with consideration for literacy, educational level, and language of the clients.

Davidhizar and Brownson (1999) noted that more than half of all Americans may be unable to read and understand health-related handouts given to them. Although illiteracy is not directly correlated to cultural diversity, there is a relationship. Miles and Davis (1995) reported that the largest U.S. population group affected by illiteracy is white and native born. However, when looking at percentages of the total population, illiteracy is proportionately higher among African Americans and Hispanic Americans than in whites. See Chapter 6 for more information on literacy.

There are client education materials in a variety of languages. It is important, however, to consider that clients must be evaluated for literacy in their own native language as well as English. Depending on their educational level, clients may be illiterate in both languages (Davidhizar & Brownson, 1999).

Gender Differences in Communication

Mulac (1998) commented, "There are two abiding truths on which the general public and research scholars find themselves in uneasy agreement: (a) men and women speak the same language, and (b) men and women speak that language differently" (p. 127). These differences in gender have been referred to as a cultural phenomenon. Mulac, Bradac, and Gibbons (2001) defined culture as the social system that reinforces behavioral expectations for group members whether they are national, ethnic, or gender groups. They report that these differences in men's and women's language are the result of different experiences and socialization in our society. The consequence of this socialization may be miscommunication. Another position, sometimes viewed as an alternative to the "culture" position, suggests that the most important consequence of gender-related language differences are differences in social power or status, which favors men.

Gudykunst and Ting-Toomey (1998) identified four "stylistic modes" of verbal communication between genders.

1. *Direct versus indirect style.* This dimension represents the degree to which speakers show their intentions through explicit verbal communication. Openness, straight-forwardness, and honesty characterize the direct style, whereas the indirect style is more ambiguous, tactful, and concerned with saving face of the individuals in the interest of harmony. Male style is characterized as relatively direct, and the female style as relatively indirect. For example, males use adjectives ("It's good to . . .") and directives ("Write this down"). Females include uncertainty verbs ("I'm not sure") and questions ("What do you think?").

2. *Succinct versus elaborate style.* This dimension addresses the quantity of talk that is valued in different cultures. Salient silences and understatement often mark the succinct style. Males, for example, often use elliptical sentences ("Great picture"). Descriptive metaphors and similes and flowery expressions mark the elaborate style that is more characteristic of women. The elaborate style potentially protects relational harmony, which is especially important to women. Examples include dependent clauses (". . . Which is the reason that . . ."); and longer-length sentences ("Because the trees still have snow, it looks like . . .").

3. *Personal versus contextual style.* The personal style is individual-centered language and enhances "I" identity. In contrast, the use of contextual style is role-centered language and enhances role identity. The personal style stresses equality, whereas the contextual style stresses the speaker and hearer positions within a hierarchy. Women are more likely to use the personal style, whereas men are more likely to use the contextual style.

4. *Instrumental versus affective style.* Male use of the instrumental continuum is seen in references to quantity ("below 32 degrees Fahrenheit") and locatives ("in the center of the picture"). Women use the affective end of the continuum, referring more often to emotion ("She'll feel terrible . . ."), and focusing on people's feelings.

Results of the studies by Gudykunst and Ting-Toomey (1998) demonstrate substantial support for the hypothesis that various features of male language are perceived as relatively direct, succinct, and instrumental. Female language is judged as relatively indirect, elaborate, and affective.

Studies of differences in communication patterns between men and women have found that men tend to communicate on the basis of social hierarchy and competition, while women tend to be more network-oriented and collaborative (Kilbourne & Weeks, 1997). Others have noted that in master's in business administration programs, curriculum, classroom conduct, and culture have been structured to be more supportive of male communication patterns. Gefen and Straub (1997) found that women in the workplace perceived e-mail to have a higher social presence and to be more useful than men did, while men found e-mail easier to use. Therefore, they inferred that women use e-mail to form more interactive and context-building exchanges, since women seek to build a cooperative context, whereas men focus more on the message content. Another aspect of electronic communication that favors women is that the medium lets everyone speak equally, instead of one person dominating a conversation (Strauss, 1996). This suggests that men would find electronic communication easier to use for information dissemination but more difficult to use for interaction among students or co-workers.

Arbaugh (2000) reported that, based on studies of gender differences in communication and technology usage, Internet-based courses may be quite favorable to women because they provide a friendly environment. Earlier studies found that women tended to have more negative attitudes toward computing and technology than men, but recent studies show these attitudes are changing. Three main reasons for this shift in attitude are age, experience, and ownership due to affordability of personal computers.

Nurse educators need to be aware of the differences in language between males and females. Considering that a majority of nurse educators and learners in nursing are female, understanding the communication patterns of males and females facilitates educational instruction.

Nurse educators have a unique opportunity and privilege to provide instruction for patients and clients, nursing students, and nurses. To do so effectively and humanly, however, we must teach in a culturally competent manner, putting to use the types of information found in this chapter.

CASE STUDY

You take a position as clinical nursing instructor in a college with a high percentage of Native American students. Having never before interacted with people from the Native American culture, you feel uncertain about your effectiveness in teaching this group of students.

1. How can you prepare yourself to be a culturally competent teacher in this college?
2. Do you foresee any discomfort arising from possible clashes between your values, beliefs, and habits and those of some of your students?
3. How will you assess whether individual Native American students in your clinical groups differ in their learning needs from the majority of their cultural group?
4. What clinical assignments might you design that will enhance the learning experience of the Native American students?

CRITICAL THINKING EXERCISES

1. Think of some patient situations in which noncompliance with health-related instruction could be related to a nurse's failure to understand the patient's culture.
2. Could the concept of an explanatory model be adapted for use in settings other than health and illness care?

3. Debate the issue of who bears more responsibility for learning about another person's culture: an immigrant to the United States who will eventually need health care or health care providers who may have to care for immigrants?

4. What are advantages and disadvantages of using a family member as an interpreter for a foreign-language-speaking patient, compared to using a telephone-service interpreter?

IDEAS FOR FURTHER RESEARCH

1. Using an existing or new measurement tool, measure the cultural competence of newly graduated staff nurses.

2. Compare the explanatory models of patients from a variety of cultures who have the same medical diagnosis.

3. Show a couple of popular nursing or health care computer programs to learners from a variety of cultural backgrounds. Interview the learners as to their reactions to the software in terms of symbols, sounds, words and phrases, human voices, colors, and behavior stereotyping.

4. Compare scores on exams in nursing courses of ESL students who are allowed to use bilingual dictionaries and who are given extra exam time compared to those who are not given those two accommodations.

REFERENCES

AAN Expert Panel Report. (1992). Culturally competent nursing care. *Nursing Outlook, 40*(6), 277–283.

Abrums, M. E., & Leppa, G. (2001). Beyond cultural competence: Teaching about race, gender, class and sexual orientation. *Journal of Nursing Education, 49*(6), 270–275.

Arbaugh, J. B. (2000). An exploratory study of the effects of gender on student learning and class participation in an Internet-based MBA course. *Management Learning, 31*(4), 503–519.

Blumhagen, D. (1982). The meaning of hypertension. In N. Chrisman & T. Marezki (Eds.), *Clinically applied anthropology*. Boston: Reidel.

Bonder, B., Martin, L., & Miracle, A. (2001). Achieving cultural competence: The challenge for clients and health care workers in a multicultural society. *Generations, 25*(1), 35–42.

Brophy, J. E., & Good, T. H. (1984). *Teacher–student relationships: Causes and consequences*. New York: Holt, Rinehart & Winston.

Campinha-Bacote, J. (1998). *The process of cultural competence in the delivery of healthcare services* (3rd ed.). Cincinnati, OH: Transcultural CARE Associates Press.

Chachkes, E., & Christ, G. (1996). Cross-cultural issues in patient education. *Patient Education and Counseling, 27,* 3–21.

Courage, M., & Godbey, K. L. (1992). Student retention: Polices and service to enhance persistence to graduation. *Nurse Educator, 17*(2), 29–32.

Davidhizar, R. E., & Brownson, K. (1999). Literacy, cultural diversity and client education. *The Health Care Manager, 18*(1), 39–47.

Davidhizar, R. E., Dowd, S. B., & Giger, J. N. (1998). Educating the culturally diverse healthcare student. *Nurse Educator, 23*(2), 38–42.

Dunn, R., & Griggs, S. A. (1995). *Multiculturalism and learning styles: Teaching and counseling adolescents.* Westport, CT: Praeger.

Eliason, M. J., & Raheim, S. (2000). Experiences and comfort with culturally diverse groups in undergraduate pre-nursing students. *Journal of Nursing Education, 39*(4), 151–156.

Fennema, E., & Peterson, P. (1986). Teacher–student interaction and self related differences in learning mathematics. *Teaching and Teacher Education, 2*(1), 19–42.

Gefen, D., & Straub, D. W. (1997). Gender differences in the perception and use of email: An extension to the Technology Acceptance Model. *MIS Quarterly, 214,* 389–400.

Giger, J., & Davidhizar, R. (1999). *Transcultural nursing: Assessment and interventions.* St. Louis: Mosby-Year Book.

Gudykunst, W. B., & Ting-Toomey, S. (1998). *Culture and interpersonal communication.* Newbury Park, CA: Sage.

Johnston, J. (1989). Changing demographics in New York State: Implications for nursing educators and practice. *Journal of the New York State Nurses Association, 20,* 7–8, 13–15.

Keane, M. (1993). Preferred learning styles and study strategies in a linguistically diverse baccalaureate nursing student population. *Journal of Nursing Education, 32*(5), 214–221.

Kilbourne, W., & Weeks, S. (1997). A socioeconomic perspective on gender bias in technology. *Journal of Socio-Economics, 26*(1), 243–260.

Kleinman, A. (1980). *Patients and healers in the context of culture.* Berkeley, CA: University of California Press.

Klisch, M. L. (2000). Retention strategies for ESL nursing students: Review of the literature 1900–99 and strategies and outcomes in a small private School of Nursing with limited funding. *Journal of Multicultural Nursing and Health, 6*(2), 18–27.

Larke, P. J. (1990). Culturally diversity awareness inventory: Assessing the sensitivity of pre-service teachers. *Action in Teacher Education, 7*(3), 23–40.

Leininger, M. (1978). *Transcultural nursing: Concepts, theories, research, and practice.* New York: John Wiley & Sons.

Lesser, G. (1976). Cultural differences in learning and thinking styles. In S. Messick (Ed.), *Individuality in learning.* San Francisco: Jossey-Bass.

Luyas, G. (1991). An explanatory model of diabetes. *Western Journal of Nursing Research, 13*(6), 681–693.

Malu, K. F., & Figlear, M. R. (1998). Enhancing the language development of immigrant ESL nursing students: A case study with recommendations for action. *Nurse Educator, 23*(2), 43–46.

McKenna, B. (1989). *College faculty: An endangered species on campus.* Washington, DC: American Federation of Teachers.

McSweeney, J. (1993). Explanatory models of myocardial event: Linkages between perceived causes and modified health behaviors. *Rehabilitation Nursing Research, 2*(1), 40–50.

McSweeney, J. C., Allan, J. D., & Mayo, K. (1997). Exploring the use of explanatory models in nursing research and practice. *Image: Journal of Nursing Scholarship, 29*(2), 243–248.

Messick, S. (1976). Personality consistencies in cognition and creativity. In S. Messick (Ed.), *Individuality in learning.* San Francisco: Jossey-Bass.

Miles, S., & Davis, T. (1995). Patients who can't read: Implications for the healthcare system. *JAMA, 274*, 1719–1720.

Morgan, K. (2000). Cross-cultural considerations for simulation-based learning environments. *Simulations & Gaming, 31*(4), 491–508.

Mulac, A. (1998). The gender-linked language effect: Do languages differences really make a difference? In D. J. Canary & K. Kindia (Eds.), *Sex differences and similarities in communication: Critical essays and empirical investigations of sex and gender in interaction.* Mahwah, NJ: Erlbaum.

Mulac, A., Bradac, J. J., & Gibbons, P. (2001). Empirical support for the gender-as-culture hypothesis: An intercultural analysis of male/female language differences. *Human Communication Research, 27*(1), 121–152.

Pacquiao, D. F. (1996). Educating faculty in the concept of educational biculturalism: A comparative study of sociocultural influences in nursing students' experiences in school. In V. Fitzsimons & M. Kelly (Eds.), *The culture of learning: Access, retention and mobility of minority students in nursing.* New York: NLN Press.

Petaschnick J. (2001). Patient education manager faces daily challenges: Culture, language among them. *Patient Care Management, 16*(6), 9–13.

Pettus, A. M., & Allain, V. A. (1999). Using a questionnaire to assess prospective teachers' attitudes toward multicultural education issues. *Education, 114*(4), 651–657.

Purnell, L. (2000). A description of the Purnell model for cultural competence. *Journal of Transcultural Nursing, 11*(1), 40–46.

Sep, Y. M., & Jezewski, M. (2000). Korean nurses' adjustment to hospitals in the USA. *Journal of Advanced Nursing, 32*(2), 721–729.

Sommer, S. (2001). Multicultural nursing education. *Journal of Nursing Education, 40*(6), 276–278.

Strauss, S. G. (1996). Getting a clue: Communication media and information distribution effects on group process and performance. *Small Group Research, 27*(1), 115–142.

Sullivan, M. H. (1993*). A meta-analysis of experimental research studies based on Dunn & Dunn learning style model and its relationship to academic achievement and performance.* Doctoral dissertation, St John's University.

Villarruel, A. M., Canales, M., & Torres, S. (2001). Bridges and barriers: Educational mobility of Hispanic nurses. *Journal of Nursing Education, 40*(6), 245–251.

Yurkovich, E. F. (2001). Working with American Indians toward educational success. *Journal of Nursing Education, 40*(6), 259–269.

6

Literacy and Readability

The inability to comprehend written material can have devastating effects on a person's life and especially on his or her health. Unfortunately, there are many people in the United States who have low literacy skills. National surveys of adults have reported that at least 21 percent and maybe as many as 47 percent have low literacy rates (Knowlton & Jansen, 1995; National Assessments of Adult Literacy, 1992).

The 1992 National Assessment of Adult Literacy defined literacy as, "Using printed and written information to function in society, to achieve one's goals, and to develop one's knowledge and potential." This survey of adult Americans looked at three literacy domains. The first is *Prose Literacy*, which refers to understanding information from texts such as books and newspapers. The second is *Document Literacy*, or the skills needed to understand and use information in applications, maps, schedules, and so on. The third domain is *Quantitative Literacy*, which is the ability to understand numbers in printed materials or having the skills to do arithmetic. In the survey, each domain included a sampling of literacy tasks encountered in everyday life, and skills were measured along a five-point scale. Overall, 47 percent of the adult population studied was considered to have low literacy skills (Quigley, 1997). About 22 percent of adult Americans were found to be in Level 1, the lowest level of literacy. Although there is no direct conversion between the government's five literacy levels and the more traditional grade levels (reading expected at a certain grade in school), a rough estimate is that people who score in Level 1 literacy are probably reading below the 5th-grade level (Doak, Doak, & Root, 1996).

Reading Levels

We usually refer to reading level and grade level as being one and the same, but often this is not the case. The fact that an adult has completed the 8th grade, for example, does not mean he or she is reading at an 8th-grade level. Several studies conducted in health care settings have found that patients often read two to three grade levels below the last completed year of school (Bauman, 1997; Cooley et al., 1995; Davis et al., 1994). Boyd (1988) found that patient reading levels were as much as five grade levels below their last completed grade in school. It is important for health care practitioners to be aware of this discrepancy between reading level and grade level so that they don't assume that if a person has a grammar school education, for example, that he or she is reading at the 8th-grade level.

What is the literacy level of adult patients? Many studies have examined this question. Davis and colleagues (1990) measured reading levels of adults who attended four public clinics and one private practice in the southern United States. The clinics served poor and low-income families. They found that the mean reading level in the clinics was 6th grade, and the mean reading level in the private practice was 10th grade. Forty percent of the clinic patients read below the 5th-grade level. Gazmarian et al. (1999) measured the functional health literacy of 3,260 Medicare enrollees in the Midwest, Southwest, and Southeast and found that 34 percent of English-speaking and 54 percent of Spanish-speaking enrollees had inadequate or marginal health literacy. Williams et al. (1995) measured literacy levels of 2,659 patients in the South and discovered that 35 percent of English-speaking patients and 62 percent of Spanish-speaking patients had inadequate or marginal functional health literacy. They reported that 42 percent of patients were unable to understand directions for taking medicine on an empty stomach and 26 percent were unable to comprehend written information scheduling their next appointment.

Research has also identified the people who are at highest risk of low literacy. The 1992 National Adult Literacy Survey identified the demographic statistics of those Americans who placed in Level 1 (lowest) literacy:

- Older adults—The number of adults over 65 who placed in Level 1 was almost double that of the overall population.
- Less educated people—About 75 percent of people with an 8th-grade education or less scored in Level 1. About 45 percent of adults who had some high school education but not a diploma performed in Level 1. About 18 percent of those with a high school diploma performed in Level 1.
- Lower-income people—The paychecks of Level 1 adults was about $240 compared to $650 for Level 5 people.
- Members of ethnic or racial minority groups—About 40 percent of black, 54 percent of Hispanic, and 33 percent of Asian adults performed in Level 1, compared to 15 percent of whites.

In spite of the research evidence that many of our patients do not understand what we give them to read, or even what we say to them, health professionals in many settings continue to ignore the problem. Some progress is being made in writing printed educational materials (PEMs) at lower reading levels (Doak et al., 1996), but research indicates that many pamphlets, booklets, information sheets, and consent forms that patients are asked to read exceed the ability of many to understand. In 1990, Dixon and Park studied written materials used in a Midwest hospital, such as pamphlets, hospital instruction booklets, and consent forms. They found that the materials required reading levels from 9th to 13th grades. Also in 1990, Davis et al. analyzed PEMs given to patients in clinics and a private practice and discovered that the reading levels of most of the material ranged from 11th to 14th grade, with consent forms being at the 16th-grade level. In 1994, a study by Davis et al. revealed that not much progress had been made in the interceding four years. Most of the PEMs given to patients in a large southern pediatric clinic were between the 9th- and 19th-grade reading levels.

There are many factors that contribute to reading difficulty of PEMs. First are the factors that are measured in most readability formulas—long sentences and polysyllabic words. In addition, complex sentence and paragraph structure, use of technical terminology, and inclusion of abstract concepts adds to reading level. Finally, mechanical factors such as print size and type, color contrasts, and density of the text must be considered (Barnes, 1996).

Skills Needed by Patients/Clients

Printed educational materials are used for many purposes in the health care field. We provide patients with educational pamphlets or booklets to supplement the oral teaching that is done. We give instruction sheets for taking medications or carrying out treatments. We also expect patients to fill out admission forms, read and sign consent forms, and read medication labels and appointment slips.

Some studies have shown that patients and clients appreciate PEMs and even prefer them to audiovisual materials (Bernier, 1993). PEMs have also been shown to be an effective method of teaching and increasing knowledge retention (Bernier, 1993; Young & Brooks, 1986). However, if patients cannot comprehend the written materials, they are of little value. Patients who are confronted with educational materials they cannot read or comprehend may avoid the learning issue altogether, with resulting noncompliance (Hussey & Gilliland, 1989). They may also guess at what they don't understand, with possible disastrous results for their health. Low literacy contributes to the increasing cost of health care because "people with low literacy skills seem to put off disease prevention actions and to wait longer before seeking medical help" (Doak et al., 1996, p.4).

Assessing Literacy

People with low literacy often inadvertently give us clues that can lead us to a realization that they may have a reading or comprehension problem. Such clues include:

- Not even attempting to read printed material
- Asking to take PEMs home to discuss with a significant other
- Claiming eyeglasses were left home
- Stating that they can't read something because they are too tired or don't feel well
- Avoiding discussion of written material or asking no questions about it
- Mouthing words as they try to read

Although following clues may give you some leads as to a patient's literacy, and may be all you can do in some situations, actually measuring literacy levels is a better approach.

Two tests are often used to measure patient literacy, the REALM (Rapid Estimate of Adult Literacy in Medicine) and the WRAT (Wide Range Achievement Test). Both tests measure the basic reading skill of *decoding* words (recognizing letters that form words and then pronouncing the words correctly). They do not measure reading comprehension. Only two to three minutes are needed to administer the tests, which makes clinical use of the tools feasible. Some hospitals and clinics use the REALM and WRAT tests routinely to assess reading ability of patients, and they record the results in the patient's chart (Doak et al., 1996).

The REALM is a reading test that requires patients to pronounce common medical and anatomical words (see Figure 6–1). The test "contains 66 words arranged in three columns in ascending order of number of syllables and increasing difficulty" (Murphy, Davis, Long, Jackson, & Decker, 1993, p. 126). To administer the test:

1. Ask the patient to read the words aloud, starting at the top of the first list and continuing through all three lists.
2. Allow the patient 5 seconds to pronounce each word.

Reading level_____

Patient name/subject # _____   Date of birth _____   Grade completed _____

Date _____   Clinic _____   Examiner _____

List 1		List 2		List 3	
fat	_____	fatigue	_____	allergic	_____
flu	_____	pelvic	_____	menstrual	_____
pill	_____	jaundice	_____	testicle	_____
dose	_____	infection	_____	colitis	_____
eye	_____	exercise	_____	emergency	_____
stress	_____	behavior	_____	medication	_____
smear	_____	prescription	_____	occupation	_____
nerves	_____	notify	_____	sexually	_____
germs	_____	gallbladder	_____	alcoholism	_____
meals	_____	calories	_____	irritation	_____
disease	_____	depression	_____	constipation	_____
cancer	_____	miscarriage	_____	gonorrhea	_____
caffeine	_____	pregnancy	_____	inflammatory	_____
attack	_____	arthritis	_____	diabetes	_____
kidney	_____	nutrition	_____	hepatitis	_____
hormones	_____	menopause	_____	antibiotics	_____
herpes	_____	appendix	_____	diagnosis	_____
seizure	_____	abnormal	_____	potassium	_____
bowel	_____	syphilis	_____	anemia	_____
asthma	_____	hemorrhoids	_____	obesity	_____
rectal	_____	nausea	_____	osteoporosis	_____
incest	_____	directed	_____	impetigo	_____

Score	
List 1	_____
List 2	_____
List 3	_____
Raw score	_____

FIGURE 6-1   Rapid Estimate of Adult Literacy in Medicine (REALM)

TABLE 6-1 REALM Scoring Chart

Raw Score	Grade Range
0–18	3rd grade and below
19–44	4th to 6th grades
45–60	7th to 8th grades
61–66	9th grade and above

3. If the patient gets stuck on a portion of the list, ask him or her to look down each list to see if he or she can pronounce any additional words.

4. Score the test by adding up the total number of words pronounced correctly.

Table 6–1 shows the corresponding grade range for each raw score.

The REALM test can be obtained from Terry Davis, PhD, Louisiana State University School of Medicine in Shreveport; telephone 318-675-4584.

The WRAT 3 is the most recent version of the Wide Range Achievement Test. In the reading portion of this test, patients read aloud from a list of 42 words of increasing difficulty (Doak et al., 1996). The examiner instructs the patient to pronounce each word and checks off each word pronounced incorrectly. When 10 consecutive words are mispronounced, the test is stopped. The administration manual shows how to convert the raw score to a grade level score. The WRAT 3 is available from Jastak Associates, Wilmington, Delaware; telephone 800-221-9728.

Teaching Patients with Low Literacy Skills

Assessing reading ability is only the first step in the process of health education for people with low literacy skills. The second step is planning an approach to teaching that will best meet the needs of individuals in this group.

First, it is important to set objectives that are realistic for the person's level of understanding. Objectives should focus on basic essential skills that must be achieved if safety is to be maintained. The objectives should be shaped by what the person already knows about the topic as well as by what he or she still needs to learn.

Choose information that will meet the objectives and pare it down to the minimum amount that is necessary. Information overload must be avoided when teaching people with low literacy. Teach limited amounts of material during each session.

Keep instructions simple by breaking them down into smaller units. For example, if teaching about taking digoxin, first teach a little about the action of the drug, then teach how to take a pulse rate, then about the need for follow-up visits. At each step, evaluation should take place so you know the person has learned.

If possible, use more than one teaching method to reinforce the learning. Just telling a person information may be enough for some people, but many with low literacy skills also have trouble understanding verbal instruction. Reinforcing the teaching with printed educational materials may help some people. Others may learn better from a videotape or even a simple computer tutorial.

In the process of teaching, use examples and analogies to which the person can relate. Use familiar illustrations and pictures that are culturally relevant. Use repetition at appropriate times.

Finally, be creative in the way you evaluate learning. Verbal quizzes may not work well with low literate people. Instead, ask them to repeat what you have said in their own words and ask for return demonstrations. If you give them PEMs, you may ask them to underline the most important information.

Developing Printed Educational Materials

Whether you are developing a brochure, a pamphlet, or an instruction sheet, the guidelines for maintaining a low readability level and attractiveness for the low literate person are the same. You should consider the organization of the information, the linguistics, and the appearance (Bernier, 1993; Dixon & Park, 1990; Doak et al., 1996; Farrell-Miller & Gentry, 1989; Hussey, 1997).

Organizational Factors
1. Include a short but descriptive title.
2. Use brief headings and subheadings.
3. Incorporate only one idea per paragraph, and be sure the first sentence is the topic sentence.
4. Divide complex instructions into small steps.
5. Consider using a question/answer format.
6. Address no more than three or four main points.
7. Reinforce main points with a summary at the end.

Linguistic Factors
1. Keep the reading level at grade 5 or 6 to make the material understandable to most low literate persons.
2. Use mostly one or two syllable words and short sentences.
3. Use a personal and conversational style. For example, "You should weigh yourself everyday" is preferable to "The person with congestive heart failure should measure body weight every day."
4. Define technical terms if they must be used.
5. Use words consistently throughout the text. For example, stay with the word *pill* rather than switching between *pill* and *medicine*.
6. Avoid the use of idioms that might mean different things to different people. For example, the term *junk food* may not be clear to all people.
7. Use graphics and language that are culturally and age relevant for the intended audience.

8. Use active rather than passive voice; for example, "Take one pill every morning" rather than "A pill should be taken every morning."

9. Incorporate examples and simple analogies to illustrate concepts.

Appearance Factors

1. Avoid a cluttered appearance by including enough *white space.*

2. Include simple diagrams or graphics that are well labeled.

3. Use upper- and lowercase letters. All capitals are difficult for everyone to read.

4. Use 10- to 14-point type in a plain font (serif is preferred).

5. Place emphasized words in bold or underline them, but do not use capitals because they are difficult to read.

6. Use lists when appropriate.

7. Try to limit line length to no more than 50 or 60 characters.

Following these guidelines will result in PEMs that are more readable for people with low literacy and make it more likely that they will benefit from this aspect of our teaching. When you have completed the development of the printed material, let a few colleagues look at it for general appearance and organization. You should also test it for readability using one of the many formulas available.

Readability Formulas

Many readability formulas are available for use. Some are easier to use than others, and some are indicated for use with long versus short passages or for certain grade levels of material. Some require special equipment or charts. Almost all readability formulas use the measurement of number of syllables and sentence length as the basic variables that are entered into mathematical equations or plotted on a graph.

The formulas that are used most frequently and that do not require any equipment are the Flesch, the Fog, and the SMOG. The Flesch Reading Ease formula was developed by Rudolph Flesch (1948) and can be applied to materials that fall between the 5th- and 12th-grade reading levels. The formula is as follows:

1. For short writings, take *3 or 4 samples of approximately 100 words* each. For a book, take 25 to 30 samples. Each sample starts at the beginning of a paragraph.

2. Figure the *number of sentences* in the samples by counting independent units of thought marked by punctuation like periods, question marks, colons, and semicolons. The last sentence should be the one that ends closest to the 100-word count, making your sample slightly more or less than 100 words.

3. Count the *number of words* in each sentence in the sample, figuring numbers, contractions, and hyphenated words as one word each.

4. Calculate *average sentence length* (SL) by counting the number of words in each sample and dividing by the number of sentences.

5. Count the *number of syllables* in your 100-word samples. Reading aloud will help you determine the syllables, especially in numbers. For example, 1915 would have four syllables.

TABLE 6–2 Interpreting Flesch Reading Ease Scores

Reading Ease Score	Reading Difficulty Level	Grade Level
90–100	Very Easy	5
80–90	Easy	6
70–80	Fairly Easy	7
60–70	Standard	8–9
50–60	Fairly Difficult	10–12
30–50	Difficult	College
0–30	Very Difficult	Postgraduate

6. Calculate *average word length* (WL) by dividing the number of syllables by the number of words in your sample and multiplying by 100.

7. Insert your SL number and WL number into this Reading Ease formula:

$$RE = 206.835 - 0.846\ WL - 1.015\ SL$$

To interpret the Reading Ease score, consult Table 6–2, which shows that a Reading Ease score of 0 to 30 would be very difficult and require postgraduate-level reading, and a score of 90 to 100 would be considered very easy reading, at a 5th-grade reading level (Spadero, 1983). The Flesch formula assumes that about 50 percent of people who are at a grade level can comprehend the material written at that grade level.

The Fog Index was developed by Gunning in the 1970s (Spadero, 1983). It can be used to determine readability from 4th grade to college, and assumes that 75 percent of people reading at the grade level should be able to read the tested material (Davis et al., 1990). To calculate the Fog Index, use the following steps:

1. For short writings, take a sample of 100 words. For long pieces, take several samples and average the results.

2. Figure the number of sentences (S) in the sample. If the 100-word count falls more than halfway through a sentence, count this sentence in the sample, and add up the number of words (W).

3. Count the number of words containing three or more syllables (A). Do not count verbs ending in "ed" or "es" if they make the word have three syllables, and do not count capitalized words or combinations of simple words like *wallpaper*.

4. Insert your (S), (W), and (A) numbers into this Grade Level formula:

$$GL = (W/S + A) \times 0.4$$

This formula is easy to interpret because the results are already expressed as a grade level.

The SMOG formula (named after the smog found in London, the author's birthplace) was developed by McLaughlin (1969) to simplify the process of measuring readability. The process is as follows:

1. Count 10 consecutive sentences at the beginning, middle, and end of a passage, for a total of 30 sentences. Sentences are considered to be independent units of thought that end with a period, question mark, or exclamation point.

2. In these sentences, count every word that has three or more syllables. Include numbers in the way they are sounded out. For example, 1915 would have four syllables.

3. Estimate the square root of the number of polysyllabic words in the count. This can be done by calculator, or estimated by taking the square root of the nearest perfect square. For instance, if the number of words is 95, the nearest perfect square is 100. If the word count falls about midpoint between two perfect squares, choose the lower number. For example, if the number of words is 110, figure the square root of 100 rather than 121.

4. Add 3 to the estimated square root to get the SMOG grade. The SMOG grade is the grade reading level.

The SMOG formula is quick and simple if you are not intimidated by estimating a square root. This formula is based on the assumption that 100 percent of people reading at that grade level will comprehend the material, compared to the other formulas that are based on perfect comprehension by only 50 to 75 percent of people at that grade level. For this reason, SMOG grades are usually about two grades higher than the grades calculated by other formulas (Spadero, 1983).

Word processing software usually has built-in readability formulas that allow you to test the prose you have written. The process usually involves clicking on the Tools button on the tool bar, then clicking on Options (in the case of Microsoft Word) or Grammatik (in the case of Corel Word Perfect) and following a path of options that leads to readability statistics. In most cases the formulas that are used are the Flesch Reading Ease and the Flesch-Kincaid.

All readability formulas have their limitations. They are based mostly on word length and sentence length, which are only two of the variables that actually affect readability. Other factors that affect readability include the conceptual nature of the words, the number of times difficult words are repeated, the layout of the printed material, and the motivation of the learner (Jimenez, 1994). Therefore, the readability scores obtained from the formulas have to be considered in the context of the general appearance of the PEM and some knowledge of the people who will be using it.

Some authors contend that any of the readability formulas will give you a reasonable estimate of the reading level of the material. They state that the formulas produce highly correlated results, and using complicated formulas will generally not give more accurate results than simple ones (Spadero, Robinson, & Smith, 1980). Other authors assert that the correlation between formulas is relatively weak, and results can vary by as much as six grade levels (Mailloux, Johnson, Fisher, & Pettibone, 1995; Meade & Smith, 1991). Mailloux and colleagues used three formulas that appear in popular word processing software to test the Gettysburg Address and found a difference of 2.5 grade levels. Some of the discrepancy may lie in the assumptions of the formulas—some are based on the assumption that 100 percent of readers at a grade level will comprehend the material, and others assume as few as 50 to 75 percent will comprehend the material, as was explained previously. If you are using a readability formula to give you a rough estimate of the level of your writing, any formula may do. If you are going to base important patient care or policy decisions on the readability of materials, it may be wise to subject the material to several tests and compare or average the results.

Improving Readability

Readability scores can be improved by rewriting the material with shorter words and shorter sentences, if that is desired. Instead of using a three-syllable word like *interchange,* use *switch.* Three-syllable words like *diabetes* that are familiar to readers are acceptable, however (Farrell-Miller & Gentry, 1989). Use short sentences that express just one idea. Following is an excerpt from the beginning of this chapter that shows how a passage might be simplified.

> *Before:* "The inability to comprehend written material can have devastating effects on a person's life and especially on his or her health. Unfortunately, there are many people in the United States who have low literacy skills."

> *After:* "If you cannot read well, it can have a bad effect on your life. It can also affect your health. There are many people in the United States who cannot read well."

This change in wording decreases the reading difficulty according to the Flesch-Kincaid Formula from 12th grade to 4th grade. You can get the idea from this example how you can reduce the reading level of your writing.

The question is sometimes raised as to whether we should reduce the reading level of all health educational materials. After all, there are many good readers. Would they be irritated at being given materials with a low reading level? Doak et al. (1996) believe that everyone would benefit from simpler documents. A commonly seen recommendation found in the literature is that PEMs should not exceed the 6th-grade level (Scown, 2001). Some authors believe, however, that we should not reduce all PEMs to the lowest common denominator but should produce a variety of materials at a range of reading levels (Scown, 2001). An argument can be made that many well-educated good readers can benefit greatly from fairly complex informational booklets. Davis et al. (1990) have made the reasonable suggestion of producing a range of reading level materials labeled with the grade level so patients can be given appropriate materials.

Many issues were raised in this chapter: literacy, readability, developing appropriate educational materials, and teaching patients with low literacy. For some of you, and many other health professionals, this is the first time you are reading about these issues. Yet, if you are working with patients, they are issues that may be critical to the health of those you serve. It is worthwhile for all health professionals to learn about literacy and how best to communicate with all of our patients.

CASE STUDY

You want to develop a pamphlet for potential clients (and families of clients) of an inner-city medical day care program for senior citizens. The first draft of a few of the paragraphs in the pamphlet is as follows:

> This program is available for people over the age of 65 who want or need to spend part of their day in a supervised setting with activities, lunch, and some medical care provided. Medical care includes blood pressure and weight monitoring, medication supervision, podiatric care, and limited dental care. Appointments with the visiting podiatrist and dentist must be made at least two weeks in advance. Additional charges are made for medical care provided.

Activities provided during the day include such things as discussion groups, story groups, crafts, woodworking, sing-alongs, puzzles, and baking. Activities are tailored to a participant's interests and abilities. All activities are included in the basic program cost.

Transportation is provided within a five-mile radius. A handicapped accessible van goes to participants' homes, and the van driver escorts the participant from the home to the van and back again. There is an additional charge for transportation.

1. Using a readability formula, measure the grade level of this excerpt.
2. Rewrite the excerpt to bring it down to 8th-grade level and then to 6th-grade level.
3. Should the pamphlet address possible program participants or their families?
4. Plan the layout of the pamphlet (taking into consideration that more information has to be included).

CRITICAL THINKING EXERCISES

1. You work in a community hospital's medical clinic. You and your team are considering a policy of measuring patients' reading levels on admission. What factors should you consider in making this decision?
2. In the medical clinic in which you work, you note that one staff member gives PEMs to some clients but rarely gives them to clients who speak with an accent or who look very poor. What might be the basis for her actions? Should you speak to her about what you observed?
3. You are an elementary school nurse. How might you use your knowledge of literacy and readability in your work with kids and parents?
4. You are a staff development educator. Your responsibilities include educational programs for all classifications of employees in the institution. When you raise the issue of literacy and readability in teaching various groups, your director tells you not to be concerned with that. Why should you be concerned or not concerned?

IDEAS FOR FURTHER RESEARCH

1. Measure readability levels of PEMs you use in your practice.
2. Develop two versions of a pamphlet or information sheet. One should be at the 6th-grade level and one at 12th-grade level. Show them to a sample of clients with high literacy to see which pamphlet they prefer and why.
3. Survey the nursing staff of a health care institution. Ask them about how aware they are of patients' literacy levels, how they assess reading comprehension, readability of PEMs distributed, and whether they think low literacy is a problem with their population of patients.

References

Barnes, L. P. (1996). Evaluating the readability of patient education materials. *MCN, 21*, 273.

Bauman, A. (1997). The comprehensibility of asthma education materials. *Patient Education and Counseling, 32*, S51–S59.

Bernier, M. J. (1993). Developing and evaluating printed educational materials: A prescriptive model for quality. *Orthopaedic Nursing, 12*(6), 39–46.

Boyd, M. D. (1988). Patient education literature: A comparison of reading levels and the reading abilities of patients. *Advances in Health Education, 1*, 101–110.

Cooley, M. E., Moriarty, H., Berger, M. S., Selm-Orr, D., Coyle, B., & Short, T. (1995). Patient literacy and the readability of written cancer educational materials. *Oncology Nursing Forum, 22*(9), 1345–1351.

Davis, T. C., Crouch, M. A., Wills, G., Miller, S., & Abdehou, D. M. (1990). The gap between patient reading comprehension and the readability of patient education materials. *The Journal of Family Practice, 31*(5), 533–538.

Davis, T. C., Mayeaux, E. J., Fredrickson, D., Bocchini, J. A., Jackson, R. H., & Murphy, P. W. (1994). Reading ability of parents compared with reading level of pediatric patient education materials. *Pediatrics, 93*(3), 460–468.

Dixon, E., & Park, R. (1990). Do patients understand written health information? *Nursing Outlook, 38*(6), 278–281.

Doak, C. C., Doak, L. G., & Root, J. H. (1996). *Teaching patients with low literacy skills* (2nd ed.). Philadelphia: Lippincott.

Farrell-Miller, P., & Gentry, P. (1989). How effective are your patient education materials? Guidelines for developing and evaluating written educational materials. *The Diabetes Educator, 15*(5), 418–422.

Flesch, R. (1948). A new readability yardstick. *Journal of Applied Psychology, 32*(3), 221–233.

Gazmarian, J. A., Baker, D. W., Williams, M. V., Parker, R. M., Scott, T. L., Green, D. C., Fehrenbach, N., Ren, J., & Koplan, J. P. (1999). Health literacy among Medicare enrollees in a managed care organization. *JAMA, 281*(6), 545–551.

Hussey, L. C. (1997). Strategies for effective patient education material design. *Journal of Cardiovascular Nursing, 11*(2), 37–46.

Hussey, L. C., & Gilliland, K. (1989). Compliance, low literacy, and locus of control. *Patient Teaching, 24*(3), 605–611.

Jimenez, S. L. M. (1994). Evaluating the readability of written patient education materials. *The Journal of Perinatal Education, 3*(4), 59–62.

Knowlton, M., & Jansen, K. (1995). Teaching a client with low literacy skills. *Imprint, 42*(5), 67–69.

Mailloux, S. L., Johnson, M. E., Fisher, D. G., & Pettibone, T. J. (1995). How reliable is computerized assessment of readability? *Computers in Nursing, 13*(5), 221–225.

McLaughlin, G. H. (1969). SMOG grading—A new readability formula. *Journal of Reading, 12*, 639–646.

Meade, C. D., & Smith, C. F. (1991). Readability formulas: Cautions and criteria. *Patient Education and Counseling, 17*, 153–158.

Murphy, P. W., Davis, T. C., Long, S. W., Jackson, R. H., & Decker, B. C. (1993). Rapid Estimate of Adult Literacy in Medicine (REALM): A quick reading test for patients. *Journal of Reading, 37*(2), 124–130.

National Assessments of Adult Literacy. (1992). Retrieved November 8, 2001, from the World Wide Web, *http://nces.ed.gov/naal/*.

Quigley, B. A. (1997). *Rethinking literacy education.* San Francisco: Jossey-Bass.

Scown, S. J. (2001). Cancer-patient reading levels in the real world. *Patient-Centered Guides.* Retrieved November 8, 2001, from the World Wide Web, *http://www.onconurse.com/news/reading _levels.html*.

Spadero, D. C. (1983). Assessing readability of patient information materials. *Pediatric Nursing, 9*(4), 274–278.

Spadero, D. C., Robinson, L. A., & Smith, L. T. (1980). Assessing readability of patient information materials. *American Journal of Hospital Pharmacy, 37,* 215–221.

Williams, M. V., Parker, R. M., Baker, D. W., Parikh, N., Pitkin, K., Coates, W. C., & Nurss, J. R. (1995). Inadequate functional health literacy among patients at two public hospitals. *JAMA, 274*(21), 1677–1682.

Young, F. K., & Brooks, B. R. (1986). Patient teaching manuals improve retention of treatment information—a controlled clinical trial in multiple sclerosis. *Journal of Neuroscience Nursing, 18*(1), 26–28.

Part III

Teaching Strategies

7

Traditional Teaching Strategies

![image] Lecturing

There is a cartoon described by Zachry (1985) in which a teacher is telling her students, "Okay class, my job is to talk and your job is to listen. If you finish first, let me know" (p. 129). The cartoon captures the concern that many educators express about lecturing. The concern is that because students are passive listeners, they "tune out" before the end of class and miss important information.

That lecturing is under attack is not news. For many years, active learning has been in vogue while passive learning is out, and critics say there is no more passive mode of learning than lecturing. In the days of Socrates and Plato, lectures were a means of conveying facts, information, and ideas that could not readily be obtained elsewhere. Books, charts, and tapes were not available, so the lecture became an essential means of teaching. Today, we have a broad array of teaching materials and strategies from which to choose, so many would argue that we no longer need the lecture method. The criticisms of lecturing have stimulated some educators to write in defense of lecturing (Birk, 1997; Stunkel, 1998). Their thesis is that lecturing in general is good, not bad, but there are bad lectures, and lectures can be used to excess.

Following is information on when lectures should be used, how good lectures are conceived and delivered, and how we can get learners to pay attention and learn from lectures.

Purposes of Lecturing

Lectures can be an efficient means of introducing learners to new topics. The teacher can use the lecture to set the stage for a new area of learning and place the topic into the perspective of what is already known. For example, an instructor might use a formal lecture to introduce the topic of fluid and electrolyte balance and relate it to what the learners know about homeostasis and nourishment. He or she could then use other strategies to develop the topic further.

113

The lecture method can be used to stimulate students' interest in a subject. Reading about pharmacology may be a sure way to make the uninitiated learner believe that it is a very dull subject indeed. However, an enlivening introductory lecture on pharmacology that applies it to our lives and our work could enable the learner to see it as a fascinating subject that just might be interesting to study. Lecture can also be used to inspire people. A well-conceived lecture on the contributions of nurses to American society could well inspire new nursing students to emulate nurses of the past. A good lecturer can inspire an audience in a way that few textbooks can.

Another purpose of the lecture is to integrate and synthesize a large body of knowledge from several fields or sources (Parker, 1993). A knowledgeable teacher can synthesize the information more readily than can a learner who is a novice in the field. Take the topic of quality assurance, for example. A teacher can use lecture to elucidate the models of quality assurance and the many ways they can be applied in health care. It would take a learner an inordinate amount of time to pull together all of this information about quality assurance and make sense of it all.

Difficult concepts can be clarified in lectures. Concepts such as arrhythmia, compensation in acid–base balance, or increased intracranial pressure may be explained best by the lecture method, especially with the added use of graphics. Other methods are often not as effective in bringing order to the students' thinking on such subjects.

Finally, as Jones (1990) states, "the lecture is valuable where knowledge is advancing rapidly and up-to-date textbooks are not available" (p. 293). A few years ago, this was the case with AIDS and may be true in any specialty at any time. A lecturer who is a clinician working in an area where practice is changing all the time may best be able to convey both the content and the excitement of rapid clinical change through the lecture method.

Advantages of the Lecture Method

The greatest advantage of the lecture over other methods is that it is economical. The size of the class is limited only by classroom space. Formal lectures are just as effective for 200 students as they are for 20, as long as the lecturer has a microphone. Lectures are also economical in terms of student time. A great deal of information can be communicated in a one-hour lecture—usually more information than could be gained from a discussion, for instance. More pertinent information can often be taught in one hour than a student could learn from a textbook in that time. The lecturer can sift through the textbook information and pull out what is most important as well as include information from other sources that a student could take hours to locate and read.

The lecturer can supplement a textbook by enhancing a topic and making it come to life. No matter how well written, words on a page are dry and impersonal compared to words communicated by a lecturer with a wealth of personal experience and enthusiasm for the subject.

During a lecture, the teacher serves as a role model for students. The teacher is an authority on the subject and is a model of someone who has developed expertise in a field and who cares about knowledge and learning. Learners have the advantage of watching a "creative mind at work" (Frederick, 1986, p. 44). The lecturer can demonstrate critical thinking and problem solving being done by an expert.

Butler (1992) believes that many lecturers enjoy a sense of "theatre" as they are on the stage in the classroom. Good lecturers are often gifted with some of the same qualities that make a successful actor, that is, a good speaking voice, good timing, dramatic gestures, a sense of humor, and a good memory. They like being in the limelight and "playing to the audience." Therefore, for these educators, the lecture brings enjoyment, and because they are so good at it, they can bring enjoyment to the learners as well.

An advantage of the mostly one-way verbal communication that occurs during a lecture is that it helps students develop their listening abilities. Stunkel (1998) asserts that students must discipline themselves to listen, remember, track arguments, decide what to take notes on, and relate what is being said to the assigned reading. In light of all these actions, maybe lectures don't consist of such passive learning after all!

The lecture method has enough advantages to warrant its continued use. Teachers should be sure, however, that they are lecturing because it serves a good purpose and not just because they don't want to take the time to develop another teaching strategy. Teachers should also do everything they can to make sure they are good lecturers.

Disadvantages of the Lecture Method

As already mentioned, many people object to the lecture method because it places learners in the passive role of a sponge, just there to soak up knowledge. That may be true if the lecture is not planned and carried out well. Even if a student is mentally active, nothing can ensure that such activity will continue for the whole lecture. In fact, there is a significant amount of research that I will describe later, which points out that students rarely attend to the whole lecture.

Educators who decry the lecture method claim that few teachers are good lecturers and therefore few can achieve class objectives by this method, much less hold students' attention or serve as good role models. Because so many students are subjected to poor lectures throughout their college days, those who go on to become educators themselves often fall into the same bad habits.

One of the chief disadvantages of the lecture method is that by nature it lends itself to the teaching of facts while placing little emphasis on problem solving, decision making, analytical thinking, or transfer of learning (Black, 1993; Cross, Tilson, Tanenbaum, & Rodgers, 1997). That doesn't mean that these latter types of learning cannot take place in a lecture, but they are less likely to occur than when other methods are used. Cross and colleagues (1997) state that lectures result in "surface learning" (p. 340), with students memorizing information and failing to truly comprehend or tie new information to existing cognitive schemata.

Another serious drawback is that lecturing is not conducive to meeting students' individual learning needs. Students are limited to learning from an authority figure and learning by the stimulation of only one of the senses—hearing. In a formal lecture, students have no opportunity to learn from peers, to learn by manipulation of data, to discover, to learn visually or through touch, and so on. The lecture works best for auditory, linguistic learners and may disadvantage those with other learning styles.

Finally, as has been mentioned briefly already, lecturing brings with it the problem of limited attention span on the part of learners. In 1978, Stuart and Rutherford conducted a much-quoted study of the attention and concentration levels of British medical students. They found that concentration rose to a peak at 15 minutes and then fell steadily until the end of the lecture. Results were fairly uniform across several classes with different lecturers and different level students. Other researchers (Foley & Smilansky, 1980; Frederick, 1986; Schoen, 1970; Thomas, 1972) have found similar results, except some found that after a period of 20 minutes or so of decline, there was a rise in attention again in the last few minutes before the end of the lecture (see Figure 7–1). Parker (1993) attributes this loss of attention to loss of novel stimulation. He states that although people are very attentive to new stimuli in any situation, the novelty soon wears off and people become somewhat immune to the stimulus unless it is varied in some way. Thus, during a lecture, the listener is stimulated in the beginning by the lecturer's voice and content, but the person soon gets used to the stimulus and stops paying close attention.

Comparing the advantages to disadvantages of lecturing, it seems that the method is valuable and should be retained, but it should be used skillfully and supplemented with other teaching methods. By using a variety of strategies, the teacher can enhance the advantages of all of the techniques.

Organizing the Lecture

Planning the lecture well ahead of the time of delivery is time well spent because a lecture thrown together at the last minute appears to be just that. You need to take time to plan the objectives of the lecture, to gauge how much time it will take to cover the content, and to consider the difficulty of the material and the ability level of the audience. Once you are clear on the objectives and the level of depth to which you will go with the content, it is time to start a written outline.

The outline of your lecture may take several forms. The *hierarchical* or *classical* lecture is the most commonly used form, especially in nursing. In this approach, information is grouped, divided, and subdivided in typical outline form. The structure looks something like this example of a lecture on "research design":

Research Design
  I. Why we need different research designs
  II. Research designs
      A. Experimental (Clinical trials)
          1. Quasi-experimental
          2. Pre-experimental
      B. Correlational
          1. Ex Post Facto (Comparative)
          2. Retrospective and Prospective
          3. Cross-Sectional and Longitudinal
      C. Descriptive
      D. Qualitative
          1. Ethnographic
          2. Phenomenological
          3. Grounded Theory
  III. Validity and Reliability of Designs

This is the simplest lecture structure and is very easy for learners to follow, especially if the outline is visually presented on slides or transparencies. It is most appropriate for teaching of facts and introducing difficult material (Bligh, 2000).

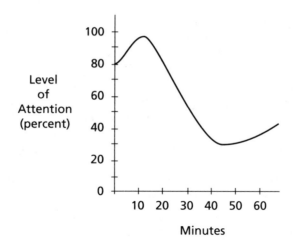

FIGURE 7-1 Attention During Lecture

The *problem-centered* format is also popular. In this structure, a problem is posed, and various hypotheses and solutions are developed. The structure might look something like this example of teaching the basic concepts of fever and its causes and treatment:

			Solutions
		Infection	Antibiotics, fluids
Problem: Fever}	**Hypotheses**:	Inflammation	Heat application
		Dehydration	Fluids and electrolytes

When problems are complex, the hypotheses and solutions may be overlapping, making the outline appear more complicated. This kind of lecture requires a lot of clarification and examples, which will be explained in the next section of this chapter.

The lecture may also follow a *comparative* structure when the objective is to differentiate between two entities. The outline may look like the example in Table 7–1 of the differ-

TABLE 7-1 A Comparative Lecture Structure

Variable	Nurse Practitioner	Physician's Assistant
Education		
Professional Status		
Autonomy		
Clinical Skills		
Prescription Privileges		
Salary		

entiation between the role of nurse practitioner and physician's assistant. The chart-type format may be actually presented to the learners to help them visualize the comparisons.

The fourth common structure for the lecture is the *thesis* format. This involves the lecturer taking a position on an issue or a particular viewpoint on a subject and then supporting or justifying that viewpoint or position with evidence or logic (Bligh, 2000; Jones, 1990). An example of a thesis approach might be a lecture on the topic of passive euthanasia, with the thesis being that, ethically, passive euthanasia is the beginning of a slippery slope.

Whatever approach is appropriate for your topic and audience, it is important that you make the structure of the lecture clear to the learners. If the learners can visualize a matrix or scaffold of some type, it makes it easier for them to "hang their ideas" on the structure, thus making memory recall easier. One approach to making the structure clear is to explain it verbally at the start of class. Another is to show the outline on a transparency, slide, or handout.

In addition to the explanation at the beginning of the class, the lecturer should continue to stress the points in the structure as the lecture unfolds. This can be done by use of *advance organizers*. An advance organizer is a statement that forms a bridge between concepts already discussed and those to come. They help learners link what they already know to what they are about to learn. An advance organizer in the lecture example of research design would be something like, "We've already talked about how a research project has to have a structure, beginning with a question that can be measured and variables that have to be defined. Now we are going to put names on some structures that can be used. They are called research designs."

At the end of the lecture, the structure and main points should be summarized. That way, the teacher ties the objectives from the beginning of the lecture to the end of the lecture, and the teacher has come full circle. If the kinds of organizing structures and techniques that have been mentioned are not followed, a disorganized lecture can occur, and many unhappy and frustrated learners will result. Table 7–2 depicts the characteristics of a disorganized lecture.

Delivering the Lecture

The planning and organizing of content are finished. Now it's time to deliver the lecture. You need to plan your delivery, rehearse, and consciously think about your techniques of delivery if you are to maximize your effectiveness.

TABLE 7-2   Characteristics of Disorganized Lectures

1. Structure or outline is not obvious to the listener. No apparent rationale for sequence of topics.
2. No mention of the objective or desired learning outcomes of the lecture.
3. Lecturer mentions the same topic at different times for no apparent purpose other than failing to complete a thought at one time.
4. No advance organizers before new concepts are introduced.
5. No transition between sections of the lecture.
6. No summary or tying thoughts together at the end.

CONTROLLING ANXIETY

If you are at all anxious about giving your lecture, you need to think about controlling your anxiety. An effective control mechanism is *imaging*. With imaging, you visualize yourself as you want to appear to your audience (Weaver & Cotrell, 1985). Do you want to appear organized and in control? Think about what that kind of person looks like in front of a class-room and picture yourself acting that way. Do you want to convey the image of a scholar and expert in your field? How does a scholarly expert act or talk? That is how you need to picture yourself in your mind. Having this preferred image in your mind can increase your self-concept and your confidence.

SPONTANEITY

The most valuable advice I can give about lecture technique is to avoid reading to the class. Reading kills all spontaneity and can be anesthetizing. To avoid the temptation to read (and it is a great temptation if you are anxious), do not write your lecture out in full sentences. If your notes are in the form of lists and phrases, you will have to think during the delivery, and spontaneity will increase. If you review your notes before the lecture and rehearse the deliv-ery at home, you will feel secure enough without a written script in front of you. I would not recommend trying to do without any notes. Organization of the lecture could suffer if you forget the order in which you planned your content. It is possible for any educator to draw a blank for a moment and be unable to recall what comes next; notes are a lifesaver in such instances.

VOICE QUALITY

If your voice is not loud enough for everyone in the class to hear easily, use a microphone if possible. You can also learn how to project your voice with a few pointers from a speech teacher and some practice. It is very frustrating for the audience if they have to strain to hear you, either because your voice is always too soft or because you drop off your voice volume at the end of a sentence.

In addition to volume, beware of lecturing in a monotone. There is no surer way to bore an audience or put them to sleep than with a monotone voice. You should vary the pitch and volume of your voice as your speak. If such variation does not come naturally to you, pay attention to people who do well with variations in their speech and analyze what they are doing. Observation of these techniques is a good way to learn them. If you are genuinely enthusiastic about your material, that enthusiasm will help to overcome any tendency to a monotone voice.

BODY LANGUAGE

You can add to the dramatic quality of your lecturing by your movements. Do not stand glued to one spot in back of a podium. Move to the side occasionally or stand in front of the podium (this proves you are not bound to your notes) or even sit on the desk for a while. Use your hands for emphasis, but don't move them to the point that they detract from your message. Be aware of your body language. Keeping your arms folded or wringing your hands or playing with a piece of chalk or a paper clip can all indicate to your audience that you are nervous.

If you have ever been in a class with a teacher who has annoying mannerisms, you know how distracting that can be. Common mannerisms are pacing, clicking fingers, jingling coins in a pocket, brushing hair off the face, and using two fingers to represent quotation marks. Verbal habits may be even more intolerable for the audience. There are lecturers who frequently say "uh" or "okay?" or "and so forth." It is easy to fall into habits like these and hard to break them. In fact, we are usually unaware of them unless some brave soul points them out to us. Watching yourself on a videotape or listening to yourself on audiotape can be enlightening.

Maintain eye contact with the class. Move your eyes around the class at times and avoid looking at just one side of the room. Our natural tendency is to focus our attention on the portion of the class that looks most interested or where heads are nodding in agreement. Often, the obviously interested students sit together, and the lecturer ends up speaking primarily to them without even being aware of it. You must make a conscious effort to maintain eye contact with all parts of the audience.

SPEED OF DELIVERY

The pacing of a lecture affects both the learners' comprehension and enjoyment of the material. Too slow a pace can induce boredom, but too fast a pace can result in writer's cramp for students as they struggle to take notes and to understand what is being said. A pause now and again helps the students to catch up and gives both them and you a few seconds to reflect on what has been said. It also gives the class a chance to ask questions that may be necessary to clarify the material. Some teachers like to hand out printed lecture notes so that students don't have to do so much writing, and the pace of the class can be faster.

GETTING OFF ON THE RIGHT FOOT

The way you begin a lecture sets the tone for all that follows. Try to avoid just walking into the class and immediately launching into the lecture. A little casual conversation for a minute or two in the beginning helps you to relax and to establish some rapport with the audience. Then try to give an opening "attention getter." Davis (1993) recommends starting with a "provocative question, startling statement, unusual analogy . . . powerful quote, or mention of a recent news event" (p. 112). You might start a lecture on hemodialysis with a statistic on how much money is spent on dialysis in the United States in one year or how long people live on hemodialysis. A lecture on congestive heart failure (CHF) might begin with an anecdote about how telenursing is revolutionizing CHF home monitoring. A good opening puts the audience in a positive frame of mind for what is to come.

CLARIFYING DURING THE LECTURE

Clarifying confusing or difficult concepts during a lecture is essential. Too often, students complain that when they ask a teacher to clarify a difficult concept, all they get is repetition of what has already been said. Clarification can be done effectively by means of examples and analogies rather than repetition. When Davis (1965) observed master lecturers in his timeless and interesting study, he noted that popular master lecturers used abundant examples. Whether from real life or hypothetical, examples not only clarify but also help to apply concepts. For example, in a lecture about research hypotheses, a score of examples from actual research could be used to explain the need for hypotheses, how they are developed, and the types that exist. Stories are lengthy examples and can also be effective. A story about a physically disabled child's typical day can make a great impression on listeners and help them to remember specific information about handicaps and their effects on activities of daily living.

Analogies can also be used for clarification. Likening an atherosclerotic vessel to a blocked drainpipe or relating the immune reaction to the mobilization of an army can help learners move more easily from the known to the unknown.

FACILITATING RETRIEVAL FROM MEMORY

There are several techniques that you can use during the delivery of a lecture that will help listeners to later remember the information. One method is repetition. Although, as was just mentioned, repetition does not help to clarify muddy points, it does help to fix information in memory and make it more likely to be retrieved at a later time. Repetition can be overdone, but simple repetition of important ideas at transitional points in the lecture can be effective. Elaboration is another form of repetition (Parker, 1993). In elaboration, repeated points are fleshed out in more detail when mentioned the second time in the lecture. Although many teachers feel they cannot spare the time to repeat information, if it means the difference between people really learning and remembering the material or forgetting it soon after, it is worth the time.

Imagery is another mechanism by which information can be lodged in memory for later retrieval. The brain encodes information in the form of either words or mental pictures (Parker, 1993). As Parker asserts, we retrieve mental pictures from long-term memory better than we retrieve words. You can use either actual graphics to help encode mental pictures, or you can call upon the learners' imaginations to form pictures. For example, you can help learners use their imagination to form images of human body physiology such as the closing of a heart valve or the movement of the lens of the eye.

Types of Lectures

There are a number of variations on the lecture theme that can be used if they fit the learning situation. For example, you cannot use the exact same lecture approach for a class that meets in a seminar room versus a lecture hall. Likewise, adaptation is needed for a lecture delivered via distance learning versus traditional classroom lectures.

Lecture variations include the traditional oral essay (Frederick, 1986). In this lecture type, the teacher is an orator and is the only speaker. The class consists of a complete polished exposition on a topic that can be inspirational and informative. Unfortunately, this type of lecture is often overused, resulting in passive and sometimes bored learners. Some teachers use the oral essay exclusively, not because it is the best way to teach the material, but because they fear loss of control of the learning situation if they get the class too involved. They also fear not being able to "cover" all of the material (Steinert & Snell, 1999).

The participatory lecture (Frederick, 1986) begins with learners brainstorming ideas on the lecture topic based on what they have read in preparation. It progresses with the teacher organizing the students' ideas and fleshing them out with expertise. Students feel some ownership of the topic and are able to attach new information to existing mental schemata.

The lecture with uncompleted handouts (Butler, 1992) involves a somewhat traditional oral essay format. However, the learners are supplied with handouts containing the lecture outline in some detail with blank spaces for learners to fill in information. The handout helps learners focus attention on important points and yet not have to take notes on every single piece of information.

The feedback lecture (Cross et al., 1997) actually consists of mini-lectures interspersed with 10-minute small group discussions structured around questions related to the lecture content. This approach gives the learners the opportunity to manipulate the lecture content and apply it immediately, thus enhancing learning and memory recall.

The mediated lecture is a term describing the use of media such as films, slides, or Web-based images along with traditional lecture. This approach can be used for Web-based courses as well as classroom courses. Using images of some type can add an emotional component to the lecture and assist in changing attitudes.

In the remainder of the chapter, discussion, questioning, and audiovisual strategies will be discussed. It should become clear how these additional traditional teaching techniques can be used in conjunction with lectures.

Discussion

Class discussions may be formal or informal. In a formal discussion, the topic is announced in advance and the class is asked to prepare to take part in the discussion by reading certain materials or watching a videotape and so on. Informal discussions may take place spontaneously at any point during the class including at the end of a lecture when the teacher asks, "Are there any questions?"

Purposes and Advantages of Discussion

The most obvious purpose of discussions is to give learners an opportunity to apply principles, concepts, and theories and, in that process, to transfer their learning to new and different situations. This approach presupposes that the learners have already been introduced to a body of information on which they can base their discussion. For example, a group of nurses may have heard an in-service lecture on management styles or read some articles on management theories. They may then come together for a discussion about management as it takes place on specific patient care units.

Another purpose is clarification of information and concepts. The group who was discussing management theory may have a difficult time grasping a particular complex theory. Discussion of the theory with explanations from the instructor and the group members may help to clarify obscure points. The discussion method, perhaps more than any other, helps the teacher gauge learners' understanding as learning is taking place. Misconceptions and hazy thinking can be assessed and corrected immediately.

Through discussions, students can learn the process of group problem solving. The discussion group may be divided into subgroups so that each can work on some aspect of the problem, or the entire group can work together to fully define the problem and then work toward a solution. From this interaction, participants learn how different people apply the steps of the problem-solving process, and they learn to draw on the expertise of group members, capitalizing on each other's strengths. An example of group problem solving with beginning nursing students might be a discussion of ways to reduce anxiety in hospitalized adults; with upper-level nursing students, it could be a discussion of ways to improve the image of the nursing profession. With a group of parents of asthmatic children, a discussion could be held on ways of balancing the child's need for exercise with the need to prevent exertional attacks.

Discussions with nurses or nursing students about professional, societal, or ethical issues can help participants develop and evaluate their beliefs and positions. In the give and take with other group members, they learn whether their position is clear, logical, and defensible.

They get immediate feedback on the position they have taken. At the same time, they are listening to the arguments of others, analyzing and weighing them, accepting or rejecting them. In other words, participants are getting practice in using critical thinking skills. With practice, they realize what they have to say and how they have to say it if they are to make their point and have an impact on the group.

Attitudes can be changed through discussion. As Bligh (2000) points out, the effectiveness of discussion in changing attitudes and values has been so well documented through earlier research conducted from the 1940s through the 1970s that no one spends time anymore trying to prove it. As people hear varying viewpoints and begin to look at issues and situations through the eyes and experiences of others, their own attitudes develop. Therefore, if you identify the need to change attitudes among individuals, discussion strategies should be considered.

Finally, an advantage of the discussion method is that many students like it and may even prefer it to other methods (Beishline & Holmes, 1997; Harvey & Vaughan, 1990).

Disadvantages of the Discussion Method

One drawback to discussions is that they take a lot of time. There is no doubt that discussion is an inefficient way to communicate information. Methods such as lecture or computer-assisted instruction are superior in terms of time efficiency.

Conventional wisdom tells us that the discussion method is effective only with small groups, which makes it an expensive strategy. McKeachie's (1999) investigations revealed that although small classes are more effective in general, discussions can be held with groups of all sizes. Bernstein (1994), for example, tested an effective method called the Expert Panel in which about 12 students per class prepared to take the part of the experts in a large class discussion. The 12 were responsible for asking and answering questions from the large group. Students from the class rotated through positions on the expert panel. Another approach is to divide a large class into smaller discussion groups. The disadvantage to this procedure is that the teacher cannot be the moderator and facilitator for all groups at the same time. There is no doubt that small group discussion is more effective in most situations because more students can take an active role.

We have all experienced the extreme frustration of being in a discussion group in which one person or a few people monopolized the discussion. This is always a danger of this method unless the group leader controls the situation. If only a few members are participating, the others are relegated to a passive role, and learning is especially inhibited if the vocal few are not contributing valuable viewpoints or conclusions.

Finally, many discussions are valuable only if the participants come prepared with the necessary background information. The contribution of uninformed opinions and misinformation benefits no one, and the discussion becomes simply a sharing of each other's ignorance.

Discussion Techniques

Good discussions do not usually happen spontaneously; they require careful planning. The teacher must develop objectives and choose appropriate topics. Not all class material lends itself to the formal discussion method. For example, it would be difficult to hold a lively dis-

cussion about the immune response. Topics that are most suitable for discussion are controversial issues, clinical or professional problems, and emotionally laden topics such as death
and dying. It is possible to have discussions about factual material, but those discussions are
usually short and take place after information has been conveyed by lecture or reading.

After choosing a topic, the teacher may use any or all of the following techniques to
facilitate an effective discussion.

- *Make your expectations clear.* The learners should know exactly what they have to do
  to prepare for the discussion and to what degree they are expected to participate.
  Preparation may involve reading a chapter or an article, watching a video, or recalling some personal experience that would be pertinent.

- *Set the ground rules.* The rules may include time limits for various aspects of the discussion, prohibitions against interrupting someone, or limits on the number of
  times any one person may speak.

- *Arrange the physical space.* Ideally, the classroom will permit chairs to be arranged so
  everyone can sit in a circle. The more eye contact among participants, the better the
  possibilities for a good discussion. Forming a circle also makes it easier for all to
  hear. If a large class must be broken into smaller discussion groups, the room
  should be large enough to allow space between groups.

- *Plan a discussion starter.* Davis (1993) has several suggestions for getting started.
  They include referring to study questions that you handed out at a prior meeting,
  asking the participants to come to the discussion with some opening questions prepared, posing a question yourself and giving the group a few minutes to think about
  it, and asking participants to pose the dumbest question they can think of.

- *Facilitate, don't discuss.* If you are taking the role of leader, you should refrain from
  doing much talking. You need to be free to watch the group process, keep the discussion moving, and make sure everyone is engaged in the process. Being relatively
  quiet will not be easy for teachers who are used to being the information source and
  resident expert in the classroom, but you cannot be an effective facilitator and participate fully in the discussion at the same time.

- *Encourage quiet group members.* Helping quiet or shy people to participate is a
  challenge. It helps to make eye contact with them and smile. You may direct simple
  questions to them or draw on their personal experiences or expertise. You might
  say, "Mary, what do you think of what Felipe has just said in light of your experience in the orthopedic unit last week?" Educators disagree on whether reticent
  people should be forced or required to speak during a discussion. My experience
  has been that if you direct easy questions to them or draw on experiences as
  described above, quiet group members are not too threatened. It is also important
  to direct questions and comments to a variety of people, not just singling out the
  quiet ones.

- *Don't allow monopolies.* It is just as challenging to keep some people quiet as it is to
  encourage others to talk. You should discourage members who are talking too
  much and not letting others take part. Avoiding eye contact with them may work to
  some extent. Sometimes you have to be blunt and say, "We've been hearing a lot
  from Sarah, now let's hear what some of the rest of you think."

- *Direct the discussion among group members.* Part of the leader's role is to direct the discussion between and among members of the group; most comments should not be addressed directly to the leader. If every participant looks at and talks to the leader, the leader is going to be much too verbal. Instead, you should make it clear that if Member A has something to say about what Member B has just contributed, Member A should address the comment to Member B. Your interventions should serve only to support the group process and occasionally introduce comments or questions that will move the discussion along and accomplish the objectives.

- *Keep the discussion on track.* If people are going off on a tangent and don't seem to be finding the way back, you should make a comment like, "We seem to have strayed a little from our topic. Let's pick up on that last point that Letitia was talking about."

- *Clarify when confusion reigns.* In the course of the discussion, the leader may need to clarify participants' statements in order to avoid confusion and misinformation. Such clarification should be used sparingly but is sometimes necessary. Rewording what a person has said may also help other group members to learn the art of clear self-expression. If rewording a member's comment seems demeaning, you can instead ask the person to give an example of what he or she is talking about.

- *Tolerate some silence.* It is perfectly acceptable and even desirable to have periods of silence in a discussion. Although many people are uncomfortable with silence in a group setting, silence gives everyone a chance to think about what has been said and to organize his or her thoughts. During a lull in the talking, a quiet student may get up the nerve to say something.

- *Summarize when appropriate.* A summary may be in order when moving from one aspect of a topic to another and is certainly needed at the end of the discussion period.

These are some of the techniques you can use to lead effective in-person discussions. Experienced educators also develop their own techniques that work for them. Most of these techniques also can be applied to online threaded discussions in Web-based courses. Although not every discussion will meet your expectations, with conscientious planning and leading, most group discussions can be fruitful.

Questioning

Asking questions is such an integral part of teaching that many teachers take it for granted. They ask questions to assess learner comprehension but don't give much thought to using questioning as a teaching strategy. No one would argue that nurses need to be able to ask and answer questions that demonstrate reasoning, analysis, and problem solving. Yet unless educators model good questioning skills, students are left to pick up that skill on their own.

Research has shown that although educators tend to ask their students a lot of questions, most of those questions are very low level, requiring only recall of factual material. They don't ask many questions that require higher-order thinking (Savage, 1998; Tanenbaum, Tilson, Cross, & Rodgers, 1997; Wink, 1993a). Educators can benefit from a structured program designed to teach them to formulate high-level questions (Wink, 1993a), and it is hoped that when teachers begin asking questions that elicit critical thinking, it will prompt students to develop the same questioning skills in their own practice.

Awareness of the effectiveness of questioning as a teaching strategy seems to have begun with Socrates. In the Socratic method of teaching, a teacher asks a series of questions that are designed to first make the students aware of their ignorance. Each answer by a student is met with another question from the teacher. Each question is designed to bring the student closer to reasoning out the fundamental truth about an issue. Although few educators today use the Socratic method, instructors would do well to put more emphasis on questioning as a means of teaching reasoning and critical thinking.

Functions of Questioning

The use of questioning places learners in an active role. They are asked to recall, to form links between previously isolated information, to analyze statements or beliefs, to evaluate the worth of ideas, and to speculate about what would happen "if." As questions are asked, learners start to mentally formulate answers if they think they may be called on in class. They cannot sit and daydream, because they never know if a question is going to come their way.

Questions can be used to assess a baseline of knowledge—to find out what a group already knows about a subject. They can also help the teacher to assess understanding and retention of information. If learners are having trouble grasping concepts or following the teacher's thought processes, questioning can quickly uncover their problems.

Questioning can also be used to review content. If the instructor wants to spend five minutes at the beginning of class reviewing content from a previous class, it might be more enlightening to do so by means of questioning rather than lecturing.

Motivation to learn can increase as learners hear questions for which they would like to know the answers. A really good question can arouse learners' curiosity. When a teacher poses a problem or dilemma and raises questions about it, learners may be motivated to come up with solutions.

Knowledgeable teachers use questions to guide learners' thought processes in a certain direction. Suppose a teacher wants to explore the chain of infection in hospitals. Her first question might be, "Why is there a higher rate of infections among hospitalized people than people who are ill at home?" This might be followed by, "Yes, patients can get infections from each other, but what about some other sources of infection?" Then, "Contaminated equipment can be responsible, too. Is there anything else?" After exploring all of the sources of infections, the instructor would try to elicit the concept of a *reservoir* of pathogens by asking, "What term could you use to describe the existence of a ready supply of pathogens in the hospital?" Questions could continue that would elicit the other links in the chain of infection. In so guiding learners' thinking on a subject, the teacher extends their knowledge while encouraging them to think logically and deepening their understanding of a subject.

Levels of Questions

Questions can be formulated that stimulate specific levels of cognitive activity in learners. Educators have devised several classification systems for questions. Here, we will examine three of the most common classifications.

Questions can be classified as being either *convergent* or *divergent* (Wink, 1993b). Convergent questions require the learner to recall or integrate information they have learned. This requires fairly low-level cognitive activity. Convergent questions have specific, usually short, and expected answers. Examples of convergent questions are, "Compare what happens in a bronchiole during pneumonia versus an asthma attack," and "Explain why neuromuscular hyperactivity occurs in hypoparathyroidism." Divergent questions ask the learner to generate new ideas, draw implications, or formulate a new perspective on a topic. There is no single correct answer. This process requires a higher level of cognitive activity. An example of a divergent question is, "What might happen if you relocate an elderly person with dementia to another type of residence from where he or she is presently living?"

In the process of classifying questions, you must always be aware that a single question could be placed in more than one category, depending on the context. The question about relocating an elderly demented person could simply be a convergent question if the student had previously been taught the effects of relocation on the elderly. It is a divergent question only if the learner has not encountered that exact information before and is being asked to weigh a number of factors and hypothesize about what might happen.

Questions can be categorized also as *lower-order* questions or *higher-order* questions (Barden, 1995). Lower-order questions are those that require the learner to recall information they have read or memorized. Higher-order questions require more than recall. To answer a higher-order question, the learner would have to be able to comprehend or think critically about the information. Barden contends that question classifications that have more than these two levels are probably not valid. She believes that although hierarchical classifications, like the next one to be discussed, are theoretically helpful, in practice it is too difficult to determine whether a learner is answering a question at the comprehension, analysis, or synthesis levels, for example.

The most popular classification system is based on Bloom's taxonomy (Bloom, 1956). Although this taxonomy was written to classify educational objectives, it nicely explains cognitive levels of questions also. Thus, many educators refer to questions that elicit thinking at the levels of knowledge, comprehension, application, analysis, synthesis, and evaluation. Table 7–3 lists Bloom's cognitive levels, explains them, and gives some sample words and phrases that could be used in questions at that level. Following are examples of questions at each cognitive level:

Knowledge
What is the definition of bronchodilator?
At what age do infants begin to crawl?

Comprehension
What does the nursing process have in common with the scientific method?
Why does intravenous tubing have to be free of air?

Application
Given these arterial blood gas results, what nursing interventions are needed?
How would you take a blood pressure reading on a person with third-degree burns of all extremities?

TABLE 7-3   Question Classification Using Bloom's Taxonomy

Level of Bloom's Taxonomy	Level of Thinking	Terms and Phrases Used in Questions
Knowledge	Involves recall of memorized data	Define, How, What, List, When, Where
Comprehension	Includes understanding and interpretation of information	Compare, Contrast, Explain, Give an example, Put in your own words, Why
Application	Requires using information in new situations	Apply, Consider, Use this information, How would you
Analysis	Involves breaking the whole into parts and showing relationships	Classify, Explain your reasons, What evidence, What hypotheses, What if
Synthesis	Requires combining elements into a new structure	Create, Generalize, Plan, Predict
Evaluation	Includes assessing a situation based on criteria	Appraise, Decide, Evaluate, Justify, Judge, How would you rate

Analysis
What is the major premise of Kubler–Ross's theory of death and dying?

What data would you need to support this nursing diagnosis?

Synthesis
Given all of the data in this case study, what nursing diagnoses can be developed?

Think of a way we could research the relationship between those variables.

Evaluation
Of the two possible solutions to this problem, which would be more appropriate?

Which leadership style would make the best use of the employees' abilities?

You can see that Bloom's taxonomy forms more of a hierarchy than the other classifications. For this reason, it is also more difficult to use. There is often a fine line between whether a question is at the level of analysis or synthesis or whether it is an analysis question or an evaluation question. The advantage of using this complex tool, however, is that it helps the educator to realize the types of higher-order thinking that can be drawn upon in helping learners to be critical thinkers.

Types of Questions

Besides varying the cognitive levels of questions, instructors can choose from seven types of questions to achieve different purposes.

1. *Factual questions.* When the teacher asks a factual question, it demands a simple recall answer. It might be a Yes/No question, asking for a one-word response, or it might ask for a sentence length response. Factual questions can be used to assess learners' understanding or to simply find out if they are paying attention.

2. *Probing questions.* When the teacher wants a learner to further explain an answer, or dig deeper into a subject, he or she may use a probe or cue such as "Can you

explain that?" or "Can you tell us a little more about why you have taken that position?" Such questions are also helpful in assessing learners' thought processes. House, Chassie, and Spohn (1990) delineate five types of probing questions: *extension probes* that ask learners to elaborate on a response; *clarification probes*, used when learners' responses are unclear; *justification probes* that ask learners to justify their responses; *prompting probes* that help a responder who is unsure of an answer or gives an incorrect answer; and *redirection probes* to elicit a variety of responses from the group of learners.

3. *Multiple-choice questions.* Such questions can be oral as well as written. "Is NPH insulin a short-, intermediate-, or long-acting insulin?" is an oral multiple-choice question. If you use this type, be careful not to include too many options, or it becomes confusing. Multiple-choice questions usually test recall and can be used to begin a discussion.

4. *Open-ended questions.* This broad category encompasses all questions that require learners to construct an answer. Questions such as "When should fetal monitoring be used?" and "When should you use clean versus sterile dressing technique?" are open-ended questions.

5. *Discussion-stimulating questions.* Once discussion about a subject has been initiated, the teacher can use various questions to promote it. Questions such as "What do the rest of you think of that statement?," "Do you agree with John's position?," and "Has anyone else had that experience?" help to move the discussion along.

6. *Questions that guide problem solving.* A teacher needs to phrase and sequence questions carefully in order to guide learners through problem-solving thinking. Typical questions might be "What information do we need before we can solve this problem?," "What other options do we have?," and "What would be the effect of that action?"

7. *Rhetorical questions.* It is sometimes appropriate to ask questions for which you expect no answers at the time. Such questions can be used to stimulate thinking in the class and may guide learners into asking some of their own questions as they study a topic. What is used as a rhetorical question in one session may become a source of discussion in a later session.

There is value in asking learners a variety of types of questions at different cognitive levels. In view of the high-level thinking required of nurses in most work situations, it would seem beneficial to accustom learners to formulating a high percentage of questions and answers at the application through evaluation levels.

Questioning Techniques

Incorporating good questioning procedures into classes requires planning and forethought. The first prerequisite is to establish an atmosphere in which students feel fairly relaxed and free to ask questions. Research has supported the belief that students who perceive their teacher as supportive are more likely to ask questions than those who believe their teacher is not supportive (Schell, 1998). It takes time before learners decide that the teacher really wants them to talk and will not humiliate them if they come up with the wrong answer.

The following questioning techniques will help educators become more confident and proficient in asking questions that will help to meet educational objectives.

- *Prepare some questions ahead of time.* If your questions are to meet the objectives for the class session and be at the appropriate cognitive level, they require careful preparation. Not every question can be planned, because it is difficult to tell how learners will respond and which directions their answers will take, but the introductory questions for the major topics should be planned.

- *State questions clearly and specifically.* A vague or poorly worded question will probably elicit silent stares. A question like "What are the legal principles that should guide your nursing care?" is so broad and nonspecific that learners would probably be unsure of how to answer. Instead, the same objectives might be achieved with the question "You read about the legal principle of *respondeat superior*. Can you give me an example of a malpractice suit in which this principle applies?"

- *Tolerate some silence.* If there is no immediate answer to your question, avoid jumping right in to answer the question yourself. Research indicates that teachers generally allow only one second before repeating the question or answering it (House et al., 1990; Johnson, 1997). Increasing the wait time to three to five seconds increases the number and depth of appropriate responses, and a greater variety of students will enter the discussion.

- *Listen carefully to responses.* Look at the speaker and pay careful attention. Do not interrupt, and do not ask follow-up questions or evaluate the response until the speaker is finished.

- *Use the "beam, focus, build" technique* (Wigle, 1999, p. 62). When you "beam," you send the question out to the whole class. Then you "focus" by calling on one student to answer the question. Finally, you "build" if you then redirect the question to other students, asking them to share their ideas. Do not be afraid of calling on particular students as long as you include everyone in the class over time and you handle wrong answers diplomatically.

- *Provide feedback.* The teacher's response to a learner's answer is very important. A nod, a smile, or a comment that shows the answer is correct are all appropriate. You should be careful, though, not to give too rapid a reward. If the teacher immediately says, "Right" after the first learner gives an answer, those in the group who are slower thinkers may be prevented from formulating and offering their own answers. Instead, allow a few seconds of silence while looking around at the other learners or ask, "Can anyone add to that answer?"

- *Handle wrong answers carefully.* Sometimes answers are not totally wrong, and you can acknowledge the accuracy of the correct part while clarifying the inaccuracy. For example, you might say, "Yvette, you are correct in saying that indwelling catheters often need to be irrigated after bladder surgery, but using force is not the best way to go." If an answer is totally wrong, you might say, "I'm sorry Edward, but that's not quite it," or you can give no response, get a few more answers, and let the class decide which responses are the correct ones. By all means, avoid embarrassing learners in front of their peers, especially if the person seems very quiet or shy.

Stimulating Learners to Ask Questions

One of the outcomes of questioning as a teaching strategy should be that learners learn how to ask questions. In fact, learners should be rewarded just as much for asking good questions as they are for giving good answers. As Elder and Paul (1998, p. 297) state, "Thinking is driven not by answers but by questions."

Teachers can stimulate student questioning by guiding their thinking along a path that will lead to the development of questions and hypotheses about a subject. But this guidance must take place in an atmosphere where it is safe to take risks and to ask questions that might seem stupid.

Teachers also have to monitor their teaching behaviors to ensure that they are not unknowingly discouraging questions. Nonverbally, teachers may indicate their unwillingness to entertain questions or their dislike of questions by avoiding eye contact, blatantly ignoring raised hands, or appearing distracted or impatient while a learner is talking. A teacher may also use seemingly innocuous statements such as "Can you hold that question until I'm finished?" or "Unless anyone has any burning questions or brilliant insights, we'll end here." Although these statements may be appropriate at rare times, their habitual use will soon convey the message that the teacher doesn't really want to be interrupted with questions, and any questions that *are* asked had better be good. Being aware of such behavior can help teachers change their verbal and nonverbal patterns.

When learners do ask questions, there are a few strategies that encourage them or others to ask more questions. These include thanking or praising the person for asking the question and, after answering it, asking the questioner if you have answered the question. All educators have probably at one time or another answered a question that wasn't really asked, just because we missed the point of the question that was asked. Also, when responding to a question, talk to the whole class, not just the questioner. This approach serves to keep the whole group involved and shows the questioner that the question was important.

Developing your skill in asking and answering questions is well worth the time and effort. Socrates would tell you that there is nothing more important for a teacher to do.

Using Audiovisuals

If used appropriately, audiovisuals can greatly enhance teaching and can add interest and stimulation to the classroom. If used inappropriately, audiovisuals simply become time fillers and entertainers, serving no real purpose. A range of traditional audiovisuals can be used effectively, from pictures and charts to overhead transparencies, slides, and videotapes. It is important for the educator to know what media are available, how to select them, and how to use them effectively.

Selecting Media

How does an educator begin to select the appropriate media, and how and when should they be used? These decisions are based on a number of factors. The chief determinants are the learning objectives. Some objectives may best be met by using lectures, some by discussion, some by individual student assignments, and some through traditional media. If several methods would be suitable, it may be best to opt for variety. Lectures/discussions can be broken up with some audiovisuals to provide interest and stimulation. Technologies should never be used simply because they fill time or make it easier for the teacher to entertain the learners, but if the educational objectives can be met in an entertaining way, why not take advantage? After all, education can also be fun.

Let's see how a teacher might make a decision about use of media based on course objectives. Suppose that a nursing instructor has to teach a four-hour unit on diabetes mellitus and related nursing care. The objectives of this unit are:

1. Explain the pathophysiology of diabetes
2. Identify assessments that should be made on the diabetic patient
3. Write a teaching plan for a newly diagnosed Type 2 diabetic
4. Evaluate the nursing care provided for a diabetic patient

The teacher decides to lecture about pathophysiology, using overhead transparencies to explain the pathologic chain of events. Assessment could be taught by means of lecture, but the instructor decides to hold the students responsible for reading the material in the textbook and then shows slides illustrating some of the abnormalities that may be discovered on assessment of the diabetic patient. Because the class has 40 students, the instructor decides that it would be impossible to assist each student in writing a teaching plan, so students are asked as a group to contribute to a teaching plan while it is being written on an overhead transparency. Finally, the instructor decides to show a videotape of a nurse who is caring for a diabetic patient recovering from ketoacidosis and plans to have the students evaluate the care given by the nurse. With this mix of teaching methods, all of the objectives can be met, and met more effectively and more interestingly than would be possible without audiovisuals.

Another factor to consider in deciding on media use is availability of both materials and technical assistance. What hardware and software are available? If it is not available, can it be purchased, produced, or rented? Will you have to learn to operate the equipment, or will someone else be able to run it? Is there someone to assist with producing software? The answers to these questions will help in making decisions on media use.

The level, ability, and number of learners are also important considerations, especially if you want to assign audiovisuals for individual use. How motivated are the learners to use audiovisual equipment on an individual basis? Is it too large a group to make individual media use feasible? Is the software appropriate for the level of the learners? If the material is either too complex or too simplistic, the learners will be frustrated or turned off.

Types of Traditional Audiovisuals

The most commonly used audiovisual media are handouts, chalkboards or whiteboards, overhead transparencies, slides, and videotapes. This section examines each briefly, including how it can best be used and the advantages and disadvantages of each.

HANDOUTS

Printed materials or handouts have been around for a long time and can be used to communicate facts, figures, and concepts. It may save a lot of time to give information in handout form rather than spend class time lecturing on it. If handouts are distributed before a given class, learners can review them in preparation for class discussion. Printed materials also ensure that all learners have access to the same information and can review that information whenever necessary. If the handout is not going to be referred to in the class session, it is best to distribute it at the end of the class period to prevent distraction during class.

Handouts in the form of pamphlets are particularly useful for reinforcing patient teaching. You can develop your own pamphlet or order them from professional organizations such as the American Heart Association or the American Diabetes Association. Whether you develop the handout or use a commercial one, be sure that the handouts meet the criteria for readability as outlined in Chapter 6.

CHALKBOARDS OR WHITEBOARDS

Chalkboards or the newer laminate white (or gray) boards are universally used in education. Although they have several uses, their outstanding feature is that they allow for spontaneity in the classroom. New ideas or solutions to problems can be jotted down as they are mentioned. If learners are suddenly confused about something, the point can be illustrated on the board. If learners cannot visualize an object, it can be quickly sketched. Chalk/whiteboards are especially useful for working out mathematical problems, for spelling new words, for outlining material to be covered in class, and for having several students placing their ideas on the board at the same time. Creative use of the board can add dimension to almost any class.

To be used properly, the chalk- or whiteboard must be placed where the entire class can see it easily and where glare is minimal. It must be kept clean between uses. You should write only on the upper two thirds of the board because learners often have difficulty seeing the bottom of the board over each other's heads. Printing or diagrams should be large enough to be seen from the back of the room, and not too much information should be on the board at one time. If the board is covered with information, chances are you are using the wrong method and should switch to handouts or an overhead projector. You should not waste class time putting material on the board that could have been prepared ahead of time on the board, handouts, transparencies, or slides.

Among the drawbacks of the chalkboard are the mess made by chalk (not a problem with whiteboards and felt pens), the fact that material on the board usually cannot be saved until the next class, and the fact that the board may not be visible to very large groups. Also, while writing on the chalk/whiteboard, your back is to the class, which may cause you to lose the flow of contact with the learners and interfere with their ability to hear you. Finally, this method is not good for the instructor who has poor handwriting, since the information may be lost to students who cannot decipher it.

OVERHEAD TRANSPARENCIES

Transparencies are sheets of acetate placed on an overhead projector that enlarges and projects the image onto a screen. Transparencies are easy to make, use, store, and transport and can be an asset to any teacher.

Transparencies can be used similarly to a chalk/whiteboard for writing down spontaneous ideas, outlining class content, or doing math problems, but their use surpasses that of a chalk/whiteboard. Transparencies can be prepared beforehand to save class time and to help organize and illustrate content. Diagrams and drawings can be drawn or copied onto transparencies. Concepts can be illustrated and lectures can be outlined. Charts and graphs can be presented. Cartoons can be projected for humor and illustration.

One of the nice features of the overhead projector is that it stands in front of the audience and you can face the class while using it; thus, eye contact can be maintained. The room does not have to be dark, although it is helpful to dim the lights around the screen. The projector is easy to use, requiring only manipulation of the on–off switch and a focus knob. Small portable projectors are available for teachers who go out on guest lectures and want to take their own audiovisual equipment.

It is easy to make your own transparencies if you keep a few points in mind. First, make sure you are using the right equipment. Some transparency sheets are designed to be used with marking pens, whereas others are designed for thermofax machines or copying machines. If you try drawing with a felt-tip pen on the wrong type of sheet, you may find that your ink bubbles up or disappears. If you try running the wrong type of sheet through a copy machine, the transparency can melt and damage the inner workings of the machine. If you are going to draw by hand on the transparency, you have a choice of permanent or nonpermanent colored pens. If you want to reuse the transparency, you must obviously use a nonpermanent pen.

Here are some tips for making effective transparencies:

- Keep the amount of information on each sheet to a minimum. A guideline is no more than six words per line and no more than six lines per transparency (Farley, 1990).
- Each letter should be at least one fourth inch high. Never make a transparency from a typed page. No one sitting a few rows back will be able to read the print.
- Be sure that every word or image can be seen from the back of the room.
- If placing a picture or diagram on the transparency, fill most of the sheet, with only one image per sheet.
- To protect transparencies over time, either mount them into a cardboard frame (commercially available) or slide them into a plastic sleeve (the type you can place in a three-ring notebook).

You can draw or print on the transparency with pens as described above, which is wonderful for in-class use. If you want to prepare the transparency ahead of time, it is preferable to design the transparency on a computer using large-size fonts, or using a program designed to make slides and transparencies such as Microsoft PowerPoint. When using PowerPoint, you can produce color transparencies if you have a color printer.

Many commercially produced transparencies are available through textbook publishing companies. The publisher provides transparencies that illustrate the major concepts of the book. Before purchasing large sets of transparencies, evaluate how much use will actually be made of them. If only a small percentage in the set is really valuable to you, it might be more economical to make your own.

Just a few more tips about actually using the overhead transparency projector:

- Turn the projector on before you actually need it to make sure it works. Keep a spare bulb in an accessible place in case the bulb has burned out (which is guaranteed to happen at the most inopportune time).
- When you stand by the projector, you may be blocking the learners' view. Move off to the side occasionally to enable better viewing.

- If you have finished referring to one transparency and will not be using the next one for a while, turn the projector off or place a blank piece of dark paper on the projector surface to reduce distraction and light glare.
- Leave each transparency on the screen long enough for learners to read or copy all of the information. It is very frustrating for the audience to have a transparency whisked away before they can finish reading it.
- If your transparency has several points listed on it, you may want to reveal only one point at a time, to keep the audience from reading ahead. Keep a piece of paper available to cover up future points on the transparency.

SLIDES

You may use slides to show pictures or project diagrams, charts, and word concepts. Slides can be effective promoters of discussions, can help to make abstractions concrete, and can lend realism to an otherwise academic discussion. Occasionally, you may want learners to see a magazine picture or chart but don't want to spend the time passing the magazine around the group. In a case like this, making slides of the material can be the answer. Any graphics that would help illustrate a lecture can be made into clear and colorful slides.

The advantages of slides over some other media are that they are not too expensive to make or buy, they are compact and easy to store, and they are easy to update and reorganize to fit changing class needs. The teacher can control the speed of slide presentation so that each frame can be discussed for the desired length of time. A remote-control extension allows you to walk around or stand in front of the class and still control the slides. It is also easy to back up to previous frames if a question arises pertaining to them. Slide projectors are lightweight and easy to carry.

The disadvantages of slides are that they can easily get smudged with fingerprints because they are so small, and they can get bent inside a malfunctioning projector. Projector bulbs don't last too long and are expensive to replace. Reduced room light is necessary to get a clear image on the screen, which makes it difficult for learners to take notes.

To prepare your own slides, you will probably need some advice or help from a media specialist in your institution. It is easy to plan out slides with words or graphics using a computer program like Microsoft PowerPoint or other presentation software. From that point, however, you may need assistance in turning your computer file into slides. In some institutions, the production staff will make the slides for you if you give them the computer file or the pictures from which you want to make the slides. Make sure that you obtain permission to use copyrighted materials, if necessary. Prepared slides are also available from many sources, including drug companies, medical and surgical supply companies, and various public health organizations.

VIDEOTAPES

Most institutions have equipment not only to play videotapes but also to produce them. So, in all settings, both educational and clinical, commercially made videos can be shown and in-house filming can usually be done. Showing commercially produced videos as a teaching method in academic settings has been found to produce learning outcomes similar to those resulting from lectures (McAlpine, 1996). It is feasible to add video clips to Web-based courses as well.

In academic settings, videotape technology can also be used to film students while they role-play interviewing, communication, and counseling skills (Burnard, 1991). Playback of the videos for individual feedback or group critique can be very instructional. Research in medical schools has shown that using videotaping for teaching interviewing skills is more effective than other teaching strategies (Beckman & Frankel, 1994).

In clinical settings, videotapes have been found to be an effective means of health education that meets accreditation requirements by the Joint Commission on Accreditation of Health Care Organizations. For example, one medical center found that preoperative teaching for outpatient surgery could be conveniently and advantageously done by giving hospital-produced videos to patients to view at home (Maller, Twitty, & Sauve, 1997). Other agencies have also found this to be a cost-effective method of patient education that is acceptable to the public and results in learning outcomes similar to that achieved by in-person teaching (Hoberty, Becker, Hoberty, & Diaz, 1998; Hurtado & Hovell, 1993).

Videotape technology has several advantages over other traditional media. On a videotape, a teacher can still maintain eye contact with the class and provide something of a personal touch, even though the performance is not live. Also, motion enhances the realism of the situation and often increases interest.

All learners watching a videotape are exposed to the same teaching, even though they may be in different locations. This helps maintain consistency and quality for the teaching of each individual learner. In academic settings, this consistency reduces the problem of slightly different information and emphasis being given for different class sections taking the same examinations.

When videotapes are used for individual learning, they can be used at the learner's own pace. The learner can replay and freeze frames according to his or her needs. In classroom settings, the teacher may choose to freeze the action and discuss what has just been played before proceeding.

The disadvantages of videotape technology include the fact that communication is only one-way and learners cannot interact with the medium; they become passive recipients of information. This effect can be minimized by instructor involvement before, during, or after showing the videotape.

The cost of good videotaping equipment can be high, and further costs are involved if technicians are required for producing tapes. Producing professional-quality videos for health education can be a costly enterprise. The rule of thumb is that it costs $1,000 per minute of final video, and duplication costs about $2.00 per tape (Maller et al., 1997). Long-term savings are achieved, however, by saving staff educator time and reducing incidence of illness or complications.

Audiovisuals, in general, are a boon to education. When used in conjunction with other teaching strategies, they add interest and quality to a class. When used for patient education, they can provide quality health teaching.

The Interactive Lecture

It should be clear by this point that the techniques of lecture, discussion, questioning, and audiovisuals can be effectively blended together into an interactive, illustrated lecture, utilizing the advantages of all the methods and reducing their disadvantages.

Class time can be divided into sections for lecture, informal discussion, questioning, more lecturing combined with various audiovisuals, and so on. Changing tactics every 15 to 20 minutes may help to recapture learners' interest at points when attention naturally seems to wander. Learners become periodically active in the class, which eliminates some of the objections to pure lecturing. Successful interactive lectures can exemplify active learning at its best.

CASE STUDY

A community health nurse educator is planning a discussion for an Alzheimer's Caregivers Support Group. The topic is the issue of placing a family member with Alzheimer's disease in a nursing care facility.

1. What are some questions the educator can prepare to start the discussion?
2. What are some questions or comments the educator can prepare to keep advancing the discussion?
3. How should the educator react if some members of the group become emotionally upset?
4. How can the educator prevent one person from taking over the discussion to the exclusion of others who want to talk?

CRITICAL THINKING EXERCISES

You have been invited to give a 30-minute speech (i.e., lecture) to the staff nurses of a hospital on National Nurses Day. You decide to give an inspirational talk on the viewpoint that nurses are the epitome of critical thinkers and problem solvers in our society.

1. Should you organize your lecture by the hierarchical, problem-centered, thesis, or comparative format? Why and how?
2. What type of lecture would be most appropriate for the occasion (oral essay, participatory lecture, or mediated lecture) and why?
3. At the end of the lecture, a staff nurse states that she disagrees with your premise that nurses are such good critical thinkers. She states that she works with some nurses who have some problem-solving skills, but they are not necessarily good critical thinkers. How would you defend your position? Is a defense of your premise appropriate in this type of lecture?

IDEAS FOR FURTHER RESEARCH

1. Perform a qualitative study of people known to be good lecturers (see Davis, 1965). What qualities do you see that make them successful at lecturing?

2. Tape record some graduate nursing classes. Presumably at this level of education, higher-order questions should prevail. Evaluate the number, type, and level of questions that are asked. You may want to compare the findings to graduate courses in other disciplines.

3. Compare the effectiveness of printed educational handouts versus videotapes for health education.

REFERENCES

Barden, L. M. (1995). Effective questioning & the ever-elusive higher-order question. *American Biology Teacher, 57*(7), 423–426.

Beckman, H. B., & Frankel, R. M. (1994). The use of videotape in internal medicine training. *Journal of General Internal Medicine, 9*, 517–521.

Beishline, M. J., & Holmes, C. B. (1997). Student preferences for various teaching styles. *Journal of Instructional Psychology, 24*(2), 95–99.

Bernstein, J. M. (1994). Discussion and learning skills in an introductory course. *Journalism Educator, 49*(1), 39–48.

Birk, L. (1997). What's so bad about the lecture? *Education Digest, 62*(9), 58–61.

Black, K. A. (1993). What to do when you stop lecturing. *Journal of Chemical Education, 70*(2), 140–144.

Bligh, D. A. (2000). *What's the use of lectures?* San Francisco: Jossey-Bass.

Bloom, B. S. (Ed.). (1956). *Taxonomy of education objectives handbook I: Cognitive domain.* New York: Longman.

Burnard, P. (1991). Using video as a reflective tool in interpersonal skills training. *Nurse Education Today, 11*, 143–146.

Butler, J. A. (1992). Use of teaching methods within the lecture format. *Medical Teacher, 14*(1), 11–25.

Cross, D. S., Tilson, E. R., Tanenbaum, B. G., & Rodgers, A. T. (1997). The facilitated lecture. *Radiologic Technology, 68*(4), 339–342.

Davis, B. G. (1993). *Tools for teaching.* San Francisco: Jossey-Bass.

Davis, R. J. (1965). Secrets of master lecturers. *Improving College and University Teaching, 13*, 150–151.

Elder, L., & Paul, R. (1998). The role of Socratic questioning in thinking, teaching, and learning. *Clearing House, 71*(5), 297–301.

Farley, J. K. (1990). Enhancing oral presentations through visual images. *Nurse Educator, 15*(5), 3–4.

Foley, R. P., & Smilansky, J. (1980). *Teaching techniques.* New York: McGraw-Hill.

Frederick, P. J. (1986). The lively lecture—8 variations. *College Teaching, 34*(2), 43–50.

Harvey, T. J., & Vaughan, J. (1990). Student nurse attitudes towards different teaching/learning methods. *Nurse Education Today, 10*(3), 181–185.

Hoberty, P. D., Becker, K. S., Hoberty, R. J., & Diaz, P. T. (1998). Learning and patient satisfaction outcomes of two methods of providing instruction in pulmonary rehabilitation. *Journal of Rehabilitation Outcomes Measurement, 2*(6), 26–31.

House, B. M, Chassie, M. B., & Spohn, B. B. (1990). Questioning: An essential ingredient in effective teaching. *The Journal of Continuing Education in Nursing, 21*(5), 196–201.

Hurtado, S. L., & Hovell, M. F. (1993). Efficacy of health promotion videotapes in the U.S. Navy: A lesson for health educators. *Journal of Health Education, 24*(2), 107–112.

Johnson, R. (1997). Questioning techniques to use in teaching. *Journal of Physical Education, Recreation & Dance, 68*(8), 45–49.

Jones, R. G. (1990). The lecture as a teaching method in modern nurse education. *Nurse Education Today, 10*(4), 290–293.

Maller, C. E., Twitty, V. J., & Sauve, A. (1997). A video approach to interactive patient education. *Journal of PeriAnesthesia Nursing, 12*(2), 82–88.

McAlpine, L. (1996). Comparison of the effectiveness of tutored videotape instruction versus traditional lecture for a basic hemodynamic monitoring course. *Journal of Nursing Staff Development, 12*(3), 119–125.

McKeachie, W. J. (1999). *Teaching tips.* Boston: Houghton Mifflin.

Parker, J. K. (1993). Lecturing and loving it: Applying the information-processing model. *Clearing House, 67*(1), 8–11.

Savage, L. B. (1998). Eliciting critical thinking skills through questioning. *Clearing House, 71*(5), 291–293.

Schell, K. (1998). Promoting student questioning. *Nurse Educator, 23*(5), 8–12.

Schoen, J. R. (1970). Use of consciousness sampling to study teaching methods. *Journal of Educational Research, 63*(9), 387–390.

Steinert, Y., & Snell, L. S. (1999). Interactive lecturing: Strategies for increasing participation in large group presentations. *Medical Teacher, 21*(1), 37–42.

Stuart, J., & Rutherford, R. J. D. (1978). Medical student concentration during lectures. *The Lancet, 2,* 514–516.

Stunkel, K. R. (1998). The lecture: A powerful tool for intellectual liberation. *The Chronicle of Higher Education, 44*(42), A52.

Tanenbaum, B. G., Tilson, E. R., Cross, D. S., & Rodgers, A. T. (1997). Interactive questioning: Why ask why? *Radiologic Technology, 68*(5), 435–438.

Thomas, E. J. (1972). The variation of memory with time for information appearing during a lecture. *Studies in Adult Education, 4,* 57–62.

Weaver, R. L., & Cotrell, H. W. (1985). Imaging can increase self concept and lecturing effectiveness. *Education, 105*(3), 264–270.

Wigle, S. E. (1999). Higher quality questioning. *Education Digest, 65*(4), 62–63.

Wink, D. M. (1993a). Effect of a program to increase the cognitive level of questions asked in clinical postconferences. *Journal of Nursing Education, 32*(8), 357–363.

Wink, D. M. (1993b). Using questioning as a teaching strategy. *Nurse Educator, 18*(5), 11–15.

Zachry, W. H. (1985). How I kicked the lecture habit: Inquiry teaching in psychology. *Teaching of Psychology, 12*(3), 129–131.

8

Activity-Based Teaching Strategies

Activity-based teaching implies active learning on the part of the learner. All of the strategies discussed in this chapter—cooperative learning, simulations and games, case studies, problem-based learning, and self-learning modules—require the learner to do more than listen and study. Learners engaged in these strategies are involved in creating and storing up knowledge for themselves. As you will see, there is a great deal of research pointing to greater knowledge retention and a high level of performance when these types of active learning strategies are used.

Cooperative Learning

Cooperative learning is not new. In fact, it has been around in some form for centuries. Its durability is probably based on the fact that, even before any research was conducted, people knew that they could learn successfully in groups. Cooperative learning is based on the premise that learners work together and are responsible for not only their own learning but also for the learning of other group members (Lindauer & Petrie, 1997). A working definition of cooperative learning is that it involves structuring small groups of learners who work together toward achieving shared learning goals. Group projects, a common feature of many nursing courses, do not necessarily constitute cooperative learning because they often consist of individuals working in tandem to meet their own goals. To meet the criteria for cooperative learning, the learners must be aware that they are responsible not only for their own learning but also for that of others in the group.

Types of Cooperative Learning Groups

Cooperative learning groups can be structured in various ways. The basic configurations are termed formal groups, informal groups, and base groups. Table 8–1 delineates the differ-

TABLE 8-1 Types of Cooperative Learning Groups

	Formal Groups	Informal Groups	Base Groups
Purpose	To complete a specific learning task consisting of concepts or skills	To enhance understanding of a specific unit of information; to make connections to prior learning	To provide encouragement and to monitor progress throughout the learning experience
Length of Existence	One class to many weeks	No more than one class and perhaps for only a few minutes during a class	The length of the learning experience; usually long term

ences among the three types of groups. The main differences are in the length of time they exist and the specific purposes they address (Johnson, Johnson, & Smith, 1998; Stein & Hurd, 2000).

You may set up a formal cooperative learning group in a nursing research course, for example, if you assign groups of students to develop a proposal for a clinical research study (Goodfellow, 1995). An assignment like this could be done in a traditional class or a distance learning class. Students will learn from each other as they brainstorm how to approach the study. Although the group may decide to divide up some of the tasks to be accomplished, they should be held accountable for group learning as well as individual learning. Group learning can be measured by evaluating the finished project and assigning a group grade. You may also want to ask questions of each group member during the development of the project so you have some assurance that all group members are engaged in the process. Individual accountability can be established by giving quizzes on the content to be learned or reinforced during the group project. "Positive goal interdependence" can be structured by providing group rewards such as "If all members of your group score above 90 percent on the test, each of you will receive five bonus points" (Johnson & Johnson, 1999, p. 29). Formal cooperative learning is probably most useful in academic settings rather than in-service or patient education situations.

Informal cooperative learning groups can be used in any setting. An application in patient education would be a situation where you are teaching about the childbirth experience to a group of parents-to-be. After teaching them about the stages of labor, you could have groups of four turn to each other and discuss what they have just learned about the events taking place in these stages. Discussion of the facts just presented helps the group members to understand and clarify misconceptions as well as to share concerns about the experience to come.

Base cooperative learning groups could be applied easily to new staff orientation or preceptorship programs. For example, if new registered nurses are being oriented to a health care facility, and the orientation or preceptorship experience lasts for six weeks, these new employees could be asked to form groups of four or five to meet for an hour a week to share experiences, encourage each other, and monitor each other's progress. The orientees could be encouraged to continue meeting as a base group after the official orientation is completed, to support each other during the transition to the professional role. Although base groups like this are not usually held accountable for learning, you can measure their effectiveness with surveys or focus groups.

Advantages of Cooperative Learning

There are several advantages gained by setting up cooperative groups. First, group members learn to function as part of a team. For nurses, this is an invaluable lesson, because they need to be able to work collaboratively in the workplace in order to effectively meet patient needs. Second, working in a group for any length of time can teach or enhance social skills. It may be necessary to teach people new to cooperative groups some theory about group process. Anyone who has been a member of a learning group or worked with these groups knows that there is always the potential for conflict. The very fact that the members are somewhat dependent on each other for their learning and possibly for a grade sets the stage for difficulties. If one member of the group is deemed not to be pulling his or her weight in the group, there may be disgruntled members. If one or more members are dominating the group, there may be resentment. So, while learning content, the group is also learning how to deal with other people, and that is always time well spent. A third advantage is that cooperative learning groups can help to address individual learning needs and learning styles (Huff, 1997). Adding cooperative learning to other teaching strategies increases the likelihood that a variety of learning styles are being attended to. A fourth advantage of cooperative learning is the fact that critical thinking is promoted (Zafuto, 1997). As group members discuss issues, explain their reasoning, and question each other, they begin to evaluate each other's positions and reasoning and to see discrepancies and flaws in hypotheses and so on. All of these activities are excellent practice in critical thinking.

There are really no disadvantages to cooperative learning, except the belief that if you use class time in cooperative learning, you won't be able to "cover all the content." The same charge is lodged against most active learning techniques. It is true that you will not be able to spend as much time lecturing on content. But that doesn't mean that students will not learn just as much or more, as we will see when examining the research that has been conducted on cooperative learning.

Research on Cooperative Learning

Research on the effectiveness of cooperative learning has been conducted since the early 1900s. Johnson and colleagues (1998) report that at least 168 studies were conducted between 1924 and 1997. Following is a summary of research findings over those years (Billings, 1994; Courtney, Courtney, & Nicholson, 1994; Huff, 1997; Johnson & Johnson, 1999; Johnson, Johnson, & Smith, 1998; Keeler & Anson, 1995; Nastasi & Clements, 1991; Zafuto, 1997).

1. Cooperative learning produces higher achievement levels than do individualistic or competitive learning approaches.
2. Outcome measures of achievement are knowledge gain, retention of knowledge, problem solving, reading, mathematics, and procedural tasks, all of which show increases with cooperative learning.
3. Other outcomes found are increased self-esteem, improved attitude toward learning, social competence, and decreased anxiety in learning.
4. Cooperative learning has been found to be a cost-effective strategy.

5. Effectiveness of cooperative learning has been found in all age groups and levels of education, both sexes, all nationalities studied, and all economic groups.

6. Effects have been equally good for learners at all ability levels.

An added bonus, according to Johnson and colleagues (1998), is that the research done on cooperative learning has a level of validity and generalizability beyond that seen in most educational research.

Exactly why is cooperative learning so effective? Nastasi and Clements (1991) propose that there are three reasons. First, we know that an effective way to learn something is to try to teach it to someone else. Second, as learners listen to each other, they work to make sense of what each is saying, and then they build on these ideas, thus adding to their cognitive schemata. Third, as learners within a group disagree with each other, they seek to reduce cognitive dissonance and, therefore, end up synthesizing divergent ideas.

With so much evidence supporting the effectiveness of cooperative learning, one wonders why this strategy is not used more often.

Simulations

Simulations are controlled representations of reality. They are exercises that learners engage in to learn about the real world without the risks of the real world. They also can be a lot of fun. Four types of simulations will be elaborated on in this chapter. They are simulation exercises, simulation games, role-playing, and case studies. For clarification, these simulation types can be defined as:

- *Simulation exercise:* A controlled representation of a piece of reality that learners can manipulate to better understand the corresponding real situation
- *Simulation game:* A game that represents real-life situations in which learners compete according to a set of rules in order to win or achieve an objective
- *Role-playing:* A form of drama in which learners spontaneously act out roles in an interaction involving problems or challenges in human relations
- *Case study:* An analysis of an incident or situation in which characters and relationships are described, factual or hypothetical events transpire, and problems need to be resolved or solved

Simulations have been a teaching strategy for centuries. War games were used in ancient China and India and more recently in eighteenth-century Germany. Chess, a simulation game, is thought to have been developed around 800 B.C. (Wildman & Reeves, 1997). The more recent use of simulations in education began in the 1960s, when business, law, educational administration, and medicine all began to use various simulation formats.

Purpose and Uses of Simulations

Simulations are intended to help learners practice decision-making and problem-solving skills, to develop human interaction abilities, and to learn psychomotor skills in a safe and controlled setting. Learners have a chance to apply principles and theories they have heard or read about and to see how and when these principles and theories work. For example, a person with a mental health problem may have been receiving counseling about how to handle interpersonal conflicts and may be making progress in understanding interpersonal theory. Role-playing an interpersonal situation can bring that understanding to life as situations are acted out. Or, in another venue, a nursing student may have learned about the nursing process from a series of lectures and audiovisuals, but the process makes a lot more sense after the student applies it in a simulation case study drawn from the real world. An added advantage of the simulation method is that simulations are usually worked out by groups of learners. Since teamwork is the essence of nursing practice, this correlation to the work world is valuable.

Simulation techniques can be used to achieve many learning objectives. In the acquisition of communication skills, simulation techniques are an almost unparalleled effective methodology. Learners can place themselves in the shoes of others (patients, nurses, physicians, families, co-workers, or supervisors) and learn something about these people's feelings and how to interact effectively with them. As they try out communication techniques, they can get immediate feedback on how they affect other people.

Simulation is also an avenue for attitude change. People who work through a simulation exercise or game or role-playing situation may discover factors about certain people and situations that they never before realized and that will change their attitudes in the future. Constructive attitudes can lead to more productive and acceptable behavior.

Decision-making skills can be fostered by simulation. Nurses or nursing students learn to make decisions by making decisions, not just by learning the theory of decision making. When they make decisions in a simulation of reality, they can see the immediate consequences. If the results are undesirable, they can backtrack and look at the factors that led to a poor decision. An educator can assist the learner in gaining insight into why a decision was effective or ineffective.

Simulation strategies can be applied to the teaching of psychomotor skills. When nursing students or refresher-course nurses practice skills in a nursing laboratory using mannequins and hospital-type equipment, for example, they are involved in a patient care simulation. They can safely practice repetitively without worrying about harming another person.

Finally, simulations can be used to evaluate learning and competence. Written examinations can be developed in a simulation format to test the application of knowledge. Such exams may be used instead of or in addition to clinical performance testing.

Role of the Educator

The educator's role in simulations has three facets: planning, facilitating, and debriefing. Planning begins with choosing or developing an appropriate simulation that will meet learning objectives. You may be able to purchase a simulation, but more likely you will have to develop one that meets your requirements. In either case, you should pilot the simulation before using it in a classroom. If you are using a simulation game, ask other educators to go through it with you. Case studies or other simulation exercises should be read carefully while you jot down notes about how you want to guide the learners at various points or questions you want to ask during the simulation. Without a trial run or preplanning, you may come up against some unanticipated snags in the classroom. Problems may be as basic as missing pieces from a game board or as complex as students having inadequate background knowledge to enable them to proceed through a simulation.

You may want to assign some reading for the learners to do before the simulation. If the theoretical background has not been covered previously in class, learners must be held responsible for coming to class prepared for the simulation. You may want to give written simulations to the learners a few days before class so that they can familiarize themselves with the scenario and see what preparation they need beforehand.

You should function as a facilitator during the actual progress of the simulation. After introducing the activity, you should take a backseat and talk relatively little. You may coach the learners who are trying to find their way through a sticky problem, encourage creative thinking, and act as an information resource, but you should not be too quick to give advice or suggest solutions. Neither should you criticize thinking that doesn't coincide with your own. It is often a good idea to take notes during the class so that in later discussion you can refer back to specific strengths and weaknesses of the process, to interesting interpersonal exchanges, or to inconsistencies that no one else may have picked up.

The most important part of your role is the final discussion or debriefing session. If at all possible, debriefing should occur immediately following the simulation when the information is fresh in everyone's mind. First, briefly summarize what has taken place. Next, it can be valuable to have the learners explain what they did and why. Self-analysis can help learners gain insight into why they made certain decisions or took a specific course of action. A game player can explain his strategy and a role player can analyze her enactment of a role. In simulations in which emotions have run high, ventilation of feelings should be part of the debriefing. Third, you should point out how principles and concepts have been applied and how the experience ties in to the learning objectives. For example, a class may engage in a simulation exercise about a patient who has cancer but who has not been told his diagnosis. His family knows but his friends do not. The situation unfolds with a series of interactions between patient and wife, patient and friends, physician and wife, and nurse and patient. An objective of the simulation is understanding the interpersonal dynamics that occur when diagnoses are withheld from patients. You could help the class see how communication principles have been used and abused in the situation and how people react in varied ways when diagnoses are concealed.

Simulation Exercises

Simulation exercises primarily focus on process learning. Participants learn how to make decisions or solve problems or apply theory. For instance, Babic and Crangle (1987) describe a simulation exercise in which undergraduate students simulated the aging process in themselves by choosing a decrement associated with aging and simulating the resulting lifestyle for 24 hours. A simulation of a "mock convention" was developed by Helmuth (1994) to help nursing students apply leadership skills. The simulation is a very involved and lengthy one in which students simulate a portion of a professional nursing organization convention. Lev (1998) conducted an exercise in which nursing students, acting as if they were from a variety of community agencies, competed for community grant monies designed to assist chronically ill people across the life span. Students learned about resource allocation in a competitive environment. Wildman and Reeves (1997) used a simulation exercise to teach nursing students how to apply management theory to organizing the work of a hospital clinical unit. These are just a few examples of simulation exercises that appear in recent nursing literature.

Simulation exercises designed to help learners apply and master psychomotor and clinical skills are also popular. Aronson and colleagues (1997) arranged a laboratory simulation in which senior nursing students visited mannequin patients who were outfitted with tubes, dressings, intravenous lines, and the like. The situations simulated emergencies, complications, and urgent scenarios that the students had to assess and to which they had to respond. Johnson and colleagues (1999) described the use of live simulated patients as an adjunct to clinical teaching. In most cases, live simulated patients are paid laypersons who are given a script to follow. Undergraduate and graduate students learn to perform physical assessments and history taking on these patients. The U.S. Air Force developed an entire simulated hospital unit in which new graduates spent four hours providing care to nine mannequins and two live actor patients (Eaves & Flagg, 2001). In the simulation, they learned about delegation, decision making, and 15 psychomotor skills. Many other variations of simulation exercises exist, and you can develop them yourself to achieve your own learning objectives.

Simulation Games

Simulation games focus on either content or process learning. Content games focus on teaching or reinforcing factual information. An example would be crossword puzzles that aim to teach terminology or bingo games that reinforce previously learned facts. Process games are those that emphasize problem solving or application of information. An example is a simulation game such as SimCity. Bareford (2001) describes the use of the computer program SimCity to help nursing students apply critical thinking skills to community assessment and planning. (See Chapter 9 for further information regarding computer simulations.) Games that follow the format of established board games, television games, and word games are sometimes called *frame games* (Bloom & Trice, 1994) because they provide a frame on which you can build new game applications. For example, if you develop a game using the television game show *Jeopardy!* as a format, you are using a frame game. Table 8–2 lists some of the games described in published articles with enough detail that they can be used with little additional work.

An advantage of using simulation games to teach facts and application of information is that gaming is, for most people, fun. You can use games to turn routine and repetitive information such as mandatory in-service topics into stimulating and enjoyable learning times (Henry, 1997). You can also use games to evaluate learning. One of the best advantages of the gaming approach is that it increases interaction among learners and allows even quiet and reserved class members to participate in a relatively low-risk situation. Although games are considered an integral part of childhood, they are also appropriate for adult learning. Because adults learn best when they see the relevance of information, when they are actively involved in the learning process, and when they can apply problem-solving methods, games—which meet all of these goals—are a natural fit for adult education (Ingram, Ray, Landeen, & Keane, 1998).

There are also disadvantages to gaming. While some educators consider all games to be simulations to some degree, some experts disagree (Berbiglia, Goddard, & Littlefield, 1997). Games considered by some not to be simulations are things like word games; therefore, some educators feel those games may be a waste of time. Some people may also believe that games are unprofessional, and they dislike the competition that games promote. There is no doubt that when people play games, even educational games, winning is uppermost in

TABLE 8-2 Games Described in the Nursing and Health Literature

Game	Author/Date	Description
"Health Planning Game"	Clark (1986)	Simulated community planning to address health care problems
"Emergency Pursuit Game"	Schmitz, MacLean, & Shidler (1991)	Teaches emergency decision-making skills
"Basic Nutrition"	Olbrich (1997)	Crossword for nurse aides
"Bug Bingo" and "Safety Bingo"	Harris & Yuan (1997)	Bingo games for mandatory in-services on infection control and safety
"Chemotherapy Word Search"	Dick (1997)	Word search puzzle to review chemotherapy terms
"Reproductive Jeopardy"	Wirth & Breiner (1997)	Review of reproductive anatomy and physiology for grades 8–12 health education
"What If? What Else? What Then?"	Free (1997)	Critical thinking game based on clinical case situations
"Anabolic Steroid Word Search"	Nutter (1998)	Word search puzzle to review terminology related to anabolic steroid use
"Mind Your Meds"	Saethang & Kee (1998)	Board game to teach noncritical care nurses to use critical cardiovascular drugs
"Bloodborne Pathogens"	Wendt (1998)	Crossword puzzle to review bloodborne pathogen standards
"Eye Q"	Marbeiter (1998)	Crossword puzzle on anatomy and physiology of the eye
"Growth and Development"	Poston (1998)	Crossword puzzle to review growth and development
"Nutrition Pursuit"	Burns (1999)	Board game to review basic nutrition
"Cranial Nerve Wheel of Competencies"	Jones, Jasperson, & Gusa (2000)	Format is combination of several frame games to test knowledge of cranial nerve function and assessment
"Blood Clot"	Wargo (2000)	Board game to reinforce knowledge of disseminated intravascular coagulation

their minds, with learning a secondary consideration. You should also consider the fact that some people do not enjoy playing educational games, as reported by Orbach (1979) in his much-quoted work on games and motivation for learning. Finally, simulation games are usually time consuming to play and very labor intensive to develop (Bloom & Trice, 1994).

There are several factors you should consider before developing or using a game for educational purposes. Peters and colleagues (1998) raise the issue of the validity of games. People who wish to develop simulation games must be aware of the fact that if you want learners to transfer knowledge from the game to the real world, the games must be a realistic representation of that world, or you may be missing the point. There are also more mundane considerations. For example, constructing a really fun and attractive game takes time and effort. Do you have the resources to construct or buy a game board or a spinner or a timer? Can you construct the physical components of the game so that they will last over many uses? Do you have the space to play the game and to store it? Careful planning will help you to minimize the time it will take to develop the game and maximize its effectiveness (Gruending, Fenty, & Hogan, 1991).

Role-Playing

Recall from the beginning of the chapter that role-playing is a form of drama in which learners spontaneously act out roles in an interaction involving problems or challenges in human relations. The word *spontaneously* is important to understand in this activity. The participants do not have scripts to follow, nor do they rehearse. They are given a written or verbal explanation of the simulated situation and are expected to have enough general knowledge about the situation to understand the roles to which they have been assigned.

This teaching method is effective in helping people gain skill in interpersonal and therapeutic relationships and in teaching them how to handle interpersonal conflicts. It enables them to step into the shoes of others and gain some insight into the perspectives of other people. Role-playing may be a means of helping people develop the quality of empathy. It can assist them in understanding social problems of groups of people who are different from them.

Many role-playing scenarios last only about three to five minutes; it doesn't take long to illustrate one particular aspect of human interaction. The educator may take more time, though, and have several sets of participants act out the same roles or have them switch roles after a few minutes. Those who are in the audience should be observing for nonverbal behavior, response patterns, examples of implementation of principles, and so on. When the time for discussion arrives, talk should be steered away from self-criticism or peer criticism of the acting and instead focused on the enactment of the roles. The audience should be critiquing the characters that are dramatized, not the people who are doing the acting.

Role-playing has long been used to teach therapeutic communication skills. An introduction to such a simulation usually begins something like this:

> **Background Information**
> Ms. Holden is a 62-year-old woman who has been hospitalized for a week with gastrointestinal bleeding. Surgery is being considered, but Ms. Holden is reluctant to have surgery because she is concerned about who will care for her 87-year-old mother, who is at home. Ms. Holden says to you, her nurse, "I just can't seem to make a decision about this operation."

One learner would enact the role of Ms. Holden, another would take the part of the nurse, and the interaction would proceed. Videotaping the session could be helpful for reference during the discussion period.

"Land of Suria," a role-playing simulation by Dahl (1984), is a fairly well-structured simulation designed to give learners experience in communicating with people from a culture previously unknown to them. Two groups of participants take part: one group play the Surians, who are concerned about a health problem resulting from urban renewal; the other group are health care workers who have never before met the Surians but who will try to discover what their problems are. This is a good example of role-playing for the purpose of learning appreciation of transcultural interaction.

Halloran and Dean (1994) developed a role-playing simulation combined with a game format. It involves people playing the roles of the elderly with physical limitations or financial or social problems. The simulation is designed to help participants assess their awareness of and sensitivity to the problems and issues of aging.

In a staff development setting, Johnson (1997) used role-playing to teach home care nurses to assess patients, communicate with families and professionals, and to fill out paperwork accurately. The role-playing approach turned a dry subject into a fun experience.

It is relatively easy for an educator to devise role-playing simulations that will help to meet many learning objectives. Keep in mind, however, that some learners are paralyzed when they have to act in front of a group and, if forced to do so, will learn little from the experience.

Case Studies

Remember the definition with which we are working: a case study is an analysis of an incident or situation in which characters and relationships are described, factual or hypothetical events transpire, and problems need to be resolved or solved.

The case method originated at Harvard Law School in the 1870s (Wade, 1999). It took almost 100 years before case studies enjoyed much use in nursing. We now know that case studies can be used successfully to apply principles discussed in class, to encourage independent study and critical thinking, and to safely expose learners to real-world situations they will encounter in the future. When you would like to provide learners with certain decision-making clinical experiences but cannot do so for various practical reasons, a case study can be used to provide at least part of that experience vicariously.

Case studies can range from the simple and short to the complex and lengthy. I devised a series of simple case studies for a course I taught to beginning nursing students that covered basic human needs, common health problems, and related nursing care. To teach students about the concepts of urinary control, urinary retention and incontinence, prevention of urinary infection, and urinary catheter care, I used the following case study. The students were required to read a relevant chapter in their textbook before coming to class and were told we would apply the information to this case study:

Common Urinary Problems – Case Study

Mr. Johnson, 65 years old, is admitted to your unit from the emergency department with a medical diagnosis of urinary retention due to BPH (enlarged prostate gland). In the ED, a Foley catheter was inserted to empty his bladder.

1. What would you assess on Mr. Johnson?
2. What nursing care does he require?

Two days later, Mr. Johnson's Foley catheter is removed to see whether he can void, but after six hours he still has not voided.

1. What assessments should you make now?
2. What nursing action could you take at this time?
3. What will determine how long you should wait before reinserting the catheter?
4. What nursing diagnoses would best describe Mr. Johnson's problems at this time?

The following week, Mr. Johnson has surgery (prostatectomy), and after two days his Foley catheter is again removed. This time he keeps dribbling urine (lack of urinary control).

1. What assessments should you make at this time?
2. What nursing care is now required?

Placing this content about basic problems into real-life simulations helped the students see how such problems evolve and are handled from a nursing perspective. It was the beginning of their use of the nursing process.

When teaching management theory to senior nursing students and to staff nurses, I have used some published vignettes of problems and conflicts experienced by nurse managers. They involved management theory, communication principles, and change and conflict theories. These were simple cases that took about 20 minutes to complete, but they were very effective in helping students apply the conceptual theory they had studied.

Case studies often are much more complex than the above. A written case may be a page or two in length and cover quite a bit of detail. If you are going to work through a complex or lengthy case with a group of learners, they should be provided with the case ahead of time so they can do the research and analysis necessary to prepare for the in-class discussion. Some examples of published cases can be seen in Table 8–3, and an example of a fully developed case can be seen in Figure 8–1.

If you want to construct a case study for a group of learners, you should follow these steps:

1. *Develop objectives.* What do you want the participants to learn when they work through the case study?

TABLE 8-3 Published Nursing Case Studies

Topic	Author/Date	Description
Barium enema	Dowd & Davidhizar (1999)	A biology professor having a barium enema is concerned about risks of the procedure.
Childhood asthma	Jones & Sheridan (1999)	A 4-year-old is admitted to the hospital. Family has no insurance. Need for discharge teaching.
Childhood diabetes	Dailey (1992)	Newly diagnosed 10-year-old, hospitalized and returned to home and school. Need for intervention in emotional and social problems.
Childhood diarrhea	Johnson & Purvis (1987)	A 16-month-old is admitted to the hospital with diarrhea and listlessness. Need to plan nursing care and consider developmental needs.
Gastrointestinal bleeding	Conyers & Ritchie (2001)	A 48-year-old is admitted to the hospital with melena and hematemesis.
Hip fracture	Goodman (1997)	A 72-year-old female smoker who lives alone with no family in the area needs a plan of care in hospital and rehabilitation.

Mrs. X is a slim 86-year-old widow with a history of coronary artery stenosis treated with angioplasty four years ago. She has been maintained on one aspirin per day, Cardizem (diltiazem hydrochloride) 60 mg TID, and Zocor (Simvastatin) 10 mg OD. She is on a low-fat diet. She is estranged from her only brother and has no contact with any of her extended family. She lives alone in her own home in a retirement village. She says that her neighbors are unfriendly, so she doesn't "bother with them." Mrs. X comes by taxi to the office of her family physician practice with a chief complaint of severe back pain radiating to her sacral area. The pain prevents her from taking care of her house, driving, and doing much lifting. She says it also keeps her awake at night. While being examined by the nurse practitioner, she also reveals that she is always fatigued, sleeps a lot during the day, and she gets short of breath with minimal exertion.

1. What additional information do you need about Mrs. X?

2. What are the central problems that may be identified in this case?

3. What future problems could develop?

4. Would Mrs. X's problems intersect, and could her treatments possibly conflict?

5. What factors will have to be considered in developing a plan of care?

6. How might Mrs. X's social interactions (or lack of them) affect her care?

7. What health care referrals might be made for Mrs. X?

FIGURE 8-1 Case Study Example

(*Note:* The focus of this case is on the multiple health and social problems confronted by many elderly people and how those problems complicate their plan of care.)

2. *Select a situation.* Choose a topic and a scenario that fits the objectives and content you want to apply. Cases should be drawn from real-life situations. You may choose a case you actually have been involved in or consult with clinicians who can give you ideas for cases. Real cases are better than fictitious ones because of the wealth of information from which to draw; fabricated cases are sometimes too simplistic or unrealistic. If you choose a case in which you have been personally involved, you can tell the learners at the end how the actual situation was resolved. Imagine how intrigued the learners are when they hear the actual outcome compared to how they thought it would be resolved. The cases you choose should not be esoteric or unique. Unique cases are tempting because they stick in your memory, but the purpose of simulations is not to teach about uncommon happenings. Rather, it is to help learners solve typical problems that they can transfer to their world.

3. *Develop the characters.* The human factor of a case is very important in a practice profession. Give enough detail about the patient, family, or health care providers so that the interpersonal aspects of the case will be an integral part of it.

4. *Develop the discussion questions.* It is all right to ask questions with factual answers, but most of the questions should require the learner to apply principles and generate a variety of possible interventions and outcomes. Questions should be designed to promote discussion (Dailey, 1992).

5. *Lead the group discussion.* After the learners have prepared their case (either working individually or in small collaborative groups) by researching background information and thinking about answers to the discussion questions, your role is to lead the discussion of the case. Explain to the class that except for the factual questions, there is no one right answer to a case. Many problems are so complex that they have a variety of resolutions rather than a solution (Tillman, 1995). Keep the atmosphere of the class relaxed so participants will feel free to discuss their hypotheses and not feel ashamed if they are on the wrong track.

Case studies and all types of simulations can be used in academic settings and staff development settings. They are appropriate for distance learning because cases can be discussed online in threaded discussion groups or chat rooms. They may even be of use in patient or community education. For example, if you are teaching a course on diabetes or child development or teaching about a public health problem, you could use a simulation exercise, game, or case study. Simulations are a very versatile teaching strategy. Not much research has been conducted on simulation learning in recent years. However, a meta-analysis was performed on 93 studies conducted between 1969 and 1980. The researchers found no significant differences between cognitive gains from simulations compared to other teaching methods but did find significant gains in desired attitudes, thus supporting simulation as being an effective means of molding professional attitudes (Dekkers & Donatti, 1981).

Problem-Based Learning

Problem-based learning (PBL) is an approach to learning that involves confronting students with real-life problems that provide a stimulus for critical thinking and self-taught content. PBL is based on the premise that students, working together in small groups, will analyze a case, identify their own needs for information, and then solve problems like those that occur in everyday life. This type of exercise will prepare them to be good problem solvers in their future work and will condition them to be lifelong learners (Boud & Feletti, 1997). It is a teaching/learning strategy that is probably most applicable to academic settings, although it can be used in staff development courses.

Problem-based learning is thought by some people to be synonymous with the simulation case method of teaching and learning. In fact, it is not the same but a significant variation from the case method. The chief differences between PBL and the case method are:

1. PBL is conducted with small groups while case studies may be used by individuals or groups.

2. Students using PBL have little background knowledge of the subject matter in the case, whereas in the case method, students already have most of the background knowledge they need to apply to the case.

3. In PBL, the cases are usually brief and the presenting problems are ill structured, while in the case method, cases are often long and detailed, and their problems are fairly well defined.

So, yes, PBL is based on the simulation approach and does involve case studies. Much of what has been said about simulations applies to PBL. But there are also some important differences that will be addressed here.

Problem-based learning began over 30 years ago at McMaster University School of Medicine in Canada and has spread to medical schools in the United States and all over the world. It has moved from medical education to many other disciplines. The first nursing applications of PBL began in Australia, where many nursing programs are built on a PBL approach to learning (Heliker, 1994). PBL grew out of a sense of frustration with traditional medical school curricula. The emphasis on memorization of more and more content and the lack of correlation between the basic sciences and clinical content were two of the stimuli for a new approach to medical education. The identification of the need to prepare professionals with skills for lifelong learning was a third (Boud & Feletti, 1997). Nursing professionals have become interested in PBL because it helps students to see the relevance of subjects they learn and because it "sets the learning in a context in which it will be used" (Glen & Wilkie, 2000, p. 13). Heliker (1994) claims that learning in context enables learners to structure their long-term memory for easy retrieval of the information.

A typical approach to a problem-based learning unit would go something like this: A class of 20 undergraduate senior nursing students is going to use PBL for several learning units in a leadership course. After a few weeks of some lecture/discussion classes on general leadership theory, the first problem is given to them. The teacher has identified learning objectives for the exercise but does not share them with the students until the end of the process (Rendas, Pinto, & Gamboa, 1998). The problem statement is:

> A small community hospital is confronted with a severe nursing shortage. They are considering a change in the nursing care delivery system to a model that involves cross-training of personnel and increased use of assistive personnel. Rumors about a change begin to circulate around the hospital and many staff seem unhappy.

Note that the problem is ill structured. That means that more information is needed to fully understand the situation, and there is no single way to proceed (Gallagher, 1997). As Gallagher explains, on the surface a PBL problem looks simple, but looks are deceptive. The problem is well designed to achieve the learning goals.

The class is divided into four groups, with five students assigned to each. The groups begin to discuss the scenario, organizing their thoughts as to what the cause, nature, and extent of the problem is. They brainstorm as to what the key concepts are in the problem description and may develop a list of "what we know" and "what we don't know." By the end of the first class, each group should have developed a list of *learning issues* and divided up issues that various students will begin to research for the next class. For example, the following learning issues may have been identified by one of the groups:

1. Nursing shortages
   a. How often do they occur?
   b. How severe do they get?

     c. What causes them?

     d. What past solutions have been tried and do they work?

2. Nursing care delivery systems

     a. What is this one called?

     b. Is it being used anywhere?

     c. How would it work?

     d. What might cross-training involve?

     e. Are there published job descriptions for assistive personnel?

3. Can we predict how people will respond to change?

     a. How can change be handled?

     b. How should a leader deal with rumors?

     c. Is there any way to predict whether this would be a good change?

If the groups do not identify the key learning issues, the teacher guides them to these issues by means of skillful questioning.

At the next class meeting(s), the groups would fill each other in on what they have discovered about their assigned topics. The groups will begin to identify how the information that they have collected will help shed light on the problem. The list of "what we know" is updated. The learners will brainstorm about the problem, and if they feel ready, they will write a problem definition and begin to develop hypotheses as to causes of the problem. They will identify continuing learning issues (perhaps some legal issues in this case). They will consult with the teacher to toss around some ideas and make sure they are on the right track. If the group is floundering or seems to be bringing the problem to a premature close, the teacher will intervene and either provide guidance or raise questions that the group has not thought about. The teacher can role-model reasoning skills for the groups and can encourage active participation by all students (VanLeit, 1995). Some educators like to introduce new facts about the case at this point, to demonstrate how real-life problems unfold in stages (Magnussen, 2001).

During the following class meeting(s), new information that was researched is shared. The groups may be ready to generate possible solutions to the problem(s). They discuss them and look at possible outcomes. They finally reach consensus about what approach to take first (Edens, 2000). When the solutions have been proposed, the teacher leads a discussion about the processes that have been used, the conclusions reached at each stage of the process, and the variety of solutions proposed. The learning objectives are then given to the students and a discussion of how well the objectives have been met ensues. Sometimes the teacher may want to follow up with some lecturing or further independent study on the part of the students to reinforce some objectives that may need strengthening. If the problem was drawn from real life, the actual outcome of the problem can be shared with the students at this point.

Many of the advantages of PBL have been mentioned above. But there are also disadvantages. Learning how to teach by PBL and the preparation of learning materials and educational resources takes a lot of time (Matthews-Smith, Oberski, Gray, Carter, & Smith, 2001). In some cases, when students are first introduced to PBL, they may be unhappy with their role and that of the teacher. Some students feel that they are doing all the work, and they experience frustration as they learn to direct their own learning (Lunyk-Child et al., 2001). Teachers, too, may have difficulty adjusting to their role in this nontraditional format.

The research that has been conducted on PBL confirms that it is probably worthwhile going through the adjustment to PBL because it does have benefits. Most of the research has been conducted in medical schools with groups of students who have used PBL as an exclusive pedagogy in one or more courses. There are several reports that found PBL to be at least as effective or more effective than traditional methods when measured by student performance on standardized medical licensure tests and clinical performance (Colliver, 2000; Edens, 2000). However, Colliver subjected the findings of three studies to a determination of effect size and found very small effect sizes. He raised the issue of whether PBL is worth the amount of resources invested in it considering the small effect sizes. However, the medical school studies were conducted in settings where PBL was being used exclusively, and it was believed to be necessary to limit the class size to smaller numbers than usual, making it a more expensive teaching strategy. When PBL is used as one among other teaching strategies within a course, and when class size is not reduced, there are no significant costs associated with it.

In addition to the small gains in theoretical and clinical knowledge, researchers are even more confident that PBL is motivational and enjoyable for students, and that they are more satisfied with their educational experience than students in traditional classrooms (Colliver, 2000; Patel & Kaufman, 2001). White and colleagues (1999) used PBL in the bridge courses into their RN to BSN completion program. Their research indicated that the students thought the teamwork was helpful and that they liked having the responsibility for their own learning.

The applications of problem-based learning in nursing are just beginning. Celia and Gordon (2001) have reported one of the first applications of PBL to staff development in their use of problems to enhance novice nurses' ability to think critically and to prioritize patient care. Its use in staff development and graduate nursing education will grow. Problem-based learning is already being adapted to online course use (Glen & Wilkie, 2000; Price, 2000).

Self-Learning Modules

Self-learning modules are also called self-directed learning modules, self-paced learning modules, self-learning packets, and individualized learning activity packages. They began their history in the 1960s in academic settings but quickly moved to staff development, where their use has far surpassed use in schools of nursing. A self-learning module can be defined as a self-contained unit or package of study materials for use by an individual. Adult learners who are motivated to learn on their own are, perhaps, the best audience for the use of modules. Self-directed learning is based on some of the principles of adult learning such as:

1. Adults are self-motivated to learn material for which they see relevance.
2. Adults' prior experience is a resource for further learning.
3. Adults are problem focused and readily learn material they can use to solve problems (Herrick, Jenkins, & Carlson, 1998; Mast & VanAtta, 1986).

These principles are intrinsic to the development and use of self-learning modules.

There are few topics or settings in which self-learning modules would not be appropriate. They can be used to teach entire courses or sections of courses in academic settings at both undergraduate and graduate levels (Fullerton & Graveley, 1998; Holtzman, 1999; Spickerman, Lee, & Eason, 1988) and have frequently been used for bridge courses for LPNs or RNs returning to school for a higher degree. They are applied to staff development for purposes of orientation, mandatory in-service topics, and just about every specialty area imaginable and for every level of nursing staff. To get some ideas of topics that have been taught by self-learning modules, see articles by Coleman, Dracup, and Moser (1991); D'Apolito and Givens (1988); Donovan, Braddock, and Hayward (1995); Flurer and Moore (2000); Lamb and Henderson (1993); and Schmidt and Fisher (1992). Finally, nurse educators are developing modules, with some modifications, for patient education (Wong & Wong, 1985).

Components of Self-Learning Modules

What does a self-learning module consist of? The components are fairly standard:

- Introduction and instructions
- Behavioral objectives
- Pretest
- Learning activities
- Self-evaluations
- Posttest

The topic for a module is a single concept. If you were teaching a medical–surgical nursing course that incorporated problems of digestion, endocrine function, and elimination, you would have at least three modules and very likely more. For instance, the concept of elimination could be taught in one module, but it might be more effective to develop two modules—one for intestinal elimination and one for urinary elimination. Likewise, you would not develop one module for a critical care course but would have several on topics like airway maintenance, hemodynamic monitoring, fluid balance, and so on.

Behavioral objectives in a self-learning module are no different from those you have already learned about and written. They express, in clear language, what the learner will be able to do on completion of the module. These objectives need to be quite specific so that both learner and teacher know what is expected and whether it has been achieved at the end of the module. You might include overall objectives for the module at the beginning, and then repeat those objectives that are pertinent to each unit of the module at the beginning of the unit. The repetition of objectives helps learners to focus on what they are to achieve (Piskurich, 1994).

A pretest is usually but not always included in a module. If the educator is sure that none of the people using the module would be familiar with any of the information in it, a pretest is not needed. If, for example, the concept of the module is self-care information for new diabetics, it would be reasonable to assume that the new diabetic has little knowledge on this topic. Most modules written for staff development and academic settings do include a pretest because nursing students and nurses come from varied health care backgrounds and may bring prior knowledge of the topic with them.

The educator may look at the pretest results, but usually they are for learner use only. The pretest helps learners evaluate which sections of the module they might skip over and which ones they need to study in depth. One other feature sometimes seen in pretests is a section that assesses prerequisite knowledge. So, if a module has been constructed with the idea that a nurse would come to the module with knowledge of the anatomy of the respiratory system, some questions on anatomy might be placed in the pretest. If the nurse were not able to answer those questions, he or she would be directed to review the anatomy before proceeding with the module.

Learning activities make up the most creative portion of the self-learning module. Activities are designed that will help the learner achieve the objectives. The activities should also appeal to people with differing learning styles. Activities might include:

- Reading textbook chapters, articles, or pamphlets
- Reviewing handouts, charts, pictures, or diagrams
- Attending short lectures, speeches, or demonstrations
- Answering study questions and getting feedback
- Watching a video or slide presentation
- Using a computer program
- Practicing a psychomotor skill in a laboratory
- Participating in a discussion group

If possible, learners should be given a choice of activities that fit best with their learning style. For example, if the same information is available in a textbook and on videotape, learners may be told to use one or the other, depending on their preferences.

Learners should have access to an instructor during the time they are involved in learning activities. There may be logistical questions to be answered, such as where to locate some learning resources, or there may be content issues that need to be clarified. In an academic setting, it is useful to schedule group discussions as one of the learning activities, and questions can then be posed during the discussion time.

While the participants are working through the learning activities, they should be checking occasionally to see whether they are achieving the objectives that were listed at the beginning of the unit. One way for them to assess how well they are achieving the objectives is for them to use self-evaluation tools. A self-test is usually included at the end of every lesson or subconcept. It is generally some form of quiz, either multiple-choice questions or short-answer questions. If the learner does not achieve a perfect score on the self-test, he or she should reenter the module for the appropriate lesson.

Posttests are used to determine whether learners have mastered module objectives. The posttest may be an objective-item test, a case study, a written assignment such as a care plan, or a demonstration of a psychomotor skill. Failure to demonstrate mastery will result in the learner's having to repeat appropriate learning activities or being given alternative activities to meet his or her individual needs.

Developing a Module

Plans for developing a model should be undertaken weeks or months before it will be needed, because module development is a time-consuming process. One author has estimated that it takes as many as 10 to 15 hours of development for every hour spent by learn-ers in completing the self-learning module (O'Very, 1999). Less time might be spent if the module is a short and simple one.

Let's say you want to develop a self-learning module on intestinal elimination. You decide that the important content will revolve around assessment of intestinal elimination, infectious and inflammatory disorders, and obstructive disorders, with accompanying nurs-ing care.

BEHAVIORAL OBJECTIVES

The first step in the development process is writing the objectives for the module. With due deliberation, you arrive at the following objectives:

1. Perform an assessment of intestinal elimination on a live simulated patient (video-taped or performed during a scheduled appointment with the instructor) correctly, including all critical elements.
2. Explain the effects of infection and inflammation on the gastrointestinal tract.
3. Differentiate between any three infectious or inflammatory gastrointestinal disor-ders in terms of pathology, patient problems, and nursing interventions.
4. View a computer simulation of a patient with inflammatory bowel disease and list the patient's problems, your proposed interventions, and the rationale for those interventions.
5. Analyze why a given list of nursing interventions would be used for a patient with an obstructed small bowel.
6. Write and implement (on videotape or during a scheduled appointment with the instructor) a teaching plan for a patient (a friend or colleague) with a selected inflammatory disorder.

PRETEST

You have identified the basic content you want to include. Now you should decide what knowledge the learner would have to bring to the learning experience in order to progress through the module. Because this module is designed for nursing students or new graduates, you realize they may come to this situation with a variety of backgrounds, so a pretest is in order.

Part of the pretest should include questions about normal anatomy and physiology of intestinal elimination. Directions that accompany the pretest would specify that if the anatomy and physiology questions are answered incorrectly, the learner should review that information in an appropriate textbook. The pretest would also include some questions that assess knowledge of the content of the module itself. If the pretest reveals mastery of certain units of content, the learner should be informed that he or she might skip that part of the module. If you want the learner to do self-evaluation and receive instant feedback, place the answers to the pretest at the end of the module. Learners need to know what level of perfor-mance constitutes mastery of the content (usually 80 to 100 percent).

LEARNING ACTIVITIES

You now have a pretty good idea of where you want the learner to go, but you still have to decide how you are going to help the learner get there. So, you plan the content and learning activities. To address various learning styles, you may choose some learning activities that are visual, some auditory, and some tactile. Choose some activities that stress abstractions and some that focus on concrete information. Always keep in mind the amount of time the learner will have to complete the module and the learning resources that are available.

The first unit in our sample module deals with assessment of intestinal elimination, and the first objective explains the outcome behavior. You arrive at the following learning activities that will help achieve the outcome:

Unit I
1. Read pages 216 to 222 in the accompanying textbook in light of the study questions on Handout 1.
2. Select one of the following activities:
   a. View the videotape, *Assessment of Intestinal Function*.
   b. Listen to the audiotape, *Step-by-Step History Taking and Physical Assessment, Part 5*.
3. Practice doing an assessment of intestinal elimination.

All of the materials needed to complete these activities should be readily available to the learner. Written materials can be placed in a three-ring binder, with papers encased in plastic page protectors. Audiovisuals and textbooks should be accessible in a secure location.

SELF-EVALUATION

Self-evaluation guides should be developed to accompany each unit. These guides are short quizzes, based on the objectives, that enable learners to check their progress. The answers to the self-evaluation guides should be placed at the end of the module for quick feedback. Performance of less-than-mastery level means that the learner must go back into the unit and repeat the appropriate learning activities. You can also design the process so that, at the end of the page with self-evaluation answers, there are additional activities to be engaged in if mastery has not been reached.

POSTTEST

While you are writing self-evaluation test questions, take time to develop the posttest. The posttest is usually, at least in part, a written examination. It may consist of multiple-choice and matching items, essay questions, or case studies with questions. In an academic setting where the student will receive a grade for the module, it may be necessary to develop alternative forms of the posttest. If a student does not achieve mastery on the first posttest, he or she is directed to repeat portions of the module and then must repeat the posttest. Obviously, it would not be a good idea to take the same posttest again in a short period of time, so a second form of the exam should be ready. In an in-service setting, the nurse usually takes the same posttest a second time.

If you look back to the objectives for the module on intestinal elimination, you will see that more than just a written posttest is indicated in order to measure achievement of the objectives. Learners also have to perform a skill demonstration in person or on videotape and write a teaching plan and implement it in person or on videotape.

INTRODUCTION AND INSTRUCTIONS

I have left the first until last. The introduction and instructions would, of course, come first in the module. But I have found it helpful to write this section after all the material for the module has been designed. This portion of the self-learning module tells the learner how to work through the module, how to use the pretest and self-evaluation guides, where to locate resources, what procedures to use for handing in assignments or scheduling skill tests, and what the roles of the educator and learner are. O'Very (1999) stresses the importance of "selling" the module in the introduction. You must capture the interest of the learner at this point, or the person may never complete the module. The use of humor and a lively conversational tone is advised. Here is a prototype for such an introduction:

> This module is designed to teach and review information on intestinal elimination. Read the objectives of the module carefully before beginning any activities and refer back to them frequently. All learning experiences and evaluations will be based on the objectives. There will be no surprises or trick questions! After reading the objectives, take the pretest. The answers to the pretest are found at the back of the module (but no peeking ahead of time allowed!). You can find out immediately how much (or how little) you know about the contents of the module. The pretest is divided into units that correspond to the units of the module. If you get all the answers to any of the units correct, it is your option to skip the learning activities of that unit and just take the posttest (and use the rest of the time to go shopping or sailing?).
>
> All of the learning activity materials are either in this packet or in the Nursing Laboratory; each learning activity will indicate where to find materials. If you sign out a videotape or computer disk from the Lab, it must be returned within 72 hours.
>
> In each unit, there are self-evaluation guides. These guides are designed to give you feedback on how well you have learned the information in one unit before you progress to the next. The answers to the guides are also in the back of the module. If you get more than two questions wrong on any guide, go back into the module and repeat that portion where you "messed up." You'll do better the second time.
>
> The skill portions of the module require you to demonstrate the skill either in person or on videotape. See the Nursing Laboratory secretary about scheduling a videotaping session or a live demonstration with an instructor.
>
> After completing all units, you will be ready for the posttest. You must schedule the posttest with the secretary in the Nursing Laboratory. This is a 20-item test with three case studies and multiple-choice questions based on the cases. It should take you no more than 20 minutes. Good luck with the module and enjoy the learning!

PILOT TESTING

When you have completed your initial work on the module, you should pilot test it. Have one or two people work through the module. Their experience will tell you if there are unforeseen snags or flaws in the module and will give you an idea of the amount of time it will take for the learner to complete all activities. You might, for example, find that some of your directions are unclear, or that some activities are too time consuming, too difficult, or too simplistic.

Advantages and Disadvantages of Self-Learning Modules

Advantages of using modules include the ability to learn independently and at one's own pace and in one's own time. This kind of flexibility is an advantage for many learners, especially nontraditional students, practicing nurses, and patients. The fact that modules can address a variety of learning styles adds to their usefulness. In addition, modules promote active learning and provide immediate feedback on performance (Tuazon, 1992).

For educators, there are several advantages. First, in academic settings, faculty who are frustrated by not having the time to help students who are struggling with course material in a traditional learning system have that opportunity in the individualized approach. Educators in all settings are freed from having to repeat the same material year after year, which can become monotonous. The opportunities for creativity in designing modules and conducting small discussion groups can lend new interest to teaching. Also, modules make it possible for a curriculum to be standardized, if that is desired. All learners using the same module will reach the same learning outcomes. Modules can hold the curriculum constant in spite of changes in staffing and resources.

There are special advantages that apply to staff development settings. Self-learning modules can reduce travel time for conferences and reduce the amount of time that staff nurses have to be away from their units. They can also reduce the cost of in-service education. Several studies have documented considerable cost savings of modules compared to traditional in-service programs (Herrick et al., 1998; Lipe et al., 1994; Nikolajski, 1992).

Disadvantages of self-learning modules are few but include the fact that some learners may miss learning with other people and miss the interactions that take place in a classroom. For learners who tend to procrastinate, individualized learning may lead to further procrastination because of lack of structure and deadlines. In settings where the module posttest is taken without supervision, learners may be less than honest about their results and thus forgo needed learning (Suggs et al., 1998). Finally, modules take many hours to design and test.

Research on Effectiveness

A considerable amount of research has been conducted on the effectiveness of self-learning modules. Several researchers compared the amount of knowledge gained by nurses using self-learning modules to those taught by lecture and found no significant differences (Coleman et al., 1991; Schlomer, Anderson, & Shaw, 1997; Suggs et al., 1998). The fact that the knowledge gain was equal was deemed satisfactory, especially in light of the additional advantages of modules already discussed. Nikolajski (1992) compared module use to classes with lecture/slide presentations and found that both groups had significant learning gains, but the gains were greater for the lecture group. Lamb and Henderson (1993) found that in comparing groups given lectures versus those using modules, the module group had significantly higher posttest scores. Grant (1993) found that nurses preferred to use modules rather than attend lecture classes, and Lipe and colleagues (1994) reported 95 to 100 percent favorable evaluations among nurses who learned from modules. Finally, Wong and Wong (1985) measured patient satisfaction, compliance behavior, and postoperative complications in two groups of patients undergoing hip surgery. The control group was taught by traditional preoperative instruction and the experimental group by means of learning modules. The experimental group was more compliant with postoperative behaviors and was more satisfied with the instruction. There was no difference in number of complications between the groups. Research findings to date, therefore, support the continuance of self-learning modules as a teaching strategy.

All of the strategies discussed in this chapter involve active learning on the part of the learner. All have found their place in the teacher's portfolio of methods, and all have received some research support. These are powerful tools to help motivate learners, to teach critical thinking, and to help learners construct their own knowledge.

CASE STUDY

You are asked to evaluate a colleague's class. The topic of the class is care of the patient with inflammatory joint disease. Your colleague has told you he plans to use a *Jeopardy!*-type game as part of the class.

1. What questions should you have in mind even before you attend the class?
2. As you observe the conduct of the game, how will you evaluate whether the game is achieving the learning objectives?
3. What observations might give you concern about whether the game is really appropriate for this class?
4. What should you be looking for in the debriefing session?

CRITICAL THINKING EXERCISES

You are an advanced practice nurse teaching a primary care course to graduate students. The problem-based learning strategy intrigues you, and you would like to apply this strategy to your course. Starting with a unit on childhood immunizations and management of childhood illnesses, you begin to develop a problem.

1. Should the problem lead the students to focus on pathophysiology, growth and development, ethical issues, pharmacology, demographics, socioeconomic issues, parent teaching, or all of these topics? How do you decide?
2. Write a problem that focuses on the issues you chose.
3. Should you do any lecturing, or will students research all information on their own? How do you decide?
4. If the students end up spending all their time on physiological issues and ignore the psychosocial issues you wanted them to address, how will you proceed?
5. When you give a quiz on immunization and childhood diseases, the students score much lower than previous classes that were taught by the lecture method. How can you account for the low scores? Should you assume that the students did not learn the material?

IDEAS FOR FURTHER RESEARCH

1. Compare the effectiveness of teaching a psychomotor skill via a laboratory simulation exercise compared to learning the same skill by a self-learning module.

2. To analyze learners' critical thinking skills, have them "think aloud" while working through a case study. Compare the reasoning processes of novice learners versus experts.

3. Compare two variations of PBL as to effectiveness in teaching ethics content (or any appropriate topic). For example, one group may receive lectures first, followed by two PBL sessions. Another group may work independently to learn all the basic content before doing the PBL sessions.

4. To see the extent to which self-learning modules are adaptable for different learning styles, test a group of people for learning styles, and separate them into groups by type of learning style. Give the same self-learning module to each group and measure learning, learner satisfaction, and perceived ease of learning.

REFERENCES

Aronson, B. S., Rosa, J. M., Anfinson, J., & Light, N. (1997). A simulated clinical problem-solving experience. *Nurse Educator, 22*(6), 17–19.

Babic, A. L., & Crangle, M. L. (1987). Simulation techniques for education in gerontology: An exercise in experiential learning. *Educational Gerontology, 13*(2), 183–191.

Bareford, C. G. (2001). Community as client: Environmental issues in the real world. *Computers in Nursing, 19*(1), 11–16.

Berbiglia, V. A., Goddard, L., & Littlefield, J. H. (1997). Gaming: A strategy for honors courses. *Journal of Nursing Education, 36*(6), 289–291.

Billings, D. M. (1994). Effects of BSN student preferences for studying alone or in groups on performance and attitude when using interactive videodisc instruction. *Journal of Nursing Education, 33*(7), 322–324.

Bloom, K. C., & Trice, L. B. (1994). Let the games begin. *Journal of Nursing Education, 33*(3), 137–138.

Boud, D., & Feletti, G. (Eds.). (1997). *The challenge of problem-based learning* (2nd ed.). London: Kogan Page.

Burns, M. T. (1999). Nutrition Pursuit: A review game. *Journal of Nutrition Education, 31*(3), 175B.

Celia, L. M., & Gordon, P. R. (2001). Using problem-based learning to promote critical thinking in an orientation program for novice nurses. *Journal for Nurses in Staff Development, 17*(1), 12–19.

Clark, H. M. (1986). A health planning simulation game. *Nurse Educator, 11*(4), 16–19.

Coleman, S., Dracup, K., & Moser, D. K. (1991). Comparing methods of cardiopulmonary resuscitation instruction on learning and retention. *Journal of Nursing Staff Development, 7*(2), 82–87.

Colliver, J. A. (2000). Effectiveness of problem-based learning curricula: Research and theory. *Academic Medicine, 75*(3), 259–266.

Conyers, V., & Ritchie, D. (2001). Case study class tests: Assessment directing learning. *Journal of Nursing Education, 40*(1), 40–42.

Courtney, D. P., Courtney, M., & Nicholson, C. (1994). The effect of cooperative learning as an instructional practice at the college level. *College Student Journal, 28*(4), 471–477.

Dahl, J. (1984). Structured experience: A risk-free approach to reality-based learning. *Journal of Nursing Education, 23*(1), 34–37.

Dailey, M. A. (1992). Developing case studies. *Nurse Educator, 17*(3), 8–11.

D'Apolito, K., & Givens, L. (1988). Critical care orientation using self-learning modules. *Critical Care Nurse, 8*(7), 66–76.

Dekkers, J., & Donatti, S. (1981). The integration of research studies on the use of simulation as an instructional strategy. *Journal of Educational Research, 74*(6), 424–427.

Dick, C. (1997). Fun and games—Chemotherapy word search. *Canadian Oncology Nursing Journal, 7*(4), 238.

Donovan, T. J., Braddock, B. S., & Hayward, M. B. (1995). Self-instructional modules: A strategy for teaching the 12-lead ECG. *Critical Care Nurse, 15*(8), 64–68.

Dowd, S. B., & Davidhizar, R. (1999). Using case studies to teach clinical problem-solving. *Nurse Educator, 24*(5), 42–46.

Eaves, R. H., & Flagg, A. J. (2001). The U.S. Air Force pilot simulated medical unit: A teaching strategy with multiple applications. *Journal of Nursing Education, 40*(3), 110–115.

Edens, K. M. (2000). Preparing problem solvers for the 21st century through problem-based learning. *College Teaching, 48*(2), 55–60.

Flurer, N. L., & Moore, C. G. (2000). Providing mandatory safety information to hospital employees: Finding a way that is fast, fun, and effective. *Journal for Nurses in Staff Development, 16*(1), 17–22.

Free, K. W. (1997). What If? What Else? What Then?: A critical thinking game. *Nurse Educator, 22*(5), 9–12.

Fullerton, J. T., & Graveley, E. (1998). Enhancement of basic computer skills—An evaluation of an intervention. *Computers in Nursing, 16*(2), 91–94.

Gallagher, S. A. (1997). Problem-based learning: Where did it come from, what does it do, and where is it going? *Journal for the Education of the Gifted, 20*(4), 332–362.

Glen, S., & Wilkie, K. (Eds.). (2000). *Problem-based learning in nursing*. London: Macmillan.

Goodfellow, L. M. (1995). Cooperative learning strategies: An effective method of teaching nursing research. *Nurse Educator, 20*(4), 26–29.

Goodman, D. (1997). Application of the critical pathway and integrated case method to nursing orientation. *The Journal of Continuing Education in Nursing, 28*(5), 205–210.

Grant, P. (1993). Formative evaluation of a nursing orientation program: Self-paced vs. lecture-discussion. *The Journal of Continuing Education in Nursing, 24*(6), 245–248.

Gruending, D. L., Fenty, D., & Hogan, T. (1991). Fun and games in nursing staff development. *The Journal of Continuing Education in Nursing, 22*(6), 259–262.

Halloran, L., & Dean, L. (1994). Old for an evening: An experiential learning game. *Journal of Nursing Education, 33*(4), 155–156.

Harris, M. D., & Yuan, J. (1997). Creative inservices to meet mandatory education requirements. *Home Healthcare Nurse, 15*(8), 573–579.

Heliker, D. (1994). Meeting the challenge of the curriculum revolution: Problem-based learning in nursing education. *Journal of Nursing Education, 33*(1), 45–47.

Helmuth, M. (1994). Mock convention: A simulation for teaching leadership. *Journal of Nursing Education, 33*(4), 159–160.

Henry, J. M. (1997). Gaming: A teaching strategy to enhance adult learning. *The Journal of Continuing Education in Nursing, 28*(5), 231–234.

Herrick, C. A., Jenkins, T. B., & Carlson, J. H. (1998). Using self-directed learning modules: A literature review. *Journal of Nursing Staff Development, 14*(2), 73–80.

Holtzman, G. (1999). The development of a self-directed module for orientation of nursing students to multiple inpatient clinical sites. *Journal of Nursing Education, 38*(8), 380–382.

Huff, C. (1997). Cooperative learning: A model for teaching. *Journal of Nursing Education, 36*(9), 434–436.

Ingram, C., Ray, K., Landeen, J., & Keane, D. R. (1998). Evaluation of an educational game for health science students. *Journal of Nursing Education, 37*(6), 240–246.

Johnson, L. (1997). Teaching good nursing is all in the act. *Homecare Education Management, 2*(12), 198–199.

Johnson, D. W., & Johnson, R. T. (1999). *Learning together and alone* (5th ed.). Boston: Allyn & Bacon.

Johnson, D. W., Johnson, R. T., & Smith, K. A. (1998). Cooperative learning returns to college. *Change, 30*(4), 27–35.

Johnson, J. H., Zerwic, J. J., & Theis, S. L. (1999). Clinical simulation laboratory: An adjunct to clinical teaching. *Nurse Educator, 24*(5), 37–41.

Jones, A. G., Jasperson, J., & Gusa, D. (2000). Cranial nerve wheel of competencies. *The Journal of Continuing Education in Nursing, 31*(4), 152–154.

Jones, D. C., & Sheridan, M. E. (1999). A case study approach: Developing critical thinking skills in novice pediatric nurses. *The Journal of Continuing Education in Nursing, 30*(2), 75–78.

Keeler, C. M., & Anson, R. (1995). An assessment of cooperative learning used for basic computer skills instruction in the college classroom. *Journal of Educational Computing Research, 12*(4), 379–393.

Lamb, M. J., & Henderson, M. C. (1993). Comparison of two methods for teaching advanced arrhythmias to nurses. *The Journal of Continuing Education in Nursing, 24*(5), 221–226.

Lev, E. L. (1998). Allocation of resources: A student simulation. *Nurse Educator, 23*(6), 11–12.

Lindauer, P., & Petrie, G. (1997). A review of cooperative learning: An alternative to everyday instructional strategies. *Journal of Instructional Psychology, 24*(3), 183–187.

Lipe, D. M., Reeds, L. B., Prokop, J. A., Phelps, B. L., Menousek, L. F., & Bryant, M. M. (1994). Mandatory inservice programs using self-learning modules. *Journal of Nursing Staff Development, 10*(3), 167–169.

Lunyk-Child, O. I., Crooks, D., Ellis, P. J., Ofosu, C., O'Mara, L., & Rideout, E. (2001). Self-directed learning: Faculty and student perceptions. *Journal of Nursing Education, 40*(3), 116–123.

Magnussen, L. (2001). The use of the cognitive behavior survey to assess nursing student learning. *Journal of Nursing Education, 40*(1), 43–46.

Marbeiter, B. (1998). Crossword puzzle: Eye Q. *Journal of Ophthalmic Nursing & Technology, 17*(1), 31–34.

Mast, M. E., & VanAtta, M. J. (1986). Applying adult learning principles in instructional module design. *Nurse Educator, 11*(1), 35–39.

Matthews-Smith, G., Oberski, I., Gray, M., Carter, D., & Smith, L. (2001). A new module in caring for older adults: Problem-based learning and practice portfolios. *The Journal of Nursing Education, 40*(2), 73–78.

Nastasi, B. K., & Clements, D. H. (1991). Research on cooperative learning: Implications for practice. *School Psychology Review, 20*(1), 110–131.

Nikolajski, P. Y. (1992). Investigating the effectiveness of self-learning packages in staff development. *Journal of Nursing Staff Development, 8*(4), 179–183.

Nutter, J. (1998). Strategies for teaching about anabolic steroids. *Journal of Health Education, 29*(1), 40–42.

Olbrich, E. (1997). Innovative games for aide inservices. *Home Care Manager, 1*(1), 18–19, 26.

Orbach, E. (1979). Simulation games and motivation for learning. *Simulation & Games, 10*(1), 3–40.

O'Very, D. I. (1999). Self-paced: The right pace for staff development. *The Journal of Continuing Education in Nursing, 30*(4), 182–187.

Patel, V. L., & Kaufman, D. R. (2001). Medical education isn't just about solving problems. *The Chronicle of Higher Education, 47*(21), B12.

Peters, V., Vissers, G., & Heijne, G. (1998). The validity of games. *Simulation & Gaming, 29*(1), 20–30.

Piskurich, G. M. (1994, March). Developing self-directed learning. *Training & Development,* 31–36.

Poston, I. (1998). Crossword puzzles: Adjunct clinical teaching strategy. *Journal of Nursing Education, 37*(6), 266–267.

Price, B. (2000). Problem-based learning the distance learning way: A bridge too far? *Nursing Education Today, 20*(2), 98–105.

Rendas, A. B., Pinto, P. R., & Gamboa, T. (1998). Problem-based learning in pathophysiology: Report of a project and its outcome. *Teaching and Learning in Medicine, 10*(1), 34–39.

Saethang, T., & Kee, C. C. (1998). A gaming strategy for teaching the use of critical cardiovascular drugs. *The Journal of Continuing Education in Nursing, 29*(1), 32–34.

Schlomer, R. S., Anderson, M. A., & Shaw, R. (1997). Teaching strategies and knowledge retention. *Journal of Nursing Staff Development, 13*(5), 249–253.

Schmidt, K .L., & Fisher, J. C. (1992). Effective development and utilization of self-learning modules. *The Journal of Continuing Education in Nursing, 23*(2), 54–59.

Schmitz, B .D., MacLean, S. L., & Shidler, H. M. (1991). An emergency pursuit game: A method for teaching emergency decision-making skills. *The Journal of Continuing Education in Nursing, 22*(4), 152–157.

Spickerman, S., Lee, B. T., & Eason, F. R. (1988). Use of learning modules to teach nursing leadership concepts. *Journal of Nursing Education, 27*(2), 78–82.

Stein, R. F., & Hurd, S. (2000). *Using student teams in the classroom.* Bolton, MA: Anker.

Suggs, P. K., Mittelmark, M. B., Krissak, R., Oles, K., Lane, C., & Richards, B. (1998). Efficacy of a self-instruction package when compared with a traditional continuing education offering for nurses. *The Journal of Continuing Education in the Health Professions, 18,* 220–226.

Tillman, B. A. (1995). Reflections on case method teaching. *Action in Teacher Education, 17*(1), 1–8.

Tuazon, N. C. (1992). The basics of constructing learning modules. *Journal of Nursing Staff Development, 8*(6), 259–261.

VanLeit, B. (1995). Using the case method to develop clinical reasoning skills in problem-based learning. *The American Journal of Occupational Therapy, 49*(4), 349–353.

Wade, G. H. (1999). Using the case method to develop critical thinking skills for the care of high-risk families. *Journal of Family Nursing, 5*(1), 92–109.

Wargo, C. A. (2000). Blood clot: Gaming to reinforce learning about disseminated intravascular coagulation. *The Journal of Continuing Education in Nursing, 31*(4), 149–151.

Wendt, J. (1998). Clueless for inservices? Try crossword education. *Hospital Infection Control, 25*(12), 187–188.

White, M. J., Amos, E., & Kouzekanani, K. (1999). Problem-based learning—An outcomes study. *Nurse Educator, 24*(2), 33–36.

Wildman, S., & Reeves, M. (1997). The value of simulations in the management education of nurses: Students' perceptions. *Journal of Nursing Management, 5*(4), 207–215.

Wirth, L. A., & Breiner, J. (1997). Jeopardy: Using a familiar game to teach health. *Journal of School Health, 67*(2), 71–74.

Wong, J., & Wong, S. (1985). A randomized controlled trial of a new approach to preoperative teaching and patient compliance. *International Journal of Nursing Studies, 22*(2), 105–115.

Zafuto, M. S. (1997). Cooperative learning: A means to promote metacognitive and collaborative skills in heterogeneous nursing students. *Journal of Nursing Education, 36*(6), 265–270.

9

Computer Teaching Strategies

Computer use in nursing and patient education is increasing greatly as hardware costs decrease, software proliferates, and the Internet and World Wide Web (WWW) expand. Other factors that have fostered the increased use of computers are the availability of grant funds for technology, growth of software companies, increasing sophistication of software, and the need to make education more cost effective (Mallow & Gilje, 1999). Nurse educators need some technological proficiency and a comfort level with computer technology in order to use technology to enhance teaching and learning and to supply nurses and patients with the skills they need to access information.

Computer Technology and Learning

Computers are used to communicate information to students and nurses in a time-saving way, to teach critical thinking and problem solving, to provide simulations of reality, and to educate from a distance. In the clinical world, computers are used to communicate with other health care professionals, to access patient records in real-time online, to provide patient teaching, and to provide home-based care and support for the chronically ill (Bachman & Panzarine, 1998).

In the rush to build more of our educational infrastructure on technology, we should take the time to be sure our incorporation of computer use is built on learning theory and an understanding of the advantages and drawbacks of technology as a teaching strategy.

Computer use can and should address the learning principles in Chapter 2. Computers, for example, support mastery learning very well. Learners may spend as much time as they want or are allowed in learning concepts and skills, until they have achieved mastery. The computer is nonjudgmental and endlessly patient. If the learner takes four tries to get the right answer, the computer will never make him or her feel stupid. Assuming that other learners are not watching, peers or teachers need never know how long it took the person to learn the content. However, if desired, records of performance can be kept on the computer. Computers can also be available to learners for more hours than an instructor is. A computer lab in a school or hospital may be open around the clock.

In addition to mastery learning, computers can maximize time on task and can help develop *overlearning* (Vockell, 1990). Overlearning is achieved when learners practice beyond the point of mastery and responses become automatic. In a traditional classroom, the brightest students usually learn quickly and have more time to devote to overlearning. Less bright students usually take the most time to learn concepts and skills and have little time left for overlearning. Thus, they are not as prepared to move on to higher levels of learning. With computer instruction, if learners are motivated intrinsically or by attractive programming, they may continue to practice until they have overlearned the material.

Computer programs provide instant feedback, which is effective in learning. The computer can reply to the student's answers with statements like "Good job, Ann," or "Juan, you have really learned that well." Teachers do not always remember to give immediate positive feedback, but the computer never forgets. Wrong answers trigger nonpunitive feedback. The computer may say "Sorry, that's incorrect; try again Kyle," or "You need more review before proceeding." The use of the learner's name gives the impression of a human teacher providing the feedback, and many people, even educators, enjoy seeing the computer use their name once in a while.

Ribbons (1998) discusses the cognitive effects of computer use. He suggests that there are cognitive effects *with* the technology, that is, those learning effects that take place during the use of the computer program. There are also cognitive effects *of* the technology, that is, effects that remain after use of the computer. In effect, he says a *cognitive residue* remains, and it can be described as skills the learner acquires during interaction with the computer that can be transferred to other situations. For example:

> A student using a World Wide Web search engine to locate literature for an assignment may be acquiring skills in searching, accessing, and managing information resources that can be generalized to other context domains. (p. 225)

Teachers should take advantage of the cognitive residue effect by choosing programs and assignments that promote transfer of learning.

Other advantages of computer instruction include interactivity, instructional consistency, reduction of teachers' repetitive tasks, individualized instruction, time efficiency, and cost effectiveness (Grobe, 1984; Schmidt, Arndt, Gaston, & Miller, 1991; Sinclair, 1985; Tibbles, Lewis, Reisine, Rippey, & Donald, 1992; Van Dongen, 1985).

Perhaps the greatest advantage of computer instruction is that it allows a person to interact in the learning situation; he or she can respond to questions, manipulate variables, solve problems, and create plans and strategies. This type of active approach makes learning more interesting, memorable, and valuable. In addition, the learner maintains control of the learning process, its speed, order, and type, to a great extent.

Instructional consistency is achieved because there is essentially one teacher, the computer program, for all learners. All patients get the same instruction before a cardiac catheterization, for example, or all students across multiple sections of a course receive the same information. When several educators are presenting information to patients, students, or nurses, there is never a guarantee that everyone is receiving the same information in an equivalent manner.

With computer use, educators can be freed from repetitive tasks that become burdensome and boring over time. For example, teaching mandatory in-service classes like blood-borne pathogens or cardiopulmonary resuscitation (CPR) may have to be done dozens of times a year for small groups on each shift. A computer program never gets tired of repeating the same information or cracking the same jokes.

Computers can individualize learning to an extraordinary degree. Not only does the learner often work alone and have freedom to use a variety of computer programs, he or she can also work at any desired rate of speed and can branch out within programs. In a well-designed program, if learners are already familiar with a certain portion of the material, they can skip ahead or move into a more advanced track. On the other hand, if learners are having difficulty, branching within the program may permit them to review certain segments of the program or move into a tutorial lesson. Evaluation of learning is also individualized as feedback is given to the learner.

Time efficiency and cost effectiveness are important advantages of computer instruction. Research has demonstrated that learning content by computer instead of traditional methods saves time (Cohen & Dacanay, 1994; Jeffries, 2001; Kulik & Kulik, 1991; Rambo, 1994). Most of the time, studies have shown reduced learning time for students; in some cases, there is reduction in educator work time, especially in staff development education. Cost effectiveness results from the savings in workload. For example, in a physician's or nurse practitioner's office, nonlicensed personnel may set up computer programs, and the physician or nurse can answer questions later.

The drawbacks to computer instruction must also be considered. Many nurse educators do not feel comfortable enough with computer instruction to jump into this medium. They either do not have good computer skills or they don't know how to incorporate computers into their teaching role. Education for educators will eventually take care of this problem, but in the meantime, it does pose obstacles in many settings, both academic and clinical.

A second drawback is cost. It has already been stated that computer learning can be cost effective. However, the initial outlay of monies for hardware and software is costly. Without grant money, this barrier may bring computer integration to a halt. One alternative is to lease computers; another is to comparison shop for software that may not be too expensive for the budget and that will not be outdated quickly.

A third concern is the effect that computer use may have on personal and professional communication. Nurses have historically based their practice on face-to-face communication with colleagues and patients, with the subtleties of both verbal and nonverbal interaction and intuition. Mallow and Gilje (1999) raise the question, "How do messages conveyed electronically through technology change educational processes within nursing education?" (p. 250). The issue of socialization of people being brought into the profession is an important one for us to consider, especially in the context of distance learning.

Computer-Assisted Instruction

Computer-assisted instruction (CAI) takes several forms; can be used to teach nurses, students and patients; and can be developed in a number of ways. All of these topics plus research findings on the effectiveness of CAI will be discussed in this section.

Computer-assisted instruction can be very effective in the hands of an astute nurse educator. To be effective, it requires that the program be aimed toward instructional objectives and be of high quality, that learners have sufficient access to computers, that there is sufficient technological support, and that the computer is judged to be the best way to teach the given content (Khoiny, 1995).

Drill and Practice

The simplest level of CAI is *drill and practice*. In this format, students have already learned certain information, either through computer programs or other teaching methods, and are now presented with repetition and application of the information. This mode particularly lends itself to teaching mathematical calculations. The students may have received a lecture/demonstration on solving math problems in pharmacology. They are then sent to the computer, which presents problem after problem to be solved. The computer program tells the student whether the answers are correct and may go so far as to diagnose the problem if answers are incorrect. For example, it may say, "You forgot to round off to the nearest tenth, Sasha." Drill and practice may be used in learning drug names and actions, in learning medical terminology, or in any situation requiring memorization of facts and concepts. It is probably the mode in which the least amount of software has been written in nursing because of the low level of learning it represents.

Tutorials

The second mode in which CAI may be written is the *tutorial* mode. The program tutors or teaches the student a body of knowledge by presenting information and asking questions, giving hints if the student gets stuck. Tutorials are most useful in teaching material at the rule and concept level. Tutorial software can free faculty members from teaching some of the routine basic material, which becomes tedious after lecturing on it the first few times, and allows them to use their time more creatively and effectively on higher-level learning. At the same time, students may find tutorials on basic information to be more interesting and fun than some instructors' lectures!

Any information taught by means of lecture could potentially be written as a computer tutorial program. Content that may be difficult for some learners to grasp is especially suited to a tutorial, because the learner can continue to review it until mastery is achieved. A segment of a tutorial program on immobility may appear something like this:

Computer: As described, immobility takes its toll on almost every body system, and nurses must use preventive measures to protect the patient from those effects. Let's review some of the material covered. If the nurse encourages a patient to force fluids, which hazard of immobility is he or she trying to prevent?

Student: (kidney stones, renal calculi, and urinary infection)

Computer: Right! A high flow rate through the urinary system helps to prevent renal calculi and urinary infection.
    Which particular fluid would be most effective in helping to prevent urinary infection?

Student: (cranberry juice or prune juice)

Computer: Good! Juices that help produce an acidic urine reduce the chances of urinary infection in an immobile patient . . .

Tutorials thus take the form of an interactive lecture with built-in feedback and can be developed very creatively, especially if graphics are used.

Games

Software for CAI can also be written in the *game* mode. Just as board games, card games, and trivia games can be used to teach nursing, so can computer games. Relatively few nursing game programs have been written and marketed, probably because good games are not easy to devise and because software specialists have been concentrating their efforts on other modes.

Simulations

The *simulation* mode is one of the most exciting and available forms of CAI. In academic settings, simulations of real-world experiences provide students with the opportunity to learn how to solve clinical problems and make sound decisions. Computer simulations can provide students with all the details about a particular patient situation and then ask them to assess the patient, arrive at diagnoses, plan interventions, and evaluate care. They can also throw in unexpected twists and turns in the course of the patient's illness and ask for revisions of plans or quick decisions. Results of good or poor decisions can be illustrated.

The advantage of providing these learning experiences via computer is that students can all be exposed to the same learning situation, which is not the case in the clinical setting. Even more important, students can take risks and make mistakes with no danger to the patient. In a computer simulation, the student is functioning in a controlled environment where pressures characteristic of the clinical area do not occur. Of course, the disadvantage of computer simulations is that educators find out only what students might do or are capable of doing in a situation, not how they actually would perform in reality.

A computer simulation might be formatted in the following way:

- Description of a patient situation.
- Student selects (from a list) which data should be collected.
- Computer provides feedback about choices.
- Student uses the correct data to arrive at nursing diagnoses.
- Computer provides feedback on diagnoses.
- Student selects (from a list) appropriate nursing goals.
- Computer responds to each selection as to why it is or is not correct.
- Student selects (from a list) appropriate nursing actions.
- Computer responds with positive and negative effects of each action.
- Student selects (from a list) evaluation criteria that indicate success of nursing actions.
- Computer provides feedback on evaluation criteria.

This is a simplified format of a computer simulation using the nursing process. Actual programs are much more complex and involve branching or relooping, meaning that whenever students lose their grasp of a situation, they can move back to an earlier part of the program to brush up on information or retrace their actions. They may be able to branch into a tutorial mode for reinforcement of background material, or they may automatically be moved into alternate paths depending on the pattern of their responses. An example of a computer simulation used to help newly hired nurses and refresher course nurses to make clinical decisions can be found in an article by Bremner and Brannan (2000).

Multimedia Presentations

Multimedia (sometimes called hypermedia) programs may incorporate text, sound tracks, graphics, still photos, animation, video clips, and material from the World Wide Web (WWW). Programs can be saved on a laptop computer and shown to an audience with a computer projector or can be produced as a CD-ROM. It is possible for faculty or even students with a modicum of computer literacy to produce multimedia programs on almost any conceivable topic (Gibbons, Bachulis, & Allen, 1999; Jeffries, 2000; Sternberger & Meyer, 2001; Thomson, 1998).

A slightly older form of multimedia is the *interactive videodisc* (IVD) program. IVDs are interesting and fun to use. They consist of a large disc on which is recorded the written program and video clips. IVD necessitates the purchase of a videodisc player in addition to the usual computer equipment. Most programs are simulations. As the learner watches the monitor, a video clip is shown and the learner is asked to interact with the video he or she is watching. The interaction may be in the form of answering questions, touching the screen to indicate what part of the anatomy or another structure is being referred to, or selecting options from a menu of nursing actions. Interactive videodiscs are available on the topics of therapeutic communication, childbirth, physical assessment, care of patients with chronic disease, and psychomotor skills, among others (Mansen & Haak, 1996; Rambo, 1994; Urick & Bond, 1994; Walker & Ross, 1995). The biggest drawback to widespread adoption of interactive videodisc programs is the cost. Many programs cost $1,000 or more.

Evaluating Software

With large numbers of software packages on the market, some of them of questionable quality, the educator must be able to intelligently evaluate what each program has to offer and whether it will meet the desired objectives. It is helpful, as Smith (1985) suggests, to look at each program from the perspective of not only the educator, but also the learner. Table 9–1 contains the criteria that are useful in evaluating software for educational purposes.

A manual or user's guide usually accompanies programs. This documentation is generally not made available to learners but should be available to the nurse educator. The manual should be clearly written, have an easy-to-use index, and contain a trouble-shooting section to help solve common problems. The manual should also include information about the type and level of learner for whom the program is designed, objectives of the lesson material, and an estimate of the average amount of time it should take to complete the program.

Evaluate the program in terms of the objectives you want to achieve. Would the learners see this program as repetitious of what you have taught in the classroom or what is in the textbook? If so, the program may still be useful as a supplementary or remedial resource. Does the program broaden or apply what is taught in class? It should relate to the course closely enough that learners see the obvious application to what they are learning in the course.

TABLE 9-1	Criteria for Evaluating Computer-Assisted Instruction Software

Accuracy

    Is the content accurate according to published nursing knowledge?

    Is the information up to date?

Ease of Use

    Are the instructions and commands clear and easy to follow?

    Is there a user's guide?

    Is there a tutorial with the program?

    Is there telephone support service?

Design

    Is this computer program the best way to deliver the content?

    Is interactivity (learner response) built in?

    How frequently is the interactivity built in?

    Does the design help make the content interesting? Fun?

Appearance

    Are there appropriate graphics?

    Is there animation and sound?

    Do the graphics and animation serve a real purpose or are they distracting?

    Does the learner interact with the graphics or animation?

Feedback

    Does the program give the learner feedback on responses?

    Do opportunities exist to repeat material for which responses were incorrect?

    Are rationales given for learner responses?

    If the learner already knows the material, can he or she branch into an area of greater complexity?

Cost Effectiveness

    What is the purchase price? Are any discounts available?

    Can copies be made of the program?

    Are free or reduced price replacement discs available in case of damage?

    Is a site license available?

When doing a trial run through the program, take note of how user friendly the program is. If you make a mistake, is it easy to rectify, or do you have to start over? Does the program require all uppercase or lowercase letters, or is it flexible in accepting either? If free response is asked of the learner, is there flexibility in the answers that are accepted, including misspelled words? If the program is being used for patient teaching, is it written at an acceptable readability level? Are the screens simple enough in appearance? Software reviews often appear in nursing journals and can also be found on the WWW. So, some of the groundwork on evaluation of software may already be done for you.

One last word on cost effectiveness. In addition to purchase and replacement costs, consider the amount of usage the product will get. If many learners use the software and use it frequently, it may be worth a costly investment. If it saves educator or learner time, it may also be cost effective over time (Bolwell, 1988).

Computer-Assisted Instruction for Patient Education

Three forces have added a sense of urgency to the delivery of patient education. One is the expectation of accreditation organizations like the Joint Commission on Accreditation of Health Care Organizations (JCAHO) that patient education will be systematic and documented. A second is the increase in lawsuits against health care facilities and providers. Enough lawsuits have brought attention to the results of lack of patient education that malpractice insurers are encouraging physicians to provide patients with printed information and to document their actions. In some cases, insurers have offered patient education software to physicians at a discount (Gabello, 1997). A third factor fostering more deliberate patient education is the rise in consumerism in our society. With the patients' rights movement bringing the issue of participation in one's own health care to the fore, people want to be educated so they can participate intelligently (Bell, 1986).

Computer-assisted instruction is a logical progression for patient education to take. Physicians and advanced practice nurses who purchase software can generate customized patient handouts at a reasonable cost. These handouts may be more up to date than commercially printed handouts and they don't take up space in the office. Many programs offer materials that have been tested for readability and appeal and can be printed in a large font for the visually impaired or printed in other languages (Gabello, 1997).

Interactive CAI software is also available for patient education. CAI has been applied to pre- and postoperative teaching, asthmatic and cardiac education, smoking cessation, health risk appraisal, and many other topics and conditions (Huss et al., 1992; Lyons, Krasnowski, Greenstein, Maloney, & Tatarczuk, 1982; Skinner, Siegfried, Kegler, & Strecher, 1993; Tibbles et al., 1992). Huss and co-authors (1992) researched the effectiveness of interactive CAI as a method of asthma patient education compared to conventional teaching. They found that the CAI group had higher postinstruction adherence to treatment regimens.

Software is available that tailors health instructions to individual patients. This type of program requires the patient first to answer demographic and background information about health beliefs and behaviors. Then an individualized prevention plan or care plan can be generated that guides the health professional in appropriate patient counseling (Skinner et al., 1993). For instance:

> The report can tell the health professional that Ms. Smith has finally quit smoking but is now concerned about the weight she is now gaining, or report that Mr. Jones has considered having a cholesterol test but thinks he is too young to be concerned about his cholesterol level. (p. 29)

Research on tailored instructions related to cancer prevention and diet change has found the information to be better remembered and more thoroughly read than ordinary printed instructions (Skinner et al., 1993).

Computerized patient education may take place in a professional office, a clinic, a hospital, or even a patient's home. In the future, reliance on this medium will probably increase as the body of research documenting its effectiveness increases.

Computer-Assisted Instruction for Nursing Students and Nursing Staff

Application of CAI to basic nursing education is extensive. Programs are available that teach psychomotor skills, dosage computation, care planning, problem solving, critical thinking, and content on many medical conditions. Students can be assigned CAI programs as required activities for a class or as supplementary material. The computer can be brought into class to run part or all of a program during class time by means of a video/computer projector. Some students might be assigned tutorials as remedial work on their own time.

The educator must be sure that there is a proper fit between the CAI program and the learning objectives. For example, if the objective is to change attitudes toward the elderly, a tutorial about the nursing needs of the elderly would not be appropriate, but an interactive case study might be.

Nursing staff can also benefit from this technology. Staff development educators have developed computer labs where staff can come in whenever they are available to view software applicable to them. This might include software on mandatory in-service topics, advanced skills, critical thinking, leadership and management, or any nursing topic of interest to staff (Tronni & Prawlucki, 1998).

Research on Effectiveness of Computer-Assisted Instruction

The first question people would most likely ask about the effectiveness of CAI is whether people learn better by this medium rather than by traditional teaching. Studies of the comparison of learner achievement using content examinations have revealed either equal or higher performance of the CAI groups in the vast majority of cases (Cohen & Dacanay, 1994; Day & Payne, 1987; Halloran, 1995; Kulik & Kulik, 1991; Kulik, Kulik, & Cohen, 1980; Jeffries, 2000; Rickelman, Taylor-Fox, Reisch, Payne, & Jelemensky, 1988; Schmidt et al., 1991). The conclusion can be drawn that CAI is at least as effective if not more effective than traditional pedagogy for the content areas studied. One must evaluate all research of this type, that is, comparing a new or innovative strategy to a traditional one, in light of the Hawthorne effect. If students know they are being studied because they are being taught by a new pedagogy, they may be more motivated to study harder and do better. Nevertheless, the vast number of studies that have been conducted give weight to the conclusion that CAI is an effective way to achieve student learning.

A few meta-analysis reports have focused on students' attitudes toward the subject matter being taught, and whether attitudes are different between CAI and traditional methods. The majority of studies reported a difference, with attitudes toward subject matter being better with CAI, but the effect sizes were small (Cohen & Dacanay, 1994; Kulik & Kulik, 1991; Kulik et al., 1980).

Computer-Managed Instruction

Teachers can use computers to manage, prepare, organize, and evaluate educational experiences. Programs designed to construct examinations fall into this category. The nurse educator may purchase a test development program that contains a bank of possible questions and the means to select appropriate questions, test students on the computer, and, afterwards, grade the examinations and perform an item analysis. Any system of record keeping such as recording grades, keeping attendance records, and recording student profiles can also be considered computer-managed instruction. Nursing faculty may use computers to schedule clinical agencies and assignments, assign rotations, and even record anecdotal records of student performance.

The use of *authoring systems* is also part of computer-managed instruction. Writing computer programs is not the exclusive domain of programmers or instructional designers. Educators without programming skills can develop CAI through authoring packages. Authoring systems are predeveloped software packages that guide the educator through the process of development of CAI. Programmers have already laid the groundwork for the CAI program, and educators need only learn some commands in order to insert content. Text, graphics, audio, and motion may be incorporated. Some authoring packages are simple to use, but they usually result in fairly simple programs. The more sophisticated authoring programs take a greater amount of time to learn but have much more flexibility in the kind of product that is developed. The major advantages of using authoring packages are that they result in a cost-effective product and they allow the educator to personalize the product (Gerheim, 1990; Sternberger & Meyer, 2001).

Using the Computer as a Tool

People who have any computer knowledge at all usually know how to use a word processing program. That is one way we use the computer as a tool—to help us write more efficiently. Students today usually learn how to use the computer as a search tool. They have gone through school using the WWW for information, and by the time they go to college, they learn how to search library and other databases for information.

A third way nurses use the computer as a tool is for patient care management. Today's nursing students will all have some experience in using computers as part of a hospital information system. Nurses using such systems need to learn how to enter physician's orders and to order lab tests, diets, and drugs. They will be required to send messages to other departments, will have to chart medications and nurse's notes, and will be developing or refining care plans or care maps on the computer. In some hospitals and home health agencies, nurses are already carrying handheld computers for patient record access and recording purposes.

The best way to prepare nursing students and newly licensed orientees to use the computer in a health care facility is to enable them to use the computer in many different ways during their education and then to give them specific training on practice programs during their orientation to work. There are enough similarities between types of computer applications that any computer familiarity helps a person transfer that learning to new programs.

The Internet

The Internet is a mammoth complex of computer connections across continents, connecting many millions of computers. With an Internet node, or a modem, potentially anyone can connect to the Internet. Universities are Internet nodes and have free access to the Internet.

Most other institutions as well as individuals must pay for access to an Internet node. The primary uses of the Internet in nursing are e-mail, news groups, and access to the WWW.

E-mail

E-mail (electronic mail) can be used to provide greater collaboration between teachers and students and between students and students. Many faculty members have attested to the fact that e-mail has enriched the learning interactions between them and their students (Brown, 2000). Also, students report e-mail as a source of peer support, especially when they have less face-to-face contact than in traditional classrooms (Ward, 1997). E-mail can be used between patients and physicians and nurses. It can be used as a means for patients to seek referrals, for consultations, and for postdischarge follow-up.

In addition to individual e-mail use, as described above, there are mailing or subscription lists called *listservs*. A listserv is a group of people who have similar interests and want to share information and experiences regarding those interests in a type of discussion group. There are listservs for nurse educators, for nursing students, and for many nursing practice specialties. To subscribe to a listserv, send an e-mail message to the listserv address, which you can usually find on the Internet via a search engine (Bliss & DeYoung, 2002).

News Groups

News groups are similar to listservs in that they are discussion groups of people with similar interests. However, messages appear in a general mailbox that everyone views, compared to the individual mailbox messages in a listserv. Internet service providers provide access to some news groups and not others, so all news groups may not be available to you. Special programs called *news reader software* may be necessary for individuals to read e-mails sent to a news group (Mascara, Czar, & Hebda, 1999). One example of a news group of interest to nurses is *sci.med.nursing,* a group discussing all kinds of nursing issues. Both news groups and listservs are also used for online support groups for people suffering from various diseases and conditions or for people who care for them. An example of growing online support groups is the development of groups for caregivers of Alzheimer's patients. Caregivers often cannot leave their homes to attend community support groups, so an online option is very attractive (White & Dorman, 2000).

World Wide Web

The Internet also provides access to the WWW, a collection of millions of "documents" found on *Web pages* that interface to the Internet. Kiser (1999) asserts that educators should consider using the Internet and WWW in the classroom when information that is required is not in the textbook or the library. It can be a place to find specialized knowledge and multimedia presentations. For example, in teaching nurse practitioners about reading x-rays, you can find a Web site that depicts normal x-rays. Projecting this Web site on a screen in front of the classroom is better than looking at pictures in a book and easier than finding slides or actual x-ray films.

Nurse educators and learners may use the Internet to search for Web sites containing full text articles or abstracts, when doing a literature search. Many patients and members of the general public are using the Internet to find Web sites with health information. The National Library of Medicine made MEDLINE available free of cost through PubMed and found that consumer use rose from 10 percent to 30 percent of total use (Leaffer & Gonda, 2000). Nurse educators and staff nurses can teach people to use Web sites for information and supply them with quality sources.

A National Institutes of Health project was done to teach senior citizens how to access and use 22 health information resources on the Internet (Leaffer & Gonda, 2000). The method was to train 20 senior citizen trainers who then trained another 80 senior citizens. The project was considered very successful when the seniors were able to access and use the health information in their own health care.

Faculty members at one university taught students how to use the WWW as a source of information for patient teaching (Colling & Rogers, 1999). They assigned a written paper on a medical condition, taught students how to search the Web, and then had them find and describe a Web site that could be used in some way for patient teaching. Students also had to evaluate the Web site.

Two problems exist in using the WWW and teaching others to use it. One is the difficulty in finding the Web sites pertinent to your purpose. The other is the quality, or lack of it, of many Web sites.

World Wide Web Searches

The WWW has millions of sites affiliated with it, none of which are catalogued or indexed. "Surfing the Web" is an approach some people take, but it is like aimlessly walking up and down unmarked and unfamiliar supermarket aisles, hoping you will soon find the item you are seeking. Surfing may be fun at times, but when you are looking for specific information, it is a very inefficient way to proceed. To be efficient in a search for information on the Web, you must use a *search engine* that indexes Web pages for you and gives you the Uniform Resource Locator (URL) for each page. Each search engine uses different databases and different techniques for its indexing, and therefore you can use two search engines and obtain quite different results (Mascara et al., 1999). Table 9–2 contains a list of major search engines by type. Another approach is to use a metasearch engine that conducts a search of several databases from other search engines or tools (Sparks & Rizzolo, 1998). Using a metasearch engine may produce a more complete and less redundant search.

Many search engines allow you to refine a search to attempt to get exactly the sources you want. Some instruct you to place quotation marks or brackets around several words if you want the search engine to consider the words as a complete phrase. To expand or contract your search, some search engines will tell you to use AND or NOT or + and − signs, respectively. Consult the Help files or Options menu of the search engines for instructions.

Evaluating World Wide Web Sites

Of the millions of Web sites, many are high quality, many are average, and many are poor. The reason for this is that there is no monitoring or quality control system for the Internet. It's like asking everyone in your neighborhood to contribute a column to a newsletter, with no guidelines for doing so. You would get some fine and probably funny columns, but you would also be likely to get some garbage.

TABLE 9-2 Major World Wide Web Search Engines

Regular Search Engines	URL
Alta Vista	*www.altavista.com*
Hotbot	*www.hotbot.lycos.com*
Northernlight	*www.northernlight.com*
Webcrawler	*www.webcrawler.com*
Yahoo!	*www.yahoo.com*
Metasearch Engines	**URL**
Dogpile	*www.dogpile.com*
Google	*www.google.com*
Metacrawler	*www.metacrawler.com*

Note: Check the following Web site to keep updated on search engines, including changes in URLs: *www.searchenginewatch.com.*

Therefore, let the reader beware, and let the reader have some criteria in mind for sorting out the good from the garbage. Table 9–3 contains a set of criteria by which the value of Web sites may be gauged. Whether you are searching for information for a paper or health information for yourself, your students, or patients, you can apply criteria like these and have some assurance that if the site meets the criteria, there is some reliability to the information.

If you refer students or patients to Web sites, be sure to check these sites frequently. Many come and go within a matter of months. Sites that last the longest are most likely to be those affiliated with institutions like universities (domain is .edu), hospitals or other non-profit organizations (domain is .org), or companies (domain is .com) that have existed for a while as opposed to those sponsored only by individuals.

Virtual Reality

Virtual reality is a computer-based, simulated three-dimensional environment in which the participant interacts with a virtual world. The learner does not just watch or read a simulation, but participates in it as if this were a real world actually experienced (Pantelidis, 1993). The initial virtual reality programs were written for the military (flight training simulators) or for Hollywood-type applications. Today, many programs are being developed for educational purposes.

Simulations have been developed for medical schools to teach dissection and surgery. For example, a surgical simulator allows medical students to see first how a surgical procedure is performed by an experienced surgeon and then use the instruments to actually (virtually) perform the surgery themselves ("Virtual Reality," 1991). The same type of program exists to enable medical students to perform cadaver dissection and to learn how to administer epidural anesthetics (McNamara, 1996).

Relatively few programs have been developed for nursing education, but they are increasing. For example, a program exists for teaching venipuncture (Merril & Barker,

TABLE 9-3 Criteria for Evaluating the Quality of WWW Sites

Purpose
1. The potential audience should be stated (i.e., for adults, children, laypeople, or professionals).
2. The purpose of the site should be stated.

Currency
1. The site should contain up-to-date information.
2. The pages should be updated frequently and the date of revision should be noted at the end of the pages.

Credibility
1. The author's credentials should be listed and should be appropriate to the content.
2. The author's organizational affiliation should be listed, if any.
3. Anonymous sites should be handled with caution.
4. Sites sponsored by sales companies should be evaluated for their objectivity and possible conflicts of interest.

Content Accuracy
1. The facts should be verifiable as being accurate and true.
2. Links to other sites should confirm the accuracy of the first.
3. The content should be logical and scientific.
4. Content should be comprehensive and "tell the whole story."
5. References should be included in the site.

Design
1. Pages should be simple, not too cluttered with graphics or boxes.
2. An internal search engine or site map should be included for comprehensive sites.
3. It should be easy to move around the site without getting lost.
4. Links to other sites should be useful, and it should be indicated whether you can or cannot return from the linked site.

1996). Six varied patient scenarios were developed in which the nursing student selects an appropriate site for the venipuncture, manipulates a needle and syringe, and feels the resistance as the needle enters the virtual skin. The student watches the action on the computer screen but actively manipulates the needle and syringe in his or her hand. Only in virtual reality can the learner enter a virtual world and feel an object, move it, and measure its movement (McNamara, 1996).

A newer form of virtual reality program in nursing uses multimedia and CD-ROM technology with an embedded virtual reality component. A program to teach the 12-lead electrocardiogram (ECG) has been developed by Jeffries (1999). In this program, students can enter a virtual intensive care unit and get a panoramic view. They click on a patient, and ECG equipment appears. With the computer mouse, the student moves the sensors to correct placement on the patient. If the sensors or cables are placed in the wrong location, they bounce back to the top of the screen. The program proceeds with virtually running the ECG and trouble-shooting problems. The major difference between this technology and full virtual reality is that the learner does not feel tactically what is happening in the virtual world.

Applications to patient education are also beginning. To help people with Parkinson's disease to steady their gait, a virtual reality program was developed in which the patients wear eye gear that displays a path and virtual obstacles and teaches them to lift their legs with each step (Weiss & Jessel, 1998). A program to teach asthmatics to take their medication appropriately is designed to increase patient compliance (McNamara, 1996).

The advantages of virtual reality simulations over paper and pencil or other computer simulations are many. As the examples show, the ability to practice invasive procedures in a lifelike scenario is an extraordinary advantage over previous simulation formats. The control that is built into the virtual reality simulation makes it a unique opportunity to practice complex and dangerous skills in a safe environment.

Unfortunately, there is a major drawback to this medium. The cost of developing, operating, and maintaining a virtual reality system is generally prohibitive unless grant funds are obtained. The cost of the program (anywhere from $10,000 to $200,000) could be offset over time when the savings in professional time and equipment are considered (McNamara, 1996). With improved technology, experts are predicting that virtual reality will be more affordable in the future (Dysart, 1996).

Another drawback is that people assume that if they learn a skill via virtual reality, they will automatically perform well in a real setting. This assumption may not be warranted (McNamara, 1996). There is little research on the effectiveness of virtual reality in terms of transfer of training from a virtual world to the real world. The research that has been done shows conflicting results (Jeffries, 1999; Kozak, Hancock, Arthur, & Chrysler, 1993).

Variations in computer learning will continue to emerge. The wise nurse educator will continue to learn more about technology applications and keep abreast of changes that can enhance patient, student, and staff education.

CASE STUDY

You are a staff nurse at a hospital. You would like to establish a Web page at the hospital for the following purposes: (a) for recently discharged patients to ask advice, (b) for the public to access health information, and (c) for the public to get physician referrals. Your head nurse encourages you to write a proposal that she can take to nursing administrators. You know that you would need to hire staff and would like to have nursing students and faculty from area universities to participate.

1. What might such an undertaking cost?
2. How would you fund this project?
3. What legal issues might arise?
4. What technical support would you need?
5. How would you market the Web site?
6. If the proposal moves forward, how would you "sell" the idea to physicians?

CRITICAL THINKING EXERCISES

1. In an undergraduate nursing program that uses a lot of computer-assisted instruction, students are allowed as much time as they need to complete or master the programs. Does the lack of time limits pose a potential problem for these students who will later have to learn and perform under time constraints?

2. A media company has made a special offer of computer-assisted instruction software on the topic of peritoneal dialysis. As a faculty member, you have to decide whether to recommend purchase of this software. How do you decide whether this would be a wise investment?

3. The trend toward computerized patient education is advancing, yet we also are aware of the literacy problem in the United States. How can we reconcile the use of possibly intimidating computer technology with the need to reach low-literate people?

4. If you were given a large grant to purchase and develop virtual reality software in a nursing program, on what skills would you focus? Can virtual reality be applied to other aspects of nursing than just psychomotor skills?

IDEAS FOR FURTHER RESEARCH

1. Investigate whether CAI is more effective for some learning styles than others.

2. Compare the quality of student papers based on Internet sources to traditional sources.

3. Study whether academic educators have experienced a higher degree of plagiarism when students use the Internet for sources. How do they prevent it?

4. Study the satisfaction levels of patients who are taught with CAI compared with traditional teaching methods.

REFERENCES

Bachman, J. A., & Panzarine, S. (1998). Enabling student nurses to use the information superhighway. *Journal of Nursing Education, 37*(4), 155–161.

Bell, J. A. (1986). The role of microcomputers in patient education. *Computers in Nursing, 4*(6), 255–257.

Bliss, J. B., & DeYoung, S. (2002). *Working the web: A guide for nurses.* Upper Saddle River, NJ: Prentice Hall.

Bolwell, C. (1988). Evaluating computer-assisted instruction. *Nursing & Health Care, 9*(9), 511–515.

Bremner, M. N., & Brannan, J. D. (2000). A computer simulation for the entry-level RN: Enhancing clinical decision making. *Journal for Nurses in Staff Development, 16*(1), 5–9.

Brown, D. G. (Ed.). (2000). *Teaching with technology.* Bolton, MA: Anker.

Cohen, P. A., & Dacanay, L. S. (1994). A meta-analysis of computer-based instruction in nursing education. *Computers in Nursing, 12*(2), 89–97.

Colling, K. B., & Rogers, A. E. (1999). Nursing students "surf" the Web: Resources for patient teaching. *Journal of Nursing Education, 38*(6), 286–288.

Day, R., & Payne, L. (1987). Computer-managed instruction: An alternative teaching strategy. *Journal of Nursing Education, 26*(1), 30–36.

Dysart, J. (1996). Virtual reality expands healthcare horizons. *Nursing & Allied Healthweek, 1*(7), 22.

Gabello, W. J. (1997). How computers enrich patient education. *Patient Care, 31*(2), 88–113.

Gerheim, S. M. (1990). Authoring options for computer assisted nursing instruction. *Computers in Nursing, 8*(1), 29–33.

Gibbons, C., Bachulis, A., & Allen, G. (1999). A comparison of a computer and paper and pencil assignment. *Computers in Nursing, 17*(6), 286–290.

Grobe, S. J. (1984). Computer assisted instruction: An alternative. *Computers in Nursing, 2*(3), 92–97.

Halloran, L. (1995). A comparison of two methods of teaching. Computer managed instruction and keypad questions versus traditional classroom lecture. *Computers in Nursing, 13*(6), 285–288.

Huss, K., Huss, R. W., Squire, E. N., Carpenter, G. B., Smith, L. J., Salata, K., Salerno, M., & Agostinelli, D. (1992). Computer education for asthmatics: What effects? *Journal of Nursing Care Quality, 6*(3), 57–66.

Jeffries, P. R. (1999). Learning how to perform a 12 lead ECG using virtual reality. *Progress in Cardiovascular Nursing, Winter,* 7–13.

Jeffries, P. R. (2000). Development and test of a model for designing interactive CD-ROMs for teaching nursing skills. *Computers in Nursing, 18*(3), 118–124.

Jeffries, P. R. (2001). Computer versus lecture: A comparison of two methods of teaching oral medication administration in a nursing skills laboratory. *Journal of Nursing Education, 40*(7), 323–328.

Khoiny, F. E. (1995). Factors that contribute to computer-assisted instruction effectiveness. *Computers in Nursing, 13*(4), 165–168.

Kiser, K. M. (1999). Integrating the Internet into lesson plans. *Clinical Laboratory Science, 12*(4), 196–198.

Kozak, J. J., Hancock, P. A., Arthur, E. J., & Chrysler, S. T. (1993). Transfer of training from virtual reality. *Ergonomics, 36*(7), 777–784.

Kulik, C. C., & Kulik, J. A. (1991). Effectiveness of computer-based instruction: An updated analysis. *Computers in Human Behavior, 7,* 75–94.

Kulik, J. A., Kulik, C. C., & Cohen, P. A. (1980). Effectiveness of computer-based college teaching: A meta-analysis of findings. *Review of Educational Research, 50*(4), 525–544.

Leaffer, T., & Gonda, B. (2000). The Internet: An underutilized tool in patient education. *Computers in Nursing, 18*(1), 47–52.

Lyons, C., Krasnowski, J., Greenstein, A., Maloney, D., & Tatarczuk, J. (1982). Interactive computerized patient education. *Heart & Lung, 11*(4), 340–341.

Mallow, G. E., & Gilje, F. (1999). Technology-based nursing education: Overview and call for further dialogue. *Journal of Nursing Education, 38*(6), 248–251.

Mansen, T. J., & Haak, S. W. (1996). Evaluation of a health assessment skills program using a computer videodisc interactive program. *Journal of Nursing Education, 35*(8), 382–384.

Mascara, C., Czar, P., & Hebda, T. (1999). *Internet resource guide for nurses & health care professionals.* Menlo Park, CA: Addison-Wesley.

McNamara, S. (1996). Virtually amazing. *The Journal for Respiratory Care Practitioners, 9*(1), 33–38.

Merril, G. L., & Barker, V. L. (1996). Virtual reality debuts in the teaching laboratory in nursing. *Journal of Intravenous Nursing, 19*(4), 182–187.

Pantelidis, V. S. (1993). Virtual reality in the classroom. *Educational Technology, April,* 23–27.

Rambo, A. (1994). Computer technology: Implications for nurse educators. *Nursing Forum, 29*(4), 30–36.

Ribbons, R. M. (1998). The use of computers as cognitive tools to facilitate higher order thinking skills in nurse education. *Computers in Nursing, 16*(4), 223–228.

Rickelman, B., Taylor-Fox, J., Reisch, J., Payne, P., & Jelemensky, L. (1988). Effect of a CVIS instructional program regarding therapeutic communication on student learning and anxiety. *Journal of Nursing Education 27*(7), 314–320.

Schmidt, S. M., Arndt, M. J., Gaston, S., & Miller, B. J. (1991). *Computers in Nursing, 9*(4), 159–163.

Sinclair, V. G. (1985). The computer as a partner in health care instruction. *Computers in Nursing, 3*(5), 212–216.

Skinner, C. S., Siegfried, J. C., Kegler, M. C., & Strecher, V. J. (1993). The potential of computers in patient education. *Patient Education and Counseling, 22,* 27–34.

Smith, J. M. (1985). Courseware evaluation. *Computers in Nursing, 3*(3), 117–121.

Sparks, S. M., & Rizzolo, M. A. (1998). World Wide Web search tools. *Image, 30*(2), 167–171.

Sternberger, C., & Meyer, L. (2001). Hypermedia-assisted instruction: Authoring with learning guidelines. *Computers in Nursing, 19*(2), 69–74.

Thomson, M. (1998). Multimedia anatomy and physiology lectures for nursing students. *Computers in Nursing, 16*(2), 101–108.

Tibbles, L., Lewis, C., Reisine, S., Rippey, R., & Donald, M. (1992). Computer assisted instruction for preoperative and postoperative patient education in joint replacement surgery. *Computers in Nursing, 10*(5), 208–212.

Tronni, C., & Prawlucki, P. (1998). Designing a computer-based clinical learning lab for staff nurses. *Computers in Nursing, 16*(3), 147–149.

Urick, J., & Bond, E. (1994). Self-instructional laboratories revisited by high technology. *Computers in Nursing, 12*(1), 5–6.

Van Dongen, C. J. (1985). Creating relevant computer-assisted instruction. *Nurse Educator, 10*(1), 21–25.

Virtual reality: A technology in nursing education's future? (1991). *Nursing Educator's Microworld, 5*(3), 17, 19.

Vockell, E. L. (1990). Instructional principles behind computer use. *The Computing Teacher, 7*(3), 10–15.

Walker, D., & Ross, J. M. (1995). Therapeutic computing: Teaching therapeutic communications utilizing a videodisc. *Computers in Nursing, 13*(3), 103–108.

Ward, R. (1997). Implications of computer networking and the Internet for nurse education. *Nurse Education Today, 17,* 178–183.

Weiss, P. L., & Jessel, A. S. (1998). Virtual reality applications to work. *Work, 11*(3), 277–293.

White, M. H., & Dorman, S. M. (2000). Online support for caregivers—Analysis of an Internet Alzheimer mailgroup. *Computers in Nursing, 18*(4), 168–176.

10

Distance Learning

Distance learning has a long history. It began over 150 years ago in the form of correspondence or home study courses (Reinert & Fryback, 1997) and has evolved to its newest form of Web-based courses. Think of distance learning as any method used to connect teachers and learners who are geographically separated. Distance learning today encompasses correspondence courses and courses delivered by satellite, television broadcasting, or telephone lines. The technology involves two-way audio or two-way audio and video technology. Courses delivered by computer via the Internet and the World Wide Web (WWW) are proliferating.

In this chapter, the discussion will first center on the issues and factors that are common to most forms of distance learning. Then more specific information will be given about interactive television modalities and Web-based courses because those are the forms of distance education that are on the cutting edge of technology today.

Advantages and Disadvantages of Distance Learning

The literature describes the benefits and drawbacks of distance learning from the perspectives of both the learner and teacher. The foremost benefit is that people in rural areas or those who are homebound can have greater access to information and even educational degrees. Learners who used to have to travel several hours to attend courses or educational sessions can now receive the information in their homes or at a local site. Other benefits include the accessibility of a larger variety of courses, the ability to learn on one's own time frame (in some cases), the self-directed nature of the learning experience, and the opportunity to learn more about technology. For institutions providing the educational material, distance learning can result in cost savings (Billings, 2000; Chandler & Hanrahan, 2000; Mather, 2000; Reinert & Fryback, 1997; Whalen & Wright, 1999; Whitworth, 1999; Wisher & Priest, 1998).

The primary drawbacks to distance learning include lack of face-to-face contact with the teacher and technology glitches that may be as severe as the system's shutting down and

187

being inaccessible. Some learners may not be able to access the hardware and software they need, and some may struggle with learning to use the technology at the same time they are supposed to be learning content. Some may not learn well with less structure in the educational experience and some may experience feelings of alienation (Cartwright, 2000; Reinert & Fryback, 1997). Approaches to minimizing the disadvantages of distance learning will be discussed along with the specific technologies.

Clinical Education in Distance Learning

One more issue that is common to the various forms of distance learning is the provision of clinical education. If some form of video or computer technology is being used, and learners do not have to come to a campus or central clinical agency, how is clinical learning achieved? The answer is that generally learners are paired up with preceptors in clinical sites near their homes (Mills, 2000). A clinical-site coordinator is usually hired to arrange these placements. In baccalaureate and master's degree programs, site coordinators usually are hired as part-time faculty and must have at least a master's degree. In continuing education programs, the site coordinator may need only a bachelor's degree (Armstrong & Sherwood, 1994).

The role of the site coordinator varies by program. The site coordinator in programs using off-site telecommunications classrooms may help the learners become familiar with the technology. She or he may be present during broadcasting and help to facilitate the class at the remote site. The role may also encompass student recruitment, advisement, and testing. Often, the facilitator becomes a major source of professional and emotional support for the learners (Kelsey, 2000). Whether the program is being delivered by television or computer technology, the site coordinator is hired to seek out and make formal arrangements with preceptors. Orientation of preceptors and evaluation of student learning is also part of the role (Block et al., 1999; Fotos, Douglas, & Wilson, 1994).

In some undergraduate programs in which distance learning is being conducted by interactive television, part-time faculty who live near the remote sites are hired to teach clinical courses (Hoeksel & Moore, 1994). The clinical instructors are familiar with the resources in their geographic area and can provide a rich learning experience for students. Close communication between faculty on campus and clinical faculty is essential in these cases.

Interactive Television Classes

A typical interactive television (ITV) classroom contains a teaching podium with a control panel for the cameras and monitors, a microphone for the teacher, a computer hookup, a document camera (somewhat like an overhead transparency projector), and a fax machine. Also in the front of the room is a large television monitor capable of showing several remote sites at one time or showing the teacher to the remote sites. The teacher usually wears a tracking device so the camera follows him or her around the front of the room. In the back of the room are several monitors that enable the teacher to see students at the remote sites. There is a VCR attached to the front monitors for both recording and playing purposes. At each student's desk there is a microphone and a control pad that moves the camera toward the student when he or she activates the microphone. Figure 10–1 shows the layout of a typical ITV classroom.

There are variations of this equipment, but in most configurations, the plan is to allow each teaching/learning site to be visible and heard and to allow maximum interaction between teacher and students and between students and students. Each remote site is similarly equipped, so transmission can occur from any site. The full-motion video images and voices are carried over special telephone lines. Compressed video technology is less expensive to install because it can be transmitted over regular telephone lines, but the quality of the video is not as good as in full-motion video (Nichols, Beeken, & Wilkerson, 1994). The ITV classroom is very expensive to build, equip, and operate. For this reason, many distance education programs are combining or replacing ITV classroom transmission with Internet-based classes. However, for the near future, many programs will continue to rely on the ITV approach.

When first confronted with this high-tech classroom, instructors may be very intimidated. It is important that they be well oriented to the equipment and conduct at least one trial run before beginning to teach. The instructor needs to know about such basic details as paying attention to his or her clothing. Solid colors transmit the best, and the teacher should avoid very dark or very light colors. Shiny jewelry should be avoided because it can cause too much reflection and be distracting (Zalon, 2000).

The new instructor must learn about pedagogical issues that are important when teaching in an ITV classroom. For example, he or she not only must learn how to operate the equipment but also must be comfortable enough with it that it becomes almost invisible during the learning experience. As Chandler and Hanrahan (2000) state:

> The key to making technology invisible is in knowing how to manage the equipment so that the machines and the miles between the instructor and students disappear. The objective is to forget the distance so that all involved feel like they are having a conversation in the same room. (p. 79)

Students also need to be oriented to the equipment. They should be aware that they must press the microphone on the desk if they want to speak and that the camera will move to put them on the screen when they do so. If the teacher does not bring up the subject of possible student discomfort with the microphone and camera, some students will think they are the only ones who do not like being on "center stage." Discussing the possible discomfort can help students to feel freer to take the first step to pressing the microphone control.

Feelings of Alienation

We know that students at remote sites often feel alienated from the teacher and the home classroom. For this reason, the teacher in the ITV classroom must make a special effort to include students at the remote sites in the discussion and learning activities and try to develop rapport with them. For example, in the first few sessions, learners may be asked to state their name when they speak. Questions may be directed to individuals at all sites on a rotating basis, and students at all sites may be asked periodically if they are keeping up and understanding the material. A little humor goes a long way in helping everyone feel more at ease, so if gentle jokes or teasing about the geographic sites or the technology can be incorporated in

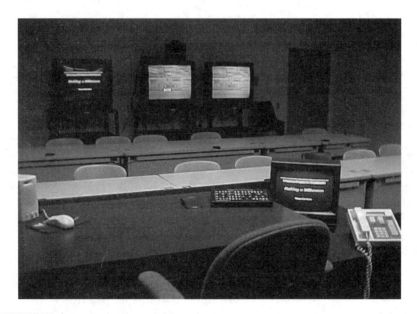

FIGURE 10-1A ITV Classroom as Seen from the Front
Courtesy of William Paterson University.

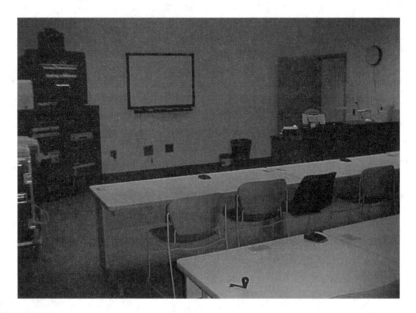

FIGURE 10-1B ITV Classroom as Seen from the Back
Courtesy of William Paterson University.

the class, it is all to the good. If at all possible, the instructor should visit each remote site at least once during the course and broadcast from that site. That practice helps to build rapport with all students, and those at the remote sites will feel less like second-class citizens.

Building some rapport among students at the various sites also leads to a positive experience in distance learning. This can be done by involving students in group projects that cross sites or having students on a listserv or chat room where they are guided by the teacher to interact with each other. Of all the forms of distance learning, ITV technology affords the most normal interaction because all learners and the teacher can hear and see each other. This is considered a distinct advantage over Web-based classes (Smith & Dillon, 1999). Video systems allow everyone involved to see body language and facial expressions and interactions between others. Smith and Dillon report that there is some evidence that "learners who see each other process information differently than learners who do not see each other" (p. 15). Certainly, there is a sense of sharing an experience and an environment that is missing in more independent learning modalities.

Class Management

In addition to paying attention to interpersonal issues, plans must be made to deal with mundane tasks like document transfer and examinations. It is desirable to either mail course materials to all students before the first class or to have materials available on a course Web site. Single handouts can be faxed to remote sites at the beginning of class sessions if there is convenient copying capability in the remote sites. Examinations, if there are any, require logistical planning. In-class written examinations must be prepared well in advance so they can be mailed to the remote sites, stored in a safe place, and distributed during the class. There must be a proctor available at all sites (this is usually the site facilitator). Often, in-class open-book tests are given or take-home exams are used.

Problems with the technology are inevitable. Therefore, the presence of a technician during broadcast times is generally considered essential even though it adds to the cost of the enterprise. Technicians can usually quickly handle minor problems like poor sound levels, cameras that don't rotate, or substandard video quality. However, it is always possible to suffer complete technological or transmission failure, so contingency plans should be discussed in the first class session. Classes should be videotaped so that if the home-site class continues after technological failure, the remote sites can play the video later (Chandler & Hanrahan, 2000).

Uses of Interactive Television

Interactive television technology can be used to deliver information to college students, staff nurses, and patients. The majority of users at present are probably colleges and universities. However, large hospitals, medical centers, and health maintenance organizations are also using ITV classrooms for staff development. Hospital conglomerates and consortiums can maximize the efficiency of some staff development programs by sending them to several sites at one time.

Programs for patients and clients in remote geographic areas are beginning to grow. For example, one large regional hospital transmitted a childbirth preparation class to a remote, small, rural hospital with very good results (Byers, Hilgenberg, & Rhodes, 1999). In the future, many public educational programs on chronic disease maintenance may be conducted in this medium.

Research on Effectiveness of Interactive Television

Distance learning of various types has been studied for the last 30 years and has generally been shown to have positive outcomes for students (Zalon, 2000). In recent years, studies of telecommunications courses have focused primarily on student satisfaction with this type of distance learning. Hoeksel and Moore (1994) reported that although their students preferred face-to-face instruction, they were generally satisfied with ITV learning. Nichols, Beeken, and Wilkerson (1994) found that student satisfaction in their course was inconsistent. Students at remote sites said the ITV course was okay, but they would not recommend it to a friend. Students at the home site also wrote rather negative comments on an evaluation, stating that "they resented having to push the microphone buttons to talk, and resented the efforts of faculty to involve those at the distant sites in discussions" (p. 186). However, on Beeken's scale, students rated the course rather highly on several variables. In 1997, Westbrook studied graduate business students to see if there were differences in satisfaction levels between on-campus and off-campus students and found none. Students at the distant sites, however, reported perceptions of significantly fewer interactions with the teacher. In a study involving 17 courses and 68 remote sites, Biner and colleagues (1997) found that "the most satisfied telecourse students were found at the sites with the fewest students" (p. 28). Block and colleagues (1999) reported that their graduate nursing students were satisfied, overall, with the distance learning experience. Kelsey (2000) studied student interactions in a telecommunications class with five remote sites. She discovered that student participation was minimal. The reasons they gave for failure to interact were technology limitations, camera shyness, fear of appearing stupid, and time constraints. Students at the remote sites reported that their most enjoyable interactions were with the site facilitators; they also relied on the site facilitators to answer most of their questions after class. Kelsey concluded that barriers to interaction led to dissatisfaction with the course. It seems likely that student satisfaction with telecommunications classes depends on the instructor as much as the medium. An experienced teacher who knows how to make all learners feel a part of the class even if they are 200 miles away will probably help to increase learner satisfaction. Also, it seems likely that the more experience learners have with ITV classes, the less dissatisfaction there will be.

A few of the above studies also focused on learning achievement in telecommunications classes. Block and colleagues (1999), Hoeksel and Moore (1994), and Nichols and colleagues (1994) found no difference in student achievement in remote-site students or home-site students. Machtmes and Asher (2000) performed a meta-analysis of 19 studies on the effectiveness of telecommunications courses that compared learning achievement in telecourses to traditional instruction. The conclusion was that there did not appear to be a difference in achievement between distance and traditional learners.

Some studies and reports have examined teacher satisfaction with telecommunications distance learning (Block et al., 1999; Hoeksel & Moore, 1994; Reinert & Fryback, 1997; Whitworth, 1999). Results vary, with some teachers reporting high satisfaction and others low satisfaction levels. Satisfaction appears to increase as more experience is gained with telecommunications classes. Sources of dissatisfaction include a sense of isolation from remote-site students and technological problems.

Distance Learning via the Internet

Classes delivered via the Internet and the WWW are usually termed *online* or *Web-based* classes. Such courses are expanding exponentially as academia, business, and health care organizations are all getting into the business of distance learning and believe that online courses can be cost effective.

Synchronous Versus Asynchronous Classes

Synchronous online learning occurs when people interact in real time electronically via the Internet or intranet. Much more common are asynchronous applications in which materials are located on a Web page that can be accessed at any time at the learners' convenience. Whether classes are synchronous or asynchronous, the role of the teacher is to guide the learners and keep them on track, while providing support and motivation (Smith & Dillon, 1999).

Development of Web-Based Courses

Developing a Web-based course is not an easy task. In most cases, the development requires the combined efforts of the instructor or content expert and an instructional designer or educational technologist. They begin by determining the course objectives and desired outcomes. Then decisions are made about how best to design the delivery of the content and activities that will produce those outcomes. Teaching strategies may consist of printed or audio-recorded lectures on the Web site, assigned readings in a textbook or in periodicals, or a variety of visuals (videos, slides, multimedia presentations). Frequently, students are asked to go to other Web sites for more information or for active learning exercises. Many different teaching strategies may be built in such as simulations, debates, problem-based learning exercises, and logs and journals. Quizzes and examinations may also be given via the Web site, and the course syllabus is accessed via the Web site. In addition, there are usually discussion forums (threaded or topic-based discussions) and e-mail between teacher and learners or between learners who may be working on group projects. A common model for online courses is one in which half of the course involves self-instruction through the use of teacher-provided online materials, simulations, and analysis of online data. The other half of the course involves either synchronous or asynchronous discussions between teacher and student or between student and student (Kozlowski, 2002; Langford & Hardin, 1999).

Good online course discussions require planning. First, you must decide if course discussions are going to be synchronous or asynchronous. The advantages and disadvantages of each may be seen in Tables 10–1 and 10–2. Another decision to be made is whether all students will participate together in one discussion or in smaller groups. Class size will weigh heavily in this determination. For example, if there are 40 students in the class, there will be many postings to the discussion page, making it difficult for the students to keep up with the volume. You may divide the class into two discussion groups to keep the postings within reasonable bounds for the students, although you will still have to read them all. This is one of

TABLE 10-1 Advantages and Disadvantages of Synchronous Discussions (Chat Rooms)

Advantages	Disadvantages
Mimics normal conversation.	All learners must be available at the same time.
Discussion takes place efficiently in "real time."	Discussion progresses quickly and depth of ideas may suffer.
Can involve professional guests.	Slow typists may not participate as much.

the reasons why online courses are usually limited to no more than 25 students (Peterson, Hennig, Dow, & Sole, 2001).

You must make your expectations and instructions clear regarding the conduct of the discussion. Instructions may include information about using the technology, requiring an antivirus program, netiquette, time frames, and grammar and spelling. Expectations about more substantive aspects of the discussion may include required readings to be done before the discussion and the citing of references to back up opinions.

Planning the content of the discussion is crucial, just as it is for in-class, face-to-face discussions. You might start with a few thought-provoking questions and have a few questions "in your pocket" to keep the discussion moving in a meaningful direction. You might also make the learners responsible for posing discussion questions related to course content.

In an academic course, students are usually evaluated and graded on their discussions. For example, they may earn points for the number of postings that meet certain standards. Expectations must be clear before evaluation begins, so that students will not think they will earn points for saying, "I agree with that last comment" (Peterson et al., 2001).

Software is available to bring course development within the capabilities of the average teacher. For example, tools like WebCT (Universal Learning Technology, Inc.), TopClass (WBT Systems), Course Wizard (Ball State University), and many others serve as authoring and management tools that help to build Web courses (Geibert, 2000; Leasure, Davis, & Thievon, 2000; Mills, 2000; Ryan, Carlton, & Ali, 1999).

Advantages and Disadvantages of Online Courses

Online courses have some unique advantages. Access to classes is even greater than with telecommunications classrooms since the learner does not have to leave home, except for

TABLE 10-2 Advantages and Disadvantages of Asynchronous Discussions (Listservs or Bulletin Boards)

Advantages	Disadvantages
Learners and teacher may log on at any time.	Procrastinators may not get involved in some of the discussion.
There is adequate time to think through responses.	Postings may become very lengthy and time consuming to read.

clinical learning. Convenience is maximized in asynchronous learning formats because the learner can learn anywhere, anytime. One of the greatest benefits of online courses is that they cause the participants to be active learners. They are not sitting and listening to a lecture but must find information via technology, discuss it, and perhaps use active learning Web sites (Niederhauser, Bigley, Hale, & Harper, 1999).

Branching within the software programs is another advantage. Branching refers to the options the learner has available to move around in the learning sequence. He or she can skip over familiar material, spend more time on the unfamiliar, and choose whatever sequence fits his or her learning style (Smith & Dillon, 1999). Pacing relates to the control of the timing of events. Some courses are totally learner controlled, with no deadlines. Such courses have lower retention rates, probably because many learners are not as self-disciplined as they need to be with independent learning (Smith & Dillon, 1999). Most online courses have some pacing built in, with the instructor determining certain deadlines and due dates. As compared to ITV classes, online classes seem to have no problem with generating interaction among learners. Through various discussion group formats, learners interact in valuable ways with each other, whether they are solving group problems or just getting feedback on their ideas (Leasure, Davis, & Thievon, 2000).

Unfortunately, there are also some drawbacks to online learning. Most people agree that although online learning has its place, it is "not an adequate substitute for the full, rich experience of the classroom" (Womack, Lyons, Roskos, Byrne, & Staggers, 1999, p. 212). Visual cues are absent, and meaning in written discussion may be slightly distorted without the body language that goes with it. Although clarification and feedback can be given, they are usually not immediate. These disadvantages, though, may be outweighed by the advantages already listed.

The technology involved in delivering online courses may be a distinct drawback. Some learners do not own or have ready access to computers. Many, especially older learners, do not have the computer literacy skills they need to master a Web-based course, even though they may think they do before they begin. Valuable course time may be lost while people try to learn the rudiments of the skills they need. For example, they may have problems in uploading files and charts to the Web (Mather, 2000). Weston and colleagues (1999) point out that although learners may have a computer and the basic skills they need, the capability of their computers may not be adequate. They may not have enough memory, correct software, or peripheral devices such as a CD-ROM, and purchasing what they need may be expensive in addition to their online charges. The various browsers learners use may present information differently and thus be confusing for them. As with any type of technology, learners who have more experience with online classes report greater ease of use and greater comfort levels (Vrasidas & McIsaac, 1999).

Disadvantages also exist for teachers. Academic faculty who have had experience with teaching online courses often say they spend more time than they do teaching traditional classes. Some of that time is devoted to typing comments on students' written work; that may take longer than jotting notes in the margins of a hard-copy paper. Some faculty report that because it so easy for students to send in drafts of their papers, they end up writing and asking for feedback on more drafts than they would in a traditional course (Cravener, 1999). Written e-mail messages may take longer than would a face-to-face conversation in the classroom, and technology glitches may also add to faculty workload.

Uses of Online Education

Presently most distance education online is taking place in colleges and universities. They are producing courses for undergraduate and graduate students, with special emphasis on RN to BSN programs and advanced practice graduate programs. Many universities and for-profit companies are also developing continuing education courses for nurses. A quick search of the Internet will reveal myriad courses for professional development in many specialties.

Although there is a great deal of health-related information on the Web, to date there are few if any online courses designed for patient teaching. It is only a matter of time, though, before health care facilities or organizations decide that online courses are an effective means of providing patient and community education.

Research on Online Courses

Research designed to test differences in level of learning between traditional and online learning have found at least equivalent learning as measured by course end examinations (Bachman & Panzarine, 1998; Billings, 2000; Leasure, Davis, & Thievon, 2000; Rosenlund, Damask-Bembenek, Hugie, & Matsumura, 1999; Yucha & Princen, 2000). Research has also found, not surprisingly, that online learning improves computer competency skills (Billings, 2000; Niederhauser et al., 1999; Ryan, Carlton, & Ali, 1999). Studies on professional socialization in distance education have demonstrated that socialization scores of distance learners are at least equivalent to the scores of learners in traditional programs (Cragg, Plotnikoff, Hugo, & Casey, 2001; Nessler, Hanner, Melburg, & McGowan, 2001). Learner satisfaction studies have shown conflicting results. Many report satisfied learners (Niederhauser, Bigley, Hale, & Harper, 1999; Soon, Sook, Jung, & Im, 2000; Womack et al., 1999). However, some found students were dissatisfied with the technology (Ryan et al., 1999; Soon et al., 2000), some with the heavy workload (Soon et al., 2000; Vrasidas & McIsaac, 1999), and some with the isolation from teacher and other students (Billings, 2000; Ryan et al., 1999). Research has just begun into the nature and quality of online discussion in Web-based courses (Teikmanis & Armstrong, 2001; VandeVusse & Hanson, 2000).

Web-Enhanced Courses

Experienced faculty who have been involved with distance learning are realizing that since traditional education and online education both have strengths and weaknesses, they can build on the strengths of both by combining them. For example, a course may be primarily online, but students may be asked to come to classes or seminars on campus two or three times during the semester; or a class may be primarily held on campus, but some work is done online throughout the semester. Web-enhanced courses may involve giving students assignments related to Web sites (not requiring them to come to class those days), having an ongoing discussion group online, or giving some course materials via a course homepage. Having some face-to-face contact with students counteracts the disadvantages of lack of personal interaction and isolation.

New ways of using the Internet or telecommunications for education are still evolving. It is important for educators to keep abreast of changing technology and its potential for learning purposes.

CASE STUDY

You are a part-time graduate student living in a rural area, and you are enrolled in a distance learning master's program. Most of your classes are transmitted via ITV from the university to a remote site 10 miles from your home. A few courses are also available on the WWW, and you always have the option of attending classes on the main campus.

Your employer will pay tuition reimbursement for your ITV classes but is reluctant to pay for Web-based courses. The reason is that employers are not sure of the quality of online courses, and they have no way of knowing if the employee is doing the work or someone else is doing it.

1. Why would an employer differentiate between the quality of ITV and Web-based courses?
2. What evidence can you collect about the quality of Web-based courses?
3. How can universities provide assurance to employers that the employee is indeed doing the work?
4. If you have the choice of all three formats, would you primarily take courses on campus, via ITV, or via the Internet?

CRITICAL THINKING EXERCISES

1. You are a director of staff development in a medical center. Some of your staff have asked you to recommend distance learning continuing education courses. Should you ever recommend continuing education courses? What are the implications of making such a recommendation?
2. How can you account for the fact that professional socialization in undergraduate distance learning programs is at least equivalent to that in traditional nursing programs? What are the factors that contribute to professional socialization?
3. Some observers have identified a "digital divide" in our country—that is, the fact that the "haves" in our society often own computers and the "have-nots" may not own computers. Those without the means to own a computer do not have ready access to health information on the WWW. How much should this issue weigh in a hospital's decision to provide most of its preventive health care information on their Web site as opposed to their previous practice of having a telephone information service?

IDEAS FOR FURTHER RESEARCH

1. In a particular community, investigate how much interest there is in receiving health information on the WWW.

2. Conduct a study to determine what percentage of patients affiliated with a health care organization are able and willing to receive Web-based information postdischarge.

3. Interview faculty as to what they believe are their roles in distance learning.

4. Survey colleges and universities to find how they support and reward faculty who develop distance learning courses or programs.

5. Observe and analyze discussion in ITV classes with several remote sites. What discussion techniques are most effective?

REFERENCES

Armstrong, M. L., & Sherwood, G. D. (1994). Site coordinators: A critical component in providing quality nursing education at distance sites. *Journal of Nursing Education, 33*(4), 175–177.

Bachman, J. A., & Panzarine, S. (1998). Enabling student nurses to use the information superhighway. *Journal of Nursing Education, 37*(4), 155–161.

Billings, D. M. (2000). A framework for assessing outcomes and practices in web-based courses in nursing. *Journal of Nursing Education, 39*(2), 60–67.

Biner, P. M., Welsh, K. D., Barone, N. M., Summers, M., & Dean, R. S. (1997). The impact of remote-site group size on student satisfaction and relative performance in interactive telecourses. *The American Journal of Distance Education, 11*(1), 23–33.

Block, D. E., Josten, L. E., Lia-Hoagberg, B., Bearinger, L. H., Kerr, M. J., Smith, M. J., Lewis, M. L., & Hutton, S. J. (1999). Fulfilling regional needs for specialty nurses through limited-cohort graduate education. *Nursing Outlook, 47*(1), 23–29.

Byers, D. L., Hilgenberg, C., & Rhodes, D. M. (1999). Telemedicine for patient education. *The American Journal of Distance Education, 13*(3), 52–62.

Cartwright, J. (2000). Lessons learned: Using asynchronous computer-mediated conferencing to facilitate group discussion. *Journal of Nursing Education, 39*(2), 87–90.

Chandler, G. E., & Hanrahan, P. (2000). Teaching using interactive video: Creating connections. *Journal of Nursing Education, 39*(2), 73–80.

Cragg, C. E., Plotnikoff, R. C., Hugo, K., & Casey, A. (2001). Perspective transformation in RN-to-BSN distance education. *Journal of Nursing Education, 40*(7), 317–322.

Cravener, P. A. (1999). Faculty experiences with providing online courses: Thorns among the roses. *Computers in Nursing, 17*(1), 42–47.

Fotos, J. C., Douglas, B. H., & Wilson, L. L. (1994). Clinical experiences for BSN students in a satellite telecommunication project. *Journal of Nursing Education, 33*(4), 181–183.

Geibert, R. C. (2000). Integrating Web-based instruction into a graduate nursing program taught via videoconferencing: Challenges and solutions. *Computers in Nursing, 18*(1), 26–34.

Hoeksel, R., & Moore, J. F. (1994). Clinical nursing education at a distance: Solving instructor interaction problems. *Journal of Nursing Education, 33*(4), 178–180.

Kelsey, K. D. (2000). Participant interaction in a course delivered by interactive compressed video technology. *The American Journal of Distance Education, 14*(1), 63–74.

Kozlowski, D. (2002). Using online learning in a traditional face-to-face environment. *Computers in Nursing, 20*(1), 23–30.

Langford, D. R., & Hardin, S. (1999). Distance learning: Issues emerging as the paradigm shifts. *Nursing Science Quarterly, 12*(3), 191–196.

Leasure, A. R., Davis, L., Thievon, S. L. (2000). Comparison of student outcomes and preferences in a traditional vs. World Wide Web–based baccalaureate nursing research course. *Journal of Nursing Education, 39*(4), 149–154.

Machtmes, K., & Asher, J. W. (2000). A meta-analysis of the effectiveness of telecourses in distance education. *The American Journal of Distance Education, 14*(1), 27–46.

Mather, M. A. (2000). In-service to go: Professional development online. *Technology & Learning, 20*(6), 18–28.

Mills, A. C. (2000). Creating Web-based, multimedia and interactive courses for distance learning. *Computers in Nursing, 18*(3), 125–131.

Nessler, M. S., Hanner, M. B., Melburg, V., & McGowan, S. (2001). Professional socialization of baccalaureate nursing students: Can students in distance nursing programs become socialized? *Journal of Nursing Education, 40*(7), 293–302.

Nichols, E. G., Beeken, J. E., & Wilkerson, N. N. (1994). Distance delivery through compressed video. *Journal of Nursing Education, 33*(4), 184–186.

Niederhauser, V. P., Bigley, M. B., Hale, J., & Harper, D. (1999). Cybercases: An innovation in Internet education. *Journal of Nursing Education, 38*(9), 415–418.

Peterson, J. Z., Hennig, L. M., Dow, K. H., & Sole, M. L. (2001). Designing and facilitating class discussion in an Internet class. *Nurse Educator, 26*(1), 28–32.

Reinert, B. R., & Fryback, P. B. (1997). Distance learning and nursing education. *Journal of Nursing Education, 36*(9), 421–427.

Rosenlund, C., Damask-Bembenek, B., Hugie, P., & Matsumura, G. (1999). The development of online courses for undergraduate nursing education. *Nursing and Health Care Perspectives, 20*(4), 194–198.

Ryan, M., Carlton, K. H., & Ali, N. S. (1999). Evaluation of traditional classroom teaching methods versus course delivery via the World Wide Web. *Journal of Nursing Education, 38*(6), 272–277.

Smith, P. L., & Dillon, C. L. (1999). Comparing distance learning and classroom learning: Conceptual considerations. *The American Journal of Distance Education, 13*(2), 6–23.

Soon, K. H., Sook, K. I., Jung, C. W., and Im, K. M. (2000). The effects of Internet-based distance learning in nursing. *Computers in Nursing, 18*(1), 19–25.

Teikmanis, M., & Armstrong, J. (2001). Teaching pathophysiology to diverse students using an online discussion board. *Computers in Nursing, 19*(2), 75–81.

VandeVusse, L., & Hanson, L. (2000). Evaluation of online course discussions. *Computers in Nursing, 18*(4), 181–188.

Vrasidas, C., & McIsaac, M. S. (1999). Factors influencing interaction in an online course. *The American Journal of Distance Education, 13*(3), 22–36.

Westbrook, T. S. (1997). Changes in students' attitudes toward graduate business instruction via interactive television. *The American Journal of Distance Education, 11*(1), 55–69.

Weston, C., Gandell, T., McAlpine, L., & Finkelstein, A. (1999). Designing instruction for the context of online learning. *The Internet and Higher Education, 2*(1), 35–44.

Whalen, T., & Wright, D. (1999). Methodology for cost-benefit analysis of Web-based tele-learning: Case study of the Bell Online Institute. *The American Journal of Distance Education, 13*(1), 24–44.

Whitworth, J. M. (1999). Looking at distance learning through both ends of the camera. *American Journal of Distance Education, 13*(2), 64–73.

Wisher, R. A., & Priest, A. N. (1998). Cost-effectiveness of audio teletraining for the U.S. Army National Guard. *The American Journal of Distance Education, 12*(1), 38–51.

Womack, D., Lyons, A., Roskos, J., Byrne, F., & Staggers, N. (1999). Student perspectives on creating completely Web-based graduate programs in nursing informatics. *Computers in Nursing, 17*(5), 212–214.

Yucha, C., & Princen, T. (2000). Insights learned from teaching pathophysiology on the World Wide Web. *Journal of Nursing Education, 39*(2), 68–72.

Zalon, M. L. (2000). A prime-time primer for distance education. *Nurse Educator, 25*(1), 28–33.

11

Teaching Psychomotor Skills

The amount of attention given to teaching psychomotor skills in nursing education has waxed and waned over the decades in the United States and in many other countries. The issue was, and continues to be, what skills professional nurses need to learn versus what skills should be learned and performed by technical and ancillary personnel. An educator's philosophy of what constitutes professional and technical nursing plays a crucial role in the amount of emphasis placed on the teaching and learning of psychomotor skills. The definition of nursing psychomotor skills used in this chapter is skills that are action oriented, that require neuromuscular coordination, and that promote patient healing and/or comfort.

History of Teaching Psychomotor Skills

For centuries, the primary focus of nursing was on "practical skills" or the "art of nursing" that emphasized hands-on "doing" for patients (Bjork, 1997; Love, McAdams, Patton, Rankin, & Roberts, 1989). Educators were concerned about students mastering skills before coming into contact with patients, so students spent many hours of their "probationary" period in a nursing arts or fundamentals of nursing laboratory practicing psychomotor skills. Skills at this time were considered to be not just motor activity, but motor activity plus attention, concern, and compassion to be shown to patients (Bjork, 1999).

In the 1960s, nurses wanted a unique identity, apart from medicine, and saw one way to achieve that as distancing nursing from the medical model and task-based practice. At the same time, nurses attempted to change to a more professional model of education, moving the site of education from the hospital to the university. The university venue brought its own pressures that further moved nursing education away from concentration on skills (Sweeney, Hedstrom, & O'Malley, 1982). For example, there was the need to incorporate many hours of liberal arts education into the curriculum, which displaced hours previously spent on nursing knowledge and skills. In addition, students were placed in a variety of clinical agencies that differed greatly from the hospital, such as clinics, schools, industry, and public health, in which few of the traditional hands-on skills were used. Those agencies that did use traditional skills each had their own procedures and equipment, so students had to make adaptations to the skills learned in the university classes and laboratories. Finally, as Sweeney and colleagues point out, some educators had a futuristic vision of nursing in which technologies were seen as changing so rapidly that there was no point in spending a lot of time teaching skills that would change by the time of graduation. The growth of staff development departments in health care agencies made it possible for many of these skills to be learned during orientation to the work site after graduation.

Finally, the proposed differentiation of technical from professional nursing caused many educators to conclude that technical nurses and technicians should perform most psychomotor skills while professional nurses would excel in planning, leading, and evaluating care and using the skills of communication and problem solving. As a result of many of these influences, schools of nursing began to ignore or dismantle their nursing arts laboratories (if they even had them), and nurses entering the work world, especially baccalaureate graduates, entered with few of the psychomotor skills that their employers still expected them to have.

The pendulum began to swing back in the 1980s when employers of new graduates became vocal about the impossibility of teaching new graduates all the skills they needed to know in a time frame that was economically feasible (Love et al., 1989). Preceptorships were developed, in part, in response to the need to have supervision of new graduate nurses who were deficient in technical skills. Students became more aware of their rights as consumers, and many expressed the need to graduate feeling confident in their ability to perform psychomotor skills.

In the 1980s, and continuing today, the interest in returning to campus laboratories to teach at least rudimentary skills has increased, and there is increased emphasis on perfecting skills in the clinical setting. Faculty are increasingly aware of the difficulty of having students practice psychomotor skills for the first time in clinical areas. Safety issues for patients, demands by informed patients for expert care, and anxiety of students having to perform for the first time in front of patients have driven educators back to campus labs.

Bjork (1999) has pointed out that with this move back to the teaching of psychomotor skills in campus laboratories, more emphasis has been placed on the motor aspects of skill learning, with deemphasis on the theoretical and caring aspects of applying skills. Alavi, Loh, and Reilly (1991) take the position that nursing skills are more than motor activity. They state that:

> Psychomotor skill competency is evidenced through performance which includes efficient and effective neuro-muscular co-ordination, knowledge of underlying theory and principles which guide its rationale for use and processes involved in its execution, with a sensitivity in carrying it out with clients so as to reflect their inherent worth and dignity. (p. 957)

Bjork and Kirkevold (2000) have developed a model of skill performance in nursing that incorporates background knowledge of the skill; motor components; and the verbal support, caring, and instruction that patients need during performance of the skill. The authors assert that learners must begin to integrate all these aspects of a skill as they learn it. If integration is left to the time when skills are performed in the clinical setting, it may not occur at all.

There seems to be general acceptance of the fact that psychomotor skills should be learned in the basic educational program in campus laboratories followed by continued practice in clinical areas, with further refining of skills during work orientations and preceptorships. The question remains: How best can skills be taught? There is a dearth of research on the teaching of psychomotor skills in nursing (Knight, 1998). Much of the research on which we depend has come from the fields of sport and exercise science, applied to nursing.

Nurse researchers need to devote effort to studying the most effective and efficient ways of teaching skills (Beeson & Kring, 1999).

Learning Psychomotor Skills

The literature describes several models of how people learn to perform psychomotor skills. The model described by Gentile (1972) is still a classic in the field. This model describes stages that learners go through. Definitions of terms related to this model and to the learning of psychomotor skills in general can be found in Table 11–1.

Phases of Skill Learning

Gentile divides skill learning into two main stages: "getting the idea of the movement" and "fixation/diversification." Within these two main phases are several cognitive and behavioral patterns.

STAGE ONE: GETTING THE IDEA OF THE MOVEMENT

The initial step in getting the idea of the movement is having a goal. That is, the learner is confronted with a clear-cut need or problem. For example, the need may be to catheterize a patient's bladder, and the goal is to learn to do so.

Many stimuli affect the learner and his or her environment at this point, some of which relate to the goal and some not. All stimuli that influence motor activity are called *regulatory stimuli* and must be attended to. The learner must devote selective attention to the regula-

---

TABLE 11–1 Terms Related to Psychomotor Skill Learning

Regulatory stimuli: External conditions that influence or regulate skill performance and to which the learner must pay attention.

Nonregulatory stimuli: External conditions that do not influence skill performance.

Closed skill: A skill performed under stable environmental conditions and stimuli.

Open skill: A skill performed under changing environmental conditions and stimuli.

Motor plan: A general mental preconception of what movements will be required to perform a skill.

Fixation: Practicing the skill in the same way each time to fix a reproducible pattern in memory.

Diversification: Practicing the skill in a variety of ways so that it can be reproduced in a modified way to meet changing environments at any time.

Arousal: A state of being stirred to action. If arousal is too high, excitability results. If arousal is too low, passivity results.

Intrinsic feedback: Awareness of performance that arises from within the individual.

Extrinsic (augmented) feedback: Awareness of performance that is supplied by an external source.

Massed practice: Continuously repeated practice sessions with very short or no rest periods between trials.

Distributed practice: Practice sessions interspersed with rest periods.

Sources: Gentile, A. M. (1987). Skill acquisition: Action, movement, and neuromotor processes. In J. H. Carr & R. B. Shepherd (Eds.), *Movement science: Foundations for physical therapy in rehabilitation* (pp. 93–154). Rockville, MD: Aspen; and Magill, R. A. (1998). *Motor learning: Concepts and applications* (5th ed.). Boston, MA: WCB McGraw-Hill.

tory stimuli in order to form an effective plan of movements that will attain the goal. Learners often have difficulty in determining which stimuli are relevant and which are not. In the case of learning urinary catheterization, the student must selectively attend to the necessary equipment; the verbal, visual, or written instructions; the position of the patient; the anxiety of the patient; the need for privacy; and so on. Stimuli that must be tuned out are irrelevant talk and noise in the environment, unnecessary equipment, and stimuli from the nurse's own body, such as an itchy nose. *Nonregulatory stimuli* are those that do not influence the skill performance, such as the color of the disinfectant.

If the skill to be learned is a closed skill, the learner's task in sorting out stimuli is not too difficult. A *closed skill* is one in which environmental conditions and relevant stimuli remain stable throughout and possibly across performances (Gentile, 1987). An example of a closed skill is handwashing and making an unoccupied bed. Most skills as they are being practiced in a laboratory are considered closed skills because lab conditions are usually held constant. When skills are performed in a clinical setting, most of them become *open skills* because they take place in a changing environment, and regulatory stimuli vary throughout the performance of the skill. A catheterization performed on a live patient is an open skill because the patient may talk, cry, or move during the procedure. Giving an injection to a squirming infant is another prime example of an open skill. Open skills, then, are more difficult for the learner because of unpredictable and changing stimuli to which attention must be given.

Once the learner recognizes and attends to the necessary stimuli, he or she will begin to plan movements to meet the environmental demands. This *motor plan* is a general mental preconception of what movements will be required to attain the goal. The learner then executes this motor plan with greater or lesser success.

STAGE TWO: FIXATION/DIVERSIFICATION

If the learner was not successful in reaching the goal of the skill, he or she would need to again go through the process of getting the idea of the movement. When the performance is successful, the learner proceeds to the stage of *fixation/diversification*. In *fixation*, the person must practice and refine the skill until it can be reproduced in the same way at any time. In *diversification*, the learner must practice performing the skill in changing environments so it can be modified as necessary at any time. Generally, closed skills result in fixation, but open skills require diversification (Magill, 1998). During this time, the learner refines his or her performance, alters it as necessary to meet new stimuli, and, in the process, fixes it in memory.

Attention

Everyone knows that we cannot pay attention to everything around us at one time. As just mentioned, learners must use selective attention when performing a skill, or they would be distracted from the priorities of the moment. But, sometimes, the problem for learners is not limiting their attention, but the difficulty of paying attention to several essential stimuli at one time. For example, teachers sometimes say that students have tunnel vision when they are learning a new task. They say things like, "You did very well with that catheterization, but you didn't talk to the patient while you were doing it." How do we account for this tunnel vision effect?

The *bottleneck theory* of attention (Allport, 1980) proposes that our information processing system can handle a limited number of stimuli at one time. Competing stimuli reach a bottleneck where some stimuli are filtered out consciously or unconsciously. People have the ability to give preference to certain stimuli at the expense of others (Schneider, Dumais, & Shiffrin, 1984).

Newer theories of attention hypothesize that humans have *limited availability of resources* (i.e., neural and mental resources) to carry out all the activities that may be attempted at one time (Magill, 1998). The amount and allocation of resources vary with the individual and are influenced by internal and external factors. One external factor is the attention demands of the task itself. *Arousal* is one important internal influencing factor. If the arousal level is too high (excitability) or too low (passivity), attention may suffer.

People learn to focus their attention to necessary stimuli through coaching and practice. Research indicates that one helpful strategy to focus attention while performing a closed skill is first to prepare by using muscle relaxation techniques and breathing control. Second, the person can use visualization or mental imagery to internally experience the skill before performing it. Third, the person can focus by concentrating on an important segment of the skill to be performed (Magill, 1998).

Feedback

Every learner needs feedback during practice sessions. Feedback may be *intrinsic* or *extrinsic*. Intrinsic feedback originates within the learner. It is like a little internal voice that tells us we performed well or we did something wrong compared to a performance standard that we have internalized.

Extrinsic feedback is supplied by the teacher or another objective source. It is sometimes called *augmented* feedback because it augments our own internal feedback. Experts in the field of motor learning have identified two forms of augmented feedback: *knowledge of results* (KR) and *knowledge of performance* (KP). Knowledge of results refers to external verbal feedback about performance outcomes. Knowledge of performance is external information about the action process involved in the performance (Swinnen, 1996). Both forms of augmented feedback are useful.

A learner should be allowed to benefit from intrinsic feedback before being given extrinsic feedback. After finishing a skill performance, the learner should have a short time in which to sense whether his or her motor plan was appropriate and whether outcomes were achieved. In fact, guiding learners to attend to intrinsic feedback is a way educators can help them learn to learn. In situations when verbal extrinsic feedback is being given, timing is important. Although the educator should give the learner time to assimilate the skill movements before giving feedback, the delay should not be too long. Research has confirmed that extrinsic feedback is most effective when no interfering activity occurs between the skill performance and the accompanying feedback (Gomez & Gomez, 1984).

Most learners fail to improve during practice without solid feedback. Recall the learning proposition from Chapter 2, "Sheer repetition without indications of improvement or any kind of reinforcement is a poor way to attempt to learn." One of the challenges of independent learning in a psychomotor skills laboratory (or for patients in their homes) is the lack of verbal extrinsic or augmented feedback. In these cases, there is heavy reliance on intrinsic feedback and on nonverbal extrinsic feedback. The learner must have a good mental representation of the skill to have it serve as a template for all performance (Milde, 1988). He or she must mentally compare present performance against the template. Videotape of the performance for later feedback with self-critique is sometimes used in skills laboratories but has been found to be of limited usefulness unless the video is viewed while comparing it to a standard printed checklist as a reference point. During self-instruction, there should be frequent reference to the original learning materials (Milde, 1988).

Practice

The second stage of Gentile's model, fixation/diversification, has important teaching implications. In this stage, the general motor pattern is practiced and refined as the learner attempts to reach an adequate skill level. Closed skills lend themselves fairly quickly to fixation, but open skills require a refinement of a variety of motor patterns to achieve diversification.

The teacher's role in this stage is to arrange for or even to supervise practice. Practice is essential in order to fix the sequential order of movements in the learner's memory, but the amount of practice needed varies with the complexity of the skill, the learner's motivation, and knowledge of related skills. Practice enables the learner to become masterful at performing the skill smoothly, with greater control, and less wasted time and motion.

Many researchers have studied timing and sequencing of skill practice. The efficacy of massed practice versus distributed practice and the relative length of practice versus rest periods have been the focus of most studies. *Massed practice* refers to repeated practice sessions with very short or no rest periods between trials. *Distributed practice* includes planned rest periods between trials. Generalizations that can be drawn from the literature (Garrison & Magoon, 1972; Magill, 1998) are:

1. People learn psychomotor skills best using a greater number of short practice sessions rather than fewer long sessions.
2. Distributed practice is generally better than massed practice.
3. Practice must be long enough for the learner to make appreciable progress; rest periods must be short enough that forgetting does not occur.

The actual length of practice and rest periods will vary with the particular skill.

It is important for educators to be aware of the fact that in spite of practice, learners do not always show steady improvement. They sometimes reach a *learning plateau* in which improvement is arrested or performance even slips. The reasons for this plateau are unclear but are thought to be due to change of motivation or attention. Some theorists believe this unpredictable behavior is related to a natural phenomenon called *nonlinear dynamics,* which postulates that behavior does not always follow an expected smooth trajectory (Wallace, 1996). Many educators have encountered this phenomenon. For instance, you may have taught diabetic patients how to draw up insulin. They seem to be learning very well and making progress, but all of a sudden, after a few successful practice sessions, everything seems to go awry and they cannot seem to do anything right. Knowing that this change in performance sometimes happens helps educators to show patience with learners.

MENTAL PRACTICE

Mental practice is a technique that has been widely studied in movement science and applied in physical education. The basic premise is that learners can improve their skill level not only by physical practice but also by mental practice. A moving model of correct performance is implanted in the mind, and that model can be pulled up and used as needed (Eaton & Evans, 1986).

After more than 50 years of use by other disciplines, nurse educators are beginning to apply what is known about mental practice (also known as mental imagery, mental rehearsal, guided imagery, and visualization) to teaching psychomotor skills in nursing. In 1967, Richardson reviewed 25 studies on the ability of mental practice to improve motor skills such as tennis drives, juggling, and card sorting. Eleven of the studies showed statistically significant relationships between the use of mental practice and improved performance. Seven more studies showed a positive trend toward the effectiveness of mental practice. Differences among study results have been attributed to the fact that people vary in their imaging abilities (Bucher, 1993).

Several nursing studies have also been conducted, with conflicting results. One study found that students who used mental practice plus physical practice to learn sterile gloving technique performed better than those who used mental practice or physical practice alone (Bucher, 1993). Doheny (1993) found no significant difference in performing intramuscular injection technique among three groups, those using physical practice only, those using mental practice only, and those using a combination of the two, and Bachman (1990) found no difference between mental practice and physical practice in registered nurses being recertified in cardiopulmonary resuscitation (CPR). These studies lend credence to the effectiveness of mental practice. If, in the future, enough nursing studies show that mental practice alone is sufficient for achieving competence in certain skills, significant changes could be made in the way psychomotor skills are taught.

Two more nursing studies have added to the information we have about mental practice. Eaton and Evans (1986) tried to determine whether "nursing students who had low ability to form images could have their imaging ability enhanced through the use of imaging exercises" (p. 193). They found that after only two brief practice sessions the abilities of subjects with previously low imagery were significantly enhanced, and in fact these subjects surpassed the high-imagery group. Speck (1990) examined the effect of guided imagery (relaxation plus mental practice) on anxiety levels of nursing students giving their first injection and found that the group that received imagery was significantly less anxious.

To use the mental practice process in teaching psychomotor skills, you first have to analyze a skill and separate it into sequential steps. Then you have to combine the procedural steps with instructions on how to implement the mental practice. Full instructions should be written out if you expect the learner to use the process at home. When meeting with the learners, first introduce the concept of mental imagery and explain how it can be useful in learning psychomotor skills. Structure the environment to reduce distracting stimuli such as noise or bright lights. If the learners seem anxious or have been rushing around prior to this session, you might have them perform some relaxation exercises such as taking deep breaths and consciously relaxing each limb. Instruct the learners to sit in a comfortable position and close their eyes. Closing the eyes is optional, because when practicing on their own the learners may have to read the instruction sheet; in a group session, it is effective in helping the learners concentrate.

Begin the instructional practice sequence in a soft voice. A typical session for a simple skill like handwashing might go something like this:

1. Close your eyes.
2. Picture yourself standing in front of a sink. The sink has one spout and both hot and cold water faucets. There is a soap dispenser on the wall above the sink to the right. There is a paper towel dispenser above the sink to the left.

3. Imagine pushing your wristwatch a few inches up your wrist.

4. You are now turning on the hot and cold water faucets.

5. Adjust the water to a comfortable warm temperature.

6. Picture yourself rinsing your hands well in this warm water.

7. Leave the water running and with your right hand get some soap from the dispenser.

8. Imagine yourself spreading the soap over all surfaces of your hands. Your hands now feel slippery.

9. Rub each part of your hands. Start with your palms, then the backs of your hands, now each finger. Look to make sure that your have enough lather; if not, get more soap.

10. Picture yourself rinsing your hands, letting the water start at your fingertips and run off your wrists. Make sure no soap is left on your hands.

11. Let the water run while you reach with your left hand for a paper towel. Dry your hands briefly and use the damp towel to turn off the water.

12. Take another paper towel to dry your hands completely.

13. Throw the paper towel in the wastebasket.

14. Now return your attention to the classroom and open your eyes.

You may encounter a few difficulties in implementing mental practice (Richardson, Wilson, Sheehy, & Young, 1984). Initially, some learners may not take the whole process seriously. After some experience with mental practice, people generally do take it seriously. A few learners may have difficulty concentrating on the imaginary skill; they may report that when they are alone their mind wanders. For these people, try having them first read the instructions and picture each step separately. Then, when they have channeled their thoughts, have them go through the whole process again with their eyes closed. Practice does make perfect, with the process of mental practice as well as with the resulting skill performance.

Whole Versus Part Learning

Teachers debate whether skills should be learned in their entirety or whether they should be broken into their component parts and taught in sections. Recent research on this topic is lacking, but based on research from the 1960s and 1970s, experts recommend the following. The part method should be used for skills that are extremely complex with many parts; the whole method should be used with skills of low complexity or where the parts are extremely interrelated or organized (Gomez & Gomez, 1984; Magill, 1998). Translating these precepts into everyday examples reveals many of both types of skills in nursing. Skills that could be taught by the whole method might include assessment of vital signs, dressing change, and nasogastric intubation. The part method might be most effective in teaching skills such as intramuscular injection (first drawing up medication, then injecting), tracheostomy care (first suctioning, then cleaning), and setting up a new intravenous line (first bottle and tubing, then calculation and regulation).

Educators should analyze each psychomotor skill according to its level of complexity and organization. It would then be fairly easy to determine which skills should be taught by which method. The experienced educator also knows which skills learners have the most difficulty mastering. These skills can be analyzed to see whether they can be separated into component parts for teaching purposes.

Approaches to Teaching Skills

Teaching psychomotor skills in a college or hospital laboratory can be done in a variety of ways. Certain structures and methods of functioning may be workable in some places but not in others, depending on a number of factors. Those factors include the type of program, the number of educators available, nature of the student body or number of practicing nurses to be taught, availability of technology, and philosophy of the program.

Independent Learning Versus Teacher Instruction

One approach to teaching skills is to use the skills laboratory primarily as a place for independent learning. In this model, the educator must do a great deal of preparation. A syllabus must be developed with instructions for how learners should proceed. Background reading material must be identified and made available. Hardware and software must be selected and prepared for use, and supplies must be ordered and made available.

Haukenes and Halloran (1984) describe a college laboratory in which self-instruction is the primary teaching method. Learners are provided with a psychomotor skills handbook containing all skills taught in the curriculum. Each skill in the book is accompanied by information about the objectives of the skill lesson, the required media and reading, the necessary practice equipment and its location, and skill-testing procedures. The learners proceed at their own pace, deciding when to visit the college lab, how much time to spend with audiovisuals and practice, and when to schedule written and performance tests. Laboratory instructors assist the students as necessary and monitor the testing procedures.

Snyder, Fitzloff, Fiedler, and Lambke (2000) describe a college laboratory in which a combination of audiovisuals and supervised practice is structured around a belief that learners must focus on the context of the skill as well as the skill itself. Therefore, faculty built a laboratory process in which students learn not only the motor aspects of a skill, but also are expected to question the appropriateness of skills to the patient context. Educators ask students to reflect on their own performance and the problem solving needed to implement the skill in a clinical setting. In the final step of the laboratory process, students are given a case scenario and perform the skill while adapting it to the scenario.

In both of the examples given above, heavy emphasis is placed on the use of media and self-instruction. The trend today is to rely more on self-instruction in skill labs and to rely less on instructor demonstrations. The reason for this is clear. In-person demonstrations by instructors are time intensive and expensive and carry a greater chance of error than media-portrayed demonstrations (Melby et al., 1997). Educators are looking for more efficient and cost-effective ways of teaching and evaluating skills.

Some research has been reported on the relative effectiveness of self-instruction, media instruction, and demonstration in teaching psychomotor skills. A study by Powell, Canterbury, and McCoy (1998) on the relative effectiveness of teaching medication administration by faculty instruction versus self-instruction using videotape found no significant difference in performance between the two groups of learners. Neither was any significant difference in groups found in a study by DeAmicis (1997), which compared the teaching of intravenous therapy skills via traditional teacher demonstration to self-instruction via interactive videodisc.

Baldwin, Hill, and Hanson (1991) compared two strategies for teaching blood pressure measurement. One group received textbook assignments, videotape, and faculty instruction and demonstration; the other group received just textbook assignments and videotape. It is no surprise that the former group that involved faculty instruction performed significantly better—after all, they had received all the same treatment plus additional teaching by faculty. It is interesting that both groups of learners had equal confidence in their ability to perform the skills. Using blood pressure measurement as the dependent variable, Beeson and Kring (1999) also tested two instructional methods. They compared traditional videotape with interactive video instruction and found no significant difference in performance.

In 1997, Melby and colleagues taught intramuscular injection techniques using two methods. One group was taught by traditional faculty demonstration while the other group was given two nursing procedure books, models, and equipment for independent study and practice. Both groups performed the skill adequately; however, students preferred faculty demonstration over independent learning.

Love and colleagues (1989) compared the use of individual self-learning modules to faculty demonstration in teaching a cluster of 10 skills. They found no significant difference in performance. A follow-up study by McAdams, Rankin, Love, and Patton (1989) involved a survey of students in the same nursing program. Students in this university program had been using self-instruction for years and were asking for more traditional faculty teaching of skills. After experiencing both methods, most of the students preferred the traditional faculty-led laboratory. Some students preferred a combination of the two methods.

Evaluation of psychomotor skill performance is also time intensive and expensive if faculty time is used, so Miller, Nichols, and Beeken (2000) compared two methods of assessment. One group of learners videotaped their own performance of a set of four skills so faculty could view and evaluate the taped performance later. In the second group, faculty evaluated student performance in real time. Faculty and student satisfaction levels were highest in the faculty-present group. Time records revealed that the videotaped method consumed about half the amount of time as the faculty-present method.

It is clear from the research that has been done on self-learning of skills versus faculty-taught skills that self-learning is more cost effective because less faculty time is involved, that both produce adequate skill learning, but that students may prefer to be taught by faculty. Research into skill teaching in staff development settings still needs to be done.

Demonstrations

As already mentioned, students often prefer instructor demonstration as a way of learning skills. But how many educators know how to give an effective demonstration? Table 11–2 contains the key elements that will help ensure good demonstration technique. New teachers sometimes find demonstrations to be anxiety provoking. Following the guidelines in the table and perhaps keeping some note cards at your side will help alleviate anxiety.

Research has shown the effectiveness of demonstrations as a teaching strategy for learning skills that are entirely new to the learner (Magill, 1998). Bandura's Social Learning Theory or Social Cognitive Theory (see Chapter 2) best explains why demonstration is an effective ped-

---

TABLE 11-2 Elements of Effective Skill Demonstrations

1. Assemble all equipment ahead of time.
2. Make sure all equipment is in working order.
3. Do a "dry run" of the procedure and time the demonstration.
4. Arrange the environment to be as realistic as possible.
5. Perform the procedure step by step, explaining as you go along.
6. When appropriate, give the rationale for your actions.
7. Refer to handouts or textbooks to show fine points that may not be visible to the audience.
8. Be sure to adhere to all relevant principles of good nursing care. For example, aseptic technique, body mechanics, and patient privacy should be followed so learners see how to incorporate them.
9. Consider performing the skill a second time (or having a learner perform a demonstration) without explanations, to show the flow of the skill.

---

agogical method for teaching skills. The basic premise of Bandura's (1977) theory is that people learn as they observe other people's behavior. The learner observes and attends to the demonstration and then retains a mental model (a type of schema) of the behavior. He or she can take out this mental model as needed for review and mental practice. One of the difficulties foreseen by Bandura is that learners do not always attend to all aspects of the demonstration; therefore, their mental model may be somewhat deficient. For this reason, a second demonstration, either by the instructor, by a student, or by videotape, may be a good idea.

Simulations

Simulation technique can be a real help in teaching psychomotor skills. Simply practicing a skill with equipment in a laboratory is a simulated experience. Nursing skills laboratories are usually stocked with equipment much like what would be found in a clinical agency, and learners often practice on mannequins or fellow learners who are simulating patients. The idea is to make the practice setting and conditions like the real world in which the skill will eventually be performed to increase the likelihood of positive transfer of learning.

In addition to simulating the setting and equipment, simulation exercises often go much farther. Elaborate scenarios may be planned in which the learners apply skills to simulated hospital or home-care situations. Students or live simulated patients may act out their reactions to the skills being "performed" on them, thus giving learners another form of feedback. An example of how a skills laboratory can be used to simulate a hospital experience can be seen in Cowan and Wiens's (1986) article, which describes how beginning students practice basic skills on live simulated patients before they begin their hospital experience. See Chapter 8 for further information on simulations.

Assessment of Psychomotor Skill Learning

Skill performance checklists are a common means of organizing skill learning and assessment. Every nurse is familiar with skill checklists because they have been around for decades of nursing education and they are used around the world. Checklists describe the step-by-step progression of skill activity needed to achieve the goal. Teachers use them while demonstrating a skill to be sure nothing is forgotten. Learners use them during self-instruction to provide guidance and feedback. Teachers also use them to evaluate skill performance. Textbooks and procedure manuals in hard-copy or computerized form make standardized skill checklists readily available, although some educators prefer to develop their own checklists.

By definition, a checklist contains a number of items that are checked off when completed. For assessment and evaluation purposes, the educator may go one step farther. Checklists may contain a rating scale with descriptors such as Adequate, Good, and Excellent or Poor, Fair, and Good, or it may be a number scale that is added to give a total score. Therefore, each element of the skill may be rated as to the expertise with which it is performed, as well as rating the overall skill performance. The educator makes a decision ahead of time as to what score or rating constitutes successful skill performance.

When evaluating performance of a particular skill, one more variation may exist. There may be some elements on the checklist considered to be absolutely essential. If the learner does not complete those critical elements or does not do them satisfactorily, they may fail the test even if all other elements are satisfactory. For example, in performing a dressing change, if the sterile field was contaminated while all else was done well, the person would fail the test. Another example would be failing to remove air from the tubing when setting up an intravenous line. This omission would constitute a failing grade.

Which Skills Should Be Taught?

An important question to be asked is which nursing skills should be taught? Patients place the highest value on skills that ensure comfort and hygiene (Knight, 1998). For many patients, a good bed bath, hair grooming, tooth brushing, positioning, and pain control are the most important skills. Nursing students, however, often consider such skills to be less important than more invasive skills that require greater technical skill. Also, according to Knight, nurses place more priority on psychosocial skills than do patients.

Sweeney, Hedstrom, and O'Malley (1982) conducted a study in which they asked baccalaureate faculty in one nursing program to rate a list of 291 skills as being essential or not essential. Ninety percent of the faculty members selected 121 of the skills as essential. Interestingly, the largest percentage of the skills was in less technical areas, such as activities of daily living and hygienic care. The authors point out that many of the skills chosen as essential were those performed in clinical areas by nurses' aides, while many of the 170 skills not chosen were more challenging skills that employers would expect new graduates to be able to perform.

Faculty opinions may have changed since this 1982 study, but there is little published research to indicate which skills are now considered essential by both faculty and employers. Alavi, Loh, and Reilly conducted one study in 1991. Faculty in a university nursing program in Australia asked 48 agencies which skills were used by practicing nurses in those agencies and the frequency with which they were used. Faculty then analyzed the skills to determine which should be incorporated in the curriculum. Faculty in schools of nursing should be in continuing discussion with clinical agencies regarding skills that are required in clinical settings and whether undergraduate programs or staff development departments will be responsible for teaching them.

Teaching psychomotor skills will always be an important element of nursing education. What will change over time is how they are taught, who teaches them, which skills will be incorporated, and where they will be taught. Those decisions should be made based on scientific rationale as well as on the educational philosophy of the institution.

CASE STUDY

As a community nurse educator, you teach CPR and first aid classes to the general public. The local police force has contracted with your agency for CPR and first aid training. Each class of new police officers will have six to eight students. Considering the educational principles discussed in this chapter, discuss the following items:

1. Would these skills be best taught through independent learning modules or through educator demonstration?
2. If the skill is taught by independent learning with educator supervision and assessment, calculate potential dollar savings compared to everything being taught by the educator.
3. If CPR and first aid are taught in a classroom, are they considered open or closed skills?
4. Considering the second stage of Gentile's model, would these skills likely result in fixation or diversification?
5. Would CPR be considered a low-complexity or high-complexity skill? Should it be taught in a whole method or part method?
6. Would you consider teaching mental practice techniques to this class?

CRITICAL THINKING EXERCISES

1. If someone is having difficulty developing intrinsic feedback during skill learning, how can you help her?
2. A nursing student tends to practice skills once and think he has mastered them when in fact he has not. How would you motivate this student to engage in more extensive practice?
3. As a staff development educator, how will you decide which skills a new graduate must validate during orientation and which can wait until a later time?
4. Suppose an undergraduate nursing program with a competency-based skills design guarantees the skill competency of their graduates. They volunteer to reteach any skills found deficient in one of their graduates. What guidelines would your staff development department use for deciding under what circumstances a new graduate would be sent back to the school for retraining?

IDEAS FOR FURTHER RESEARCH

1. Compare the effect of augmented feedback on skill learning versus no augmented feedback.
2. Study the effects of mental practice on the learning of simple skills versus complex skills.
3. Use the "think aloud technique" to study the thought process of novices versus experts who are performing a nursing psychomotor skill in the clinical setting. Perhaps examine whether novices who are taught a broad conceptualization of skills (including concern for patient anxiety and comfort, for example) focus on all aspects of a skill or just the motor aspects.
4. Interview new graduate nurses who have just completed an orientation program. How confident do they feel in performing psychomotor skills? Interview them again in two or three months to see if the confidence level has changed significantly.

REFERENCES

Alavi, C., Loh, S. H., & Reilly, D. (1991). Reality basis for teaching psychomotor skill in a tertiary nursing curriculum. *Journal of Advanced Nursing, 16*, 957–965.

Allport, D. A. (1980). Attention and performance. In G. Claxton (Ed.), *Cognitive psychology* (pp. 112–153). London: Routledge & Kegan Paul.

Bachman, K. (1990). Using mental imagery to practice a specific psychomotor skill. *Journal of Continuing Education in Nursing, 21*(3), 125–128.

Baldwin, D., Hill, P., & Hanson, G. (1991). Performance of psychomotor skills: A comparison of two teaching strategies. *Journal of Nursing Education, 30*(8), 367–370.

Bandura, A. (1977). *Social learning theory*. Englewood Cliffs, NJ: Prentice Hall.

Beeson, S. A., & Kring, D. L. (1999). The effects of two teaching methods on nursing students' factual knowledge and performance of psychomotor skills. *Journal of Nursing Education, 38*(8), 357–359.

Bjork, I. T. (1997). Changing conceptions of practical skill and skill acquisition in nursing education. *Nursing Inquiry, 4*, 184–195.

Bjork, I. T. (1999). What constitutes a nursing practical skill? *Western Journal of Nursing Research, 21*(1), 51–70.

Bjork, I. T., & Kirkevold, M. (2000). From simplicity to complexity: Developing a model of practical skill performance in nursing. *Journal of Clinical Nursing, 9*(4), 620–631.

Bucher, L. (1993). The effects of imagery abilities and mental rehearsal on learning a nursing skill. *Journal of Nursing Education, 32*(7), 318–324.

Cowan, D., & Wiens, V. (1986). Mock hospital: A preclinical laboratory experience. *Nurse Educator, 11*(5), 30–32.

DeAmicis, P. A. (1997). Interactive videodisc instruction is an alternative method for learning and performing a critical nursing skill. *Computers in Nursing, 15*(3), 155–158.

Doheny, M. O. (1993). Mental practice: An alternative approach to teaching motor skills. *Journal of Nursing Education, 32*(6), 260–264.

Eaton, S. L., & Evans, S. B. (1986). The effect of nonspecific imaging practice on the mental imagery ability of nursing students. *Journal of Nursing Education, 25*(5), 193–196.

Garrison, K. C., & Magoon, R. A. (1972). *Educational psychology.* Columbus, OH: Charles E. Merrill.

Gentile, A. M. (1972). A working model of skill acquisition with application to teaching. *Quest, 17,* 3–23.

Gentile, A. M. (1987). Skill acquisition: Action, movement, and neuromotor processes. In J. H. Carr & R. B. Shepherd (Eds.), *Movement science: Foundations for physical therapy in rehabilitation* (pp. 93–154). Rockville, MD: Aspen.

Gomez, G. E., & Gomez, E. A. (1984). The teaching of psychomotor skills in nursing. *Nurse Educator, 9*(4), 35–39.

Haukenes, E., & Halloran, M. C. S. (1984). A second look at psychomotor skills. *Nurse Educator, 9*(3), 9–13.

Knight, C. M. (1998). Evaluating a skills centre: The acquisition of psychomotor skills in nursing—A review of the literature. *Nurse Education Today, 18,* 441–447.

Love, B., McAdams, C., Patton, D. M., Rankin, E. J., & Roberts, J. (1989). Teaching psychomotor skills in nursing: A randomized control trial. *Journal of Advanced Nursing, 14,* 970–975.

Magill, R. A. (1998). *Motor learning: Concepts and applications* (5th ed.). Boston, MA: WCB McGraw-Hill.

McAdams, C., Rankin, E. J., Love, B., & Patton, D. (1989). Psychomotor skills laboratories as self-directed learning: A study of nursing students' perceptions. *Journal of Advanced Nursing, 14,* 788–796.

Melby, V., Canning, A., Coates, V., Forster, A., Gallagher, A., McCartney, A., & McCartney, M. (1997). The role of demonstrations in the learning of psychomotor skills. *NT Research, 2*(3), 199–209.

Milde, F. K. (1988). The function of feedback in psychomotor-skill learning. *Western Journal of Nursing Research, 10*(4), 425–434.

Miller, H. K., Nichols, E., & Beeken, J. E. (2000). Comparing videotaped and faculty-present return demonstrations of clinical skills. *Journal of Nursing Education, 39*(5), 237–239.

Powell, S. S., Canterbury, M. A., & McCoy, D. (1998). Medication administration: Does the teaching method really matter? *Journal of Nursing Education, 37*(6), 281–283.

Richardson, A. (1967). Mental practice: A review and discussion. *Research Quarterly, 38*(1), 95–107.

Richardson, G. E., Wilson, S. S., Sheehy, C. D., & Young, N. (1984). Educational imagery and the allied health educator. *Journal of Allied Health, 13*(1), 38–47.

Schneider, W., Dumais, S. T., & Shriffrin, R. M. (1984). Automatic and control processing and attention. In R. Parasuraman & D. R. Davies (Eds.), *Varieties of attention* (pp. 1–27). Orlando, FL: Academic Press.

Snyder, M. D., Fitzloff, B. M., Fiedler, R., & Lambke, M. R. (2000). Preparing nursing students for contemporary practice: Restructuring the psychomotor skills laboratory. *Journal of Nursing Education, 39*(5), 229–230.

Speck, B. J. (1990). The effect of guided imagery upon first semester nursing students performing their first injections. *Journal of Nursing Education, 29*(8), 346–350.

Sweeney, M. A., Hedstrom, B., & O'Malley, M. (1982). Process evaluation: A second look at psychomotor skills. *Journal of Nursing Education, 21*(2), 4–17.

Swinnen, S. P. (1996). Information feedback for motor skill learning: A review. In H. N. Zelaznik (Ed.), *Advances in motor learning and control* (pp. 37–66). Champaign, IL: Human Kinetics.

Wallace, S. A. (1996). Dynamic pattern perspective of rhythmic movement: An introduction. In H. N. Zelaznik (Ed.), *Advances in motor learning and control* (pp. 155–194). Champaign, IL: Human Kinetics.

12

Promoting and Assessing Critical Thinking

At its very minimum, the practice of nursing requires the ability to (a) draw upon one's knowledge base in nursing and related sciences, (b) perform a myriad of psychomotor skills, and (c) interact effectively with individuals and groups. But in the chaotic, ever-changing, unpredictable, uncertain world and health care arena of the twenty-first century, nurses need additional abilities if they are to provide quality care to individuals, families, and communities.

Those additional skills include—but are not limited to—the following:

- Work collaboratively with an interdisciplinary team
- Provide evidence (i.e., research) to support one's interactions
- Draw reasoned conclusions
- Document clearly and comprehensively
- Provide leadership that leads to positive change
- Be unwilling to merely accept the status quo or tradition
- Be creative
- Connect ideas, often in unique ways
- Engage in dialogue with individuals and groups
- Communicate effectively through verbal, written, and electronic means
- Manage conflicting information
- Make decisions despite gaps in information and knowledge
- Have a questioning mind
- Be characterized by a "spirit of inquiry"
- Contribute to the ongoing development of nursing science
- Be open to new perspectives, interpretations, and alternatives
- Be reflective and contemplative
- Think critically

An ability to think critically is a skill that nurses need in the practice setting and in every-day life. Indeed, there is extensive discussion about critical thinking—what it is, whether it is a discipline-specific or a "generic" skill, how it develops, how learning experiences can be designed to enhance it, and how one measures it. In addition, one of the bodies that accredit nursing education programs—the National League for Nursing Accrediting Commission (NLNAC, 2001)—requires that *critical thinking* be an outcome of such programs and that faculty document their graduates' abilities in this area.

Despite these external requirements to address students' critical thinking skills, and despite an extensive literature base on the topic, there is much uncertainty about what this phenomenon is and what responsibility nurse educators have to promote/advance it in students and graduate nurses. This chapter addresses these very issues. In addition, this chapter includes information on various approaches to measuring critical thinking in nursing students and nurses in practice.

Defining Critical Thinking

James McGregor Burns (1978) once said about the concept of *leadership* that it is "one of the most observed and least understood phenomena on earth" (p. 2). And in his extensive scholarly analysis of leadership, Bass (1990) noted that "there are almost as many different definitions of [the concept] as there are persons who have attempted to define [it]" (p. 11).

The same can be said of the concept of *critical thinking:* It is widely observed but little understood, and it has been defined in numerous ways. An analysis of some of the more significant definitions may be useful in better understanding just what critical thinking is and is not.

Nearly 50 years ago, Dressel and Mayhew (1954) described critical thinking as the ability to define a problem, select pertinent information needed to solve the problem, recognize stated and unstated assumptions, formulate or select relevant and promising hypotheses, draw valid conclusions, and judge the validity of inferences. Although this definition includes many notions that, today, are thought to be significant elements of critical thinking, it had little impact on the educational or practice arena.

A definition of critical thinking that had greater impact—perhaps because it was associated with an instrument to measure the concept—was offered in 1964 by Watson and Glaser. These scholars described critical thinking as a composite of attitudes of inquiry; knowledge of the nature of valid inferences, abstractions, and generalizations; and skills in employing and applying these attitudes and this knowledge. In addition to addressing some of the skills needed for critical thinking, Watson and Glaser introduced the idea that critical thinking also involves one's frame of mind or attitude. This is an important concept because it acknowledges that critical thinking is more than merely a "collection" of skills one uses in certain situations (e.g., nursing practice); instead, it is a perspective through which one views *all* situations.

Little significant work was done in relation to critical thinking for nearly 20 years after Watson and Glaser formulated their definition and designed their instrument (the Watson–Glaser Critical Thinking Appraisal [WGCTA]). But since the mid-1980s, many other definitions of the concept have been offered, as noted in Table 12–1.

TABLE 12-1 Definitions of Critical Thinking

Alfaro-LeFevre (1999, p. 9): "purposeful, outcome-directed (results-oriented) thinking . . . [that] requires knowledge, skills, and experience . . . [and helps one] constantly reevaluat[e], self-correct . . . , and strive to improve"

Bandman & Bandman (1995, p. 7): "reasoning in which we analyze the use of language, formulate problems, clarify and explicate assumptions, weigh evidence, evaluate conclusions, discriminate between good and bad arguments, and seek to justify those facts and values that result in credible beliefs and actions"

Beyer (1985, p. 487): "the process of determining the authenticity, accuracy, and worth of information or knowledge claims"

Brookfield (1987, pp. 5–9): "a productive and positive activity . . . a process, not an outcome . . . triggered by positive as well as negative events . . . emotive as well as rational. . . . [It involves] identifying and challenging assumptions . . . challenging the importance of context . . . try[ing] to imagine and explore alternatives . . . [and] reflective skepticism"

Ennis (1985, p. 45): "reflective and reasonable thinking that is focused on deciding what to believe or do"

Facione (1990): "purposeful, self-regulatory judgment which results in interpretation, analysis, evaluation, and inference as well as explanation of the evidential, conceptual, methodological, criteriological, or contextual considerations upon which that judgment was based"

Ford & Profetto-McGrath (1994, p. 342): the mediation "between authentic knowledge and autonomous action through a process of critical reflection"

Halpern (1994, p. 13): "those skills (or strategies) that increase the probability of achieving a desirable outcome (e.g., making a good decision, reaching a sound conclusion, successfully solving a problem)"

Hanford (1994, p. 7): "the ability to make connections, to bring to bear on an issue, question, or problem all the factors or influences that attend it"

Kurfiss (1988, p. 2): "an investigation whose purpose is to explore a situation, phenomenon, question, or problem to arrive at a hypothesis or conclusion about it that integrates all available information and that can therefore be convincingly justified"

Lipman (1988, p. 3): "skillful, responsible thinking that facilitates good judgment because it (a) relies upon criteria, (b) is self-correcting, and (c) is sensitive to context"

McPeck (1981, p. 81): "the propensity and skill to engage in an activity with reflective skepticism"

National Council for Excellence in Critical Thinking (1992, p. 201): "the intellectually disciplined process of actively and skillfully conceptualizing, applying, analyzing, synthesizing, and/or evaluating information gathered from, or generated by, observation, experience, reflection, reasoning, or communication, as a guide to belief and action"

Paul (1993, p. 91): "thinking about your thinking while you're thinking in order to make your thinking better"

Perkins (1985): "considering and seeking reasons with a non-formal bearing on the claim, pro or con, in an attempt to resolve the truth of the claim"

Scheffer & Rubenfeld (2000): "[using] habits of the mind [such as] confidence . . . contextual perspective . . . creativity . . . flexibility . . . inquisitiveness . . . intellectual integrity . . . intuition . . . open-mindedness . . . perseverance . . . [and] reflection . . . [and using the skills of] analyzing . . . applying standards . . . discriminating . . . information seeking . . . logical reasoning . . . predicting . . . [and] transforming knowledge"

Sternberg (1985): the mental processes, strategies, and representations people use to solve problems, make decisions, and learn new concepts

An analysis of these definitions suggests that (a) a critical thinker is nonbiased, reasoned, and truth oriented, (b) critical thinking involves making judgments, (c) thinking can be judged to be "critical" if it holds up to certain evaluative criteria, and (d) critical thinking is tied to belief or action (i.e., it is done for some purpose). The definitions also reinforce perspectives expressed earlier that critical thinking is a "spirit," an attitude, or an inclination to think about one's thinking.

Like many others, the author of this chapter developed a definition in 1995 that attempted to capture many elements of those developed by others:

> Critical thinking is using the powers of the mind to view the world and to act in a discerning way. It includes having a questioning attitude, examining underlying assumptions, and considering the validity of alternative solutions, in order to make reasoned judgments that are sensitive to context.

Faculty in individual schools of nursing who pursue NLNAC accreditation of their program(s) are required to define critical thinking as it relates to their program(s). Many faculty groups have adopted or adapted published definitions of critical thinking, while others have developed their own perspective on the concept. One such definition was formulated by the faculty of the School of Nursing at Fairfield University (Fairfield, Connecticut) in their *Self-Study Report for NLNAC Accreditation* (1997, p. 147):

> Critical thinking is a way of interacting with the world that is reflective, open, and generative.

Interacting with the world was described by this faculty as engaging with ideas as well as people, being curious, appreciating contextual influences, being broad rather than narrow, being aware of one's own values, being involved, being able to tolerate ambiguity and uncertainty, and not having tunnel vision. By *reflective,* this faculty meant having a sound knowledge base, examining the whole, being thoughtful, examining assumptions, being insightful, drawing conclusions that are well founded, and continuously looking at and investigating ideas and perspectives, among other things. To this faculty, being *open* meant being flexible and open to new ideas, considering alternative lines of reasoning, being creative, having intellectual curiosity, and continually rethinking issues, perspectives, and points of view, including one's own. Finally, being *generative* in one's thinking meant creating new ideas, proposing alternatives, being willing to grow and take risks, taking responsibility for initiating change, and constantly growing and learning.

One of the leading experts in the area of critical thinking, Richard Paul (1993), summarized the concept by identifying a number of aspects of critical thinking (see Table 12–2). Paul (1990) also outlined "Intellectual Standards for Disciplining the Mind"—standards that can be used as criteria to judge whether a person's thinking is critical. Those standards note that thinking judged to be "critical" is precise, deep, logical, relevant, accurate, and significant, among other criteria.

In essence, when we engage in critical thinking, we identify and evaluate the assumptions that underlie our conclusions, judgments, and actions. When we engage in critical thinking, we consider multiple perspectives, can articulate a point of view, make decisions and commitments, and consider the consequences of our decisions. Finally, when we engage in critical thinking, we justify our beliefs and actions, but we also are willing to modify our beliefs and actions as new information is received and processed.

Some authors (Ennis, 1989, 1990; Facione, 1990; Hager, 1990; Norris, 1988; Paul, 1990; Scriven, 1990) assert that critical thinking skills are generic, and there is nothing different between critical thinking in one situation (e.g., nursing) and critical thinking in another situation (e.g., child rearing). Those who advocate this position assert that while

TABLE 12-2 Aspects of Critical Thinking

Judging whether a statement is actually the application of a certain principle

Judging whether an observation statement is reliable

Judging whether an inductive conclusion is warranted

Judging whether the real problem has been identified

Grasping the true meaning of a statement

Judging whether there is ambiguity in a line of reasoning

Judging whether certain statements contradict each other

Judging whether conclusions follow necessarily

Judging whether a statement is specific enough

Judging whether something is an assumption

Judging whether a definition is adequate

Judging whether a statement made by an alleged authority is acceptable

Source: Paul, R. (1993). *Critical thinking: How to prepare students for a rapidly changing world.* Santa Rosa, CA: Foundation for Critical Thinking.

each field may have its own unique logic, to some degree, each field does not have its own skills of critical thinking.

Other experts (Barrow, 1990; McPeck, 1981) note that while having subject matter knowledge does not necessarily mean that an individual will deal intellectually with what she or he knows, knowledge of a subject is a necessary condition for critical thinking in an area. They conclude, therefore, that there are different skills for different circumstances, that subject matter knowledge is a necessary condition for critical thinking, and that critical thinking is subject specific.

A panel of nursing experts that was convened in 2000 to assist the National League for Nursing in developing a critical thinking test for nursing students seemed to agree with the latter point, as they formulated a definition of *critical thinking in nursing*. That definition reads as follows: "Critical thinking in nursing practice is a discipline specific, reflective reasoning process that guides a nurse in generating, implementing, and evaluating approaches for dealing with client care and professional concerns" (National League for Nursing, 2001, p. 2).

The point of this analysis of various definitions of the concept of critical thinking, and whether or not that definition needs to be discipline specific, is to encourage nurse educators to think carefully and, indeed, critically about the essence of the definition they use to judge learner achievement in this significant area. This is particularly important when one considers that the chosen definition will affect what is "measured," how it is measured, and what strategies will be implemented to advance students' or nurses' critical thinking.

Distinguishing Critical Thinking from Other Concepts

Critical thinking often is defined as problem solving, using the scientific method, using the nursing process, cognitive/intellectual development, or creativity. While there are elements in each of these concepts that are compatible with critical thinking, none is the same as critical thinking.

Problem solving involves drawing on knowledge and experience to address an immediate problem, where "a correct answer usually exists, and only a limited number of approaches . . . will work" (Kurfiss, 1988, p. 28). With problem solving, a long-term perspective is not necessarily taken. Critical thinking, in comparison, involves "reasoning about open-ended or 'ill-structured' problems" (Kurfiss, 1988, p. 28), and it involves a questioning spirit that operates all the time, not merely when one is presented with a problem.

The scientific method is a linear, objective approach to studying problems in order to find solutions. When using this process, one is expected to minimize bias and one's personal involvement in a situation. Critical thinking, on the other hand, is reflective, involves personal "investment," is nonlinear (i.e., "messy"), and, again, is not necessarily focused on solving a problem or answering a question.

Like the scientific method, the nursing process is a systematic, linear approach to assessing a situation, outlining a plan for solution, taking action, and evaluating results. When one engages in critical thinking, there are no "steps" to follow, it is not linear, it may not be specific to a clinical practice situation, and action is not required (i.e., one may raise questions simply to stimulate further thinking or to open new possibilities).

Critical thinking may be thought to be a component of cognitive/intellectual development, but it is not the same thing. Cognitive development has to do with how individuals reason, view knowledge, manage diversity of opinion and conflicting points of view, and relate to authorities as they come to know and understand. Critical thinking, in comparison, is not focused on the nature of knowledge, and it is not focused on relationships with "authority." It is, therefore, a narrower concept than cognitive/intellectual development.

Finally, critical thinking and creativity are related, but different, phenomena. Creativity involves imagination and spontaneity, it is artistic and free, it is original and (to some extent) intuitive, and it leads to a novel product (an idea, a solution, an invention). By comparison, critical thinking is logical, analytical, and judgmental; there may be no tangible product at the end; and it focuses not on the product but on evaluating the *worth* of a product (a solution, an expressed view, or an action) by using explicit criteria.

Nurse educators, therefore, need to be careful not to "take the easy way out" by saying that critical thinking is the same as the nursing process, problem solving, or the scientific method. Nor must they make it more than it is by confusing it with creativity or cognitive/intellectual development. Critical thinking is different from each of these concepts in a number of ways, and the educator's definition of it needs to reflect that uniqueness.

Ways We May Inhibit the Critical Thinking of Nursing Students

Someone once said, "We don't have to make human beings smart. They are born smart. All we have to do is stop doing things that make them stupid" (Anonymous). Without even realizing it, faculty may be doing things that inhibit the development of students' critical thinking (Bowers & McCarthy, 1993; Brookfield, 1993). Therefore, before we propose strategies to promote/enhance students' thinking, it is important that we discuss the things we may need to *stop* doing.

For example, educators often believe that the only way students can learn anything about nursing is if they hear it from us. As a result, many of us carefully structure our class sessions such that there are no questions for students to ask, students are not challenged to "struggle" in order to understand the material being presented, and we present complicated material in a structured, orderly way that takes the "messiness" out of it. This approach may give students a false impression that clinical situations are not as complex or difficult as they, indeed, are.

When we expect perfection and reinforce the status quo, we may be inhibiting the development of students' critical thinking. In addition, nurse faculty often make assumptions about students and learning (Miller & Malcolm, 1990, p. 71) that do little to promote critical thinking. Among those assumptions are the following: Beginning students do not know how to problem solve or think critically; mistakes are always bad, costly, and to be avoided; there is a single best way to think about and solve problems; certainty is good; and faculty know best.

In our desire to "cover as much content as possible in the time available," educators tend to use the lecture format more than may be desirable if we truly want to promote students' critical thinking. While the lecture has many advantages, it reduces students to "little more than background" (Bloom, 1953, p. 164) and is not the most effective strategy to enhance thinking. Indeed, Paul (1992, p. 3) bemoans the observation that "the professor who 'dictates,' the student who 'reiterates,' the 'talking' teacher, [and] the 'quiet' student still dominate the everyday classroom," and he asserts that if we are to help students develop their critical thinking skills, we must overcome our "addiction to coverage" (Paul, 1994a, p. 11).

Paul is not alone in his criticism of the overuse of lecture. Hanford (1994, p. 6), for example, noted "the growing overreliance on what John Goodlad has called 'frontal teaching,'" in which we try to cram facts and information into learners' heads and fail to give them adequate time to truly understand what they are supposed to be learning. He cites Ted Sizer's notion of "less is better" and suggests we "teach fewer facts and allow more time for discussing and thinking" (p. 6).

The structure of nursing curricula themselves may inhibit the development of critical thinking. When nearly every course in the curriculum is preselected for students and the sequencing of courses is carefully scripted, students do not have to think about why they are enrolling in certain courses, nor do they have to make choices from among alternatives after weighing the value of each of those alternatives.

Finally, we may do well to consider the assignments we give students. We use multiple-choice testing extensively, and although multiple-choice questions can be developed to challenge students' thinking (McDonald, 2002), they often are at a low level of complexity and do not require students to think critically at all. The guidelines to written assignments we give often are very precise, including the number of pages, the number of references to be cited, and even the sources of references. In such instances, students do not have to think about the issues they will analyze, how they will "tackle" the analysis, what their personal perspectives are on the issue, what resources they will use to substantiate their points of view, how they will judge the value of the resources used, or their own assumptions about the topic at hand.

Inhibitors may exist in clinical teaching as well. When faculty or preceptors always take responsibility for making learners' clinical assignments, we do not challenge them to think about their learning needs, the kinds of experiences that will help them meet those needs, how they can build on their own strengths, or the kinds of experiences that will help them relate theoretical learning to clinical application of that knowledge.

In far too many instances, and often without realizing it, nurse educators have put systems and practices in place that may serve to inhibit, rather than promote, students' critical thinking. Perhaps it is time for educators to question "sacred cows," challenge "traditional" practices, and create a new "status quo" in terms of our curricula, our teaching strategies, and our evaluation practices if we are to prepare students who truly can think critically. The success of our graduates in the complex, uncertain, unpredictable, ever-changing twenty-first century world may depend on it.

Strategies That Enhance Critical Thinking

A character in one of Sue Grafton's novels (1992, p. 306) noted that "Thinking is hard work, which is why you don't see a lot of people doing it." Indeed, critical thinking is not easy, and the development of such skills takes effort. But there are many strategies nurse educators can use to enhance or promote the critical thinking of students and nurses in practice. Before discussing specific teaching/learning and evaluation strategies, however, it is important to think about more foundational principles.

A critical thinking approach to education requires that teachers and learners alike view learning as a shared responsibility. It is the educator's responsibility to create an environment that supports this concept.

When learning is viewed as a shared responsibility, the teacher's role is that of mentor and facilitator. Learners define their own learning needs, take responsibility to use a variety of resources to meet those needs, and evaluate their progress toward meeting those goals. Such an environment is egalitarian and democratic, learners are empowered, and they feel as if they share in the control of the learning process.

As a mentor and facilitator, particularly one who is attempting to promote the critical thinking of learners, it is the educator's responsibility to "push" and challenge learners while supporting them. Our purpose in teaching critical thinking is to alter learners' dispositions toward being closed to alternatives and perspectives that are different from or in conflict with their own. This is very difficult, if not impossible, to do through lecture. Therefore, one strategy to promote students' critical thinking is to do less lecturing.

Discussion

Lecture should be limited to a small percentage of the class time, and educators should focus on depth of understanding more than on breadth of content. Indeed, the focus on "content" should be streamlined so that only the most significant concepts and principles are addressed. Our classes need to move from straight lecture or lecture with comments and questions that are directed to the teacher to focused interactions between teacher and student and, indeed, among students themselves. The highest level of discussion occurs when teacher and students engage in thoughtful dialogue about an unannounced topic.

During discussions that enhance critical thinking, the teacher role models critical thinking and answers questions only when learners are unable to do that for themselves. Learners' questions are answered by one another or by the teacher who "thinks out loud" to formulate a response, rather than merely answering a question as an "all-knowing" expert. An even more effective strategy is for learners to discover answers to their own questions by thinking through the question, what they know about that topic, the assumptions they may be making about it, the gaps in knowledge on the topic, and so on. The teacher, then, serves to redirect the discussion, bring out salient points, and summarize.

The use of discussion as a teaching/learning strategy is unpredictable, and it may make the classroom "a relatively chaotic affair" (Bloom, 1953, p. 164). In addition, some of what is said by learners during a discussion may be erroneous or incomplete, and it needs to be corrected by the teacher. But a discussion is a "controlled chaos," and it presents an excellent opportunity for teachers to give up control so they can help learners realize the strengths and flaws in their thinking.

Research with students (Bloom, 1953) has demonstrated that (a) discussion actively holds their thoughts to the immediate situation more than lecture does (i.e., their thoughts do not drift to unrelated topics), and (b) irrelevant and passive thoughts occur twice as frequently in lecture as in discussion. With lecture, learners' thoughts about the person speaking are less, their thoughts about themselves with respect to the topic are significantly less, and thoughts that involve synthesis of ideas and attempts to solve problems or questions raised are far less. Indeed, using discussion as a teaching/learning strategy can be most effective in promoting students' critical thinking.

Asking Effective Questions

When teachers do ask questions of learners—in the classroom, in the clinical area, in conferences, in one-on-one interactions—those questions need to be of a higher level if they are to promote critical thinking. The asking of factual questions (i.e., those with one right answer) should be minimized. In addition, teachers need to be careful with questions that have as many answers as there are different human preferences (e.g., Do you prefer "X" or "Y" or "Z"?). Neither of these types of questions promotes critical thinking.

Instead, the questions we ask of our learners should require reasoned responses, and they should help learners explore and understand various points of view. Educators should pose "questions that probe thinking for clarity; questions that hold individuals accountable for [the relevance, depth, and breadth of] their thinking; and questions that move learners from mere enactment of the nursing role to the internalization of questions they need to ask themselves to become astute practitioners" (Colucciello, 1997, p. 244).

Much has been written about using the *Socratic method* (Paul & Elder, 1995, 1996) in our classrooms, a method that relies heavily on probing, thought-provoking questions being posed by the teacher. In this method, all thoughts are treated as if they are in need of further development and refinement, regardless of how reflective they may be. The teacher responds to all comments and questions with more questions, all for the purpose of helping learners seek to understand the ultimate foundations for what is said.

Finally, one specific strategy has been identified that relies heavily on effective questioning: *structured controversy* (Johnson & Johnson, 1989; Pederson, Duckett, & Maruyama, 1990). With this approach, controversy is purposefully introduced and used to enhance thinking, as well as both cognitive and affective learning. Learner groups argue for and against an issue, much as is done in a debate, but they go one step further. After presenting the arguments, they use reasoned judgment, not merely factual knowledge, to reach a consensus that they can support with evidence. Such a strategy can be used to explore various issues facing the nursing profession, but it also can be used in the examination of patient care situations.

Text Interaction

Students in nursing programs use many textbooks as learning resources, and faculty assign extensive amounts of reading in such texts. But how do students learn to "get the most out of" all that reading? What guidance do teachers give students that encourage them to think critically about what they are reading, compare it to other things they have read or experiences they have had, be alert to inappropriate conclusions, and so on? The strategy of *text interaction* (Abegglen & Conger, 1997) may provide some assistance.

With text interaction, students interact with the readings prior to class. They raise questions about what is presented, note assumptions that are being made, point out conflicting information, recognize when conclusions are being drawn without adequate evidence having been provided, note questions they have that are not answered in the text, and so on. Indeed, the "interaction" results in much more than a mere outline of the contents of the pages read.

Teachers can use these analyses in any number of ways. For example, students can be asked to submit their "text interactions" at the beginning of class, they can be called on to share one item from their notes with the class, or they can be asked to use their notes in small group discussion with their peers. The point is to help students interact with, not merely "plow through," a textbook or an article. The goal is to help them think about what they are reading so that they develop the questioning attitude or spirit of inquiry that characterizes a critical thinker.

Problem-Based Learning

One of the newer strategies being used to promote critical thinking is *problem-based learning*. With this approach, learning occurs when individuals attempt to manage problems much like those that are found in clinical practice. In this process, individuals learn content (e.g., medications or pathophysiology) when it is needed to solve a problem, not when the teacher thinks they need to learn it. Learners typically address the problems in teams, and teachers are expert resources who are available to learners as they struggle with finding information, judging its worth, dealing with its inconsistencies or incompleteness, making decisions in uncertainty, using evidence to support conclusions, and implementing other critical thinking skills.

Problem-based learning may be used as a teaching/learning strategy in a particular course or set of courses, or it may be used as the design for the entire curriculum. In the latter instance, there may be no courses (e.g., Anatomy & Physiology, Nursing Care of Children) as we have come to know them. Instead, student teams work collaboratively to complete a series of problems through which they will learn the concepts that faculty deemed most significant. However, they will learn those concepts at different speeds, in different sequences, and in different learning circumstances. (See Chapter 8 for more information on problem-based learning.)

Concept Mapping

Concept maps are metacognitive tools that assist learners to "see" their own thinking and reasoning about a topic as they depict relationships among factors, note causes and effects, identify predisposing factors, formulate expected outcomes, and so on. Concept maps direct learners to consider the context in which a situation occurs, and they help learners make purposeful judgments.

For example, the teacher may construct a situation about a clinical problem (e.g., an elderly patient with complex health needs, whose culture is different from that of most of the learners and whose family and socioeconomic support are minimal) or a professional issue (e.g., how to use nurses most effectively in the clinical setting). Learners are then asked to diagram all the elements of the situation and show the relationships among them.

In "mapping" the professional issue noted above, learners would be expected to include concepts of licensure, specific agency or broad health policies, the educational preparation of the nursing workforce, the nature and extent of the nursing workforce's experience, finances, changing patient care needs, competencies needed by the nursing workforce, responsibilities of other health team members (including ancillary personnel), historical "traditions," and so on. The relationship of these concepts to the central one and to one another needs to be "plotted," as do the directions of those relationships, if known. For example, the map should note which factors are precursors to the situation or precede other factors, and which ones are the result or outcome of certain elements.

Mapping all these concepts requires that learners draw on an extensive knowledge base, examine assumptions that may be made about concepts or the relationships among them, and think carefully about how "all the pieces fit together." Once this is done, appropriate strategies for dealing with the situation/issue can be formulated.

Concept mapping, thus, is a way to help learners develop their critical thinking skills and to make their thinking visible. It promotes integrated thinking and points out areas where conflicting information exists, both of which are important factors in critical thinking and effective clinical practice.

Other Strategies

There are many other strategies that can be used to help students and nurses develop their critical thinking abilities. Several of these strategies have been discussed more fully in other chapters but are described here briefly.

Case studies provide learners with an open-ended problem that has more than one desirable outcome. Learners are required to judge the advantages and disadvantages of various options, compare alternative solutions, and justify their choice of actions. Use of case studies helps learners see and appreciate more than one perspective and often points out assumptions they make in the face of incomplete information.

Collaborative learning provides opportunities for teams of learners to complete assignments. In such approaches (which can be structured in an almost unlimited way), the talents of each learner are used to solve problems, learners critique each other's work, and they learn from one another. One specific collaborative strategy is that of *Dyad Testing* (Vinten & Ellett, 2001) in which pairs of learners work together to respond to test questions. In doing this, they think about the worth of each answer option, argue why each might be right or wrong, and help each other in the decision-making process.

One-minute papers (Cross, 1981) afford learners one of the easiest and most enjoyable ways to think critically on a continuous basis. At the start of each class session, participants are given a single sheet of paper with statements such as the following:

The most important/interesting thing I learned in class today was . . .

As a result of today's class discussion, I am confused about . . .

After doing the readings for class today, I have questions about . . .

I would like to spend more time discussing . . .

They are asked to respond to each statement sometime before the session ends and to submit their papers before leaving. Feedback by the educator should focus on clarifying areas of confusion, answering questions, and commenting on the quality of the responses. The latter point helps learners think about their thinking, their ability to listen and understand, and their ability to process what they are hearing.

Microthemes, one example of writing-to-learn strategies, are one- to two-page written analyses or thought papers about "controversial" topics related to the course that are completed regularly, perhaps even on a weekly basis. Initially, the teacher critiques the thinking and arguments presented in each paper, but as time goes by, learners follow the example set by the teacher to critique their own or each other's papers using preestablished standards of critical thinking (e.g., those proposed by Paul [1994b]). Through this strategy, learners not only formulate positions on issues/topics, but they are challenged to evaluate the quality of those positions and the soundness of the thinking that underlies them. Microthemes, therefore, could be an effective strategy to enhance critical thinking.

Journals are an excellent way to help learners reflect on their experiences, their values, their actions, and their interactions with others. This narrative form encourages individuals to draw on and fuse concepts learned with personal experiences, and it offers a safe way to express one's innermost fears, insights, and concerns. If journals are to be effective, however, feedback from the teacher is critical. Such feedback must be thoughtful, reflective, nonjudgmental, focused, and extensive, as it is a way for the educator to role model critical thinking. In fact, for journals to be most effective, the teacher needs to put as much time into reading and commenting on the entries as it took for learners to write them.

Self-assessment/evaluation, when it is viewed as more than the mere completion of forms, is a strategy that can be used to promote critical thinking. When self-assessment is completed periodically throughout an experience (i.e., a course, a clinical rotation, and so on), when learners are given guidance in how to complete the self-assessment, and when helpful feedback on the content and thoughtfulness of the assessment is given, self-assessment becomes a learning activity and not just a chore. Learners might be asked to identify the five personal strengths and five personal weaknesses that impacted their learning of the material, or they could discuss their growth from one assessment point to the next. They could be asked to comment on the extent to which they were aware of assumptions they and others were making when caring for patients, or reflect on the quality of the thinking displayed in their practice or project.

There are many other strategies educators can use to promote learners' critical thinking. Among them are the use of portfolios (Facione & Facione, 1996), imagery (Krejci, 1997), and concept analysis/concept clarification (Kemp, 1985; Kramer, 1993). Indeed, almost any strategy can be designed to promote the critical thinking skills and dispositions of learners, if it is thought through carefully and if it is used within a positive learning environment.

Positive Learning Environment

The use of strategies like discussion, journals, and self-assessments "force" learners to be reflective and confront things about themselves that may be uncomfortable. But since "exploration is what learning is all about" (Anonymous), it is very important that educators create a positive learning environment in which students feel safe, respected, and supported to engage in experiences that may make them uncomfortable.

A positive learning environment affirms learners' self-worth, shows support for their efforts, reflects and mirrors their ideas, and encourages interactions between and among learners. It is an environment where people listen attentively to one another, opportunities are created for interaction, and learners feel safe to share ideas and take risks. Indeed, since "students learn more from following their own wrong path than from the well-worn foot-steps of the experts" (de Tornyay, 1990, p. 51), educators need to create a place where students can "follow their own wrong path" with confidence.

Finally, in a positive learning environment, the teacher uses silence to encourage reflection, introduces controversy and then helps individuals learn how to manage it, and role models critical thinking. But teachers need to be careful when role modeling critical thinking, that they do not suggest that their way of thinking is the only way or the one right way; learners must be helped to understand that the teacher's way of thinking through problems and issues is only one approach. Of great importance is for the teacher to be able to say, "I don't know," and to not need to be on "center stage, in the spotlight."

Teachers need to provide learners with support in the form of structure, guidance, concrete examples, opportunities for direct experiences, a high degree of personalism, congruence, and the use of many senses. But if they are to promote critical thinking, they need to gradually minimize those support strategies and maximize strategies that challenge students. Indeed, "thinking critically and creatively requires [learners] to take the risk of being challenged" (de Tornyay, 1990, p. 51).

We must get learners out of the "velvet ruts of routine" (p. 47) by creating "positive turbulence" (Gryskiewicz, 2000, p. 48). Learners are challenged by freedom to choose, flexibility, self-direction, abstract thinking, reflective thinking, independent functioning, peer collaboration, diverse perspectives and values, conflicting information, vagueness, and uncertainty. They also are supported in their risk-taking by educators who "model how to take risks . . . exude organization and competence . . . minimize the pain of making a mistake . . . and provide risk-taking opportunities" (de Tornyay, 1990, p. 51). By balancing challenge and support, learners will be encouraged to advance in their thinking abilities.

Assessing Critical Thinking

There are many ways to assess or measure individuals' critical thinking skills, abilities, and tendencies, and, in fact, a "multimodal assessment program" (Facione & Facione, 1996, p. 44) is thought to be the best approach to understand learners' abilities in this area. Three fairly common standardized tests that measure generic critical thinking skills or dispositions, one standardized test that measures the broader concept of cognitive/intellectual development, and one new standardized test that is specific to nursing will be addressed here.

In the *Watson–Glaser Critical Thinking Appraisal (WGCTA)* (Watson & Glaser, 1980), critical thinking is defined as a composite of attitudes, knowledge, and skills. The WGCTA is an 80-item test that is available in Forms A and B, and it has a reported reliability between .69 and .85. Scores are reported in five specific skill areas—inference, recognition of assumptions, deduction, interpretation, and evaluation of arguments—and the test is discipline neutral.

The *California Critical Thinking Skills Test (CCTST)* (Facione, 1992) is a 34-item multiple-choice format test, available in Forms A and B, that also is discipline neutral. It measures critical thinking skills in relation to short problem statements and scenarios and has a reported reliability of .70 to .71. Scores are reported in each of the skill areas used to define critical thinking: analysis, evaluation, inference, deductive reasoning, inductive reasoning, and self-regulation.

Rather than measuring critical thinking skills, the *California Critical Thinking Dispositions Inventory (CCTDI)* (Facione & Facione, 1992) measures critical thinking *tendencies* in relation to Likert-type attitudinal prompts. It is a 75-item instrument with a reliability of .90. In addition to an overall score, individuals receive a score in each of the elements used to define critical thinking dispositions: truth-seeking, open-mindedness, analyticity, systematicity, critical thinking self-confidence, inquisitiveness, and cognitive maturity.

Less commonly used than the WGCTA, CCTST, and CCTDI is the *Learning Environment Preference (LEP) Test*. This test is based on Perry's (1970) scheme of cognitive/intellectual development and is intended to measure that broader concept. It focuses on five domains that are related to epistemology and approaches to learning: view of learning, role of the instructor, role of the student and her or his peers, the classroom atmosphere and activities, and the role of evaluation in learning. By responding to 13 items in each of these five areas (for a total of 65 items), individuals rate the significance of various aspects of a learning environment as they describe their ideal environment for learning.

The most recent standardized test, and one that has been designed specifically for nursing, is the *Critical Thinking in Clinical Nursing Practice/RN Test*, published by the National League for Nursing in 2001. This 120-item test, with a reported reliability of .88, reflects 21 critical thinking behaviors (e.g., interprets evidence, judges worth of evidence, detects bias, supports conclusions with evidence), each of which relates to the broad critical thinking skills of interpretation, analysis, evaluation, inference, and explanation. It also reflects the nursing process and nine areas of nursing content (e.g., research, cultural/spiritual systems, health promotion/illness management, and client education/empowerment).

Critical thinking need not be measured only by standardized tests, however. In addition to being used to promote critical thinking, concept maps are a way to evaluate critical thinking (Daley, Shaw, Balistrieri, Glasenapp, & Piacentine, 1999). They can be evaluated in terms of the hierarchical organization of concepts within the map, the appropriateness and validity of relationships among concepts, the number and significance of connections that are made, and the completeness of information included in the map, among other criteria. As such, they give an indication of the individual's critical thinking skill.

An individual's critical thinking can also be evaluated by observing identified indicators (Alfaro-LeFevre, 2001). Indicators are behaviors one would observe directly and include actions such as (but not limited to) the following: admits bias and inclinations, shows tolerance for different viewpoints, identifies relationships, and suspends or revises judgment as indicated by new or incomplete data. Although observation of indicators is time consuming and somewhat "subjective," it can be the most powerful and reliable way to assess critical thinking and should be used whenever possible. What one actually *does*—not merely what one *says* or what score one receives on a cognitive test—is the true measure of one's abilities, values, and so on, including one's critical thinking skills.

Finally, a learner's portfolio can be used to assess critical thinking. Such a portfolio might include papers, journals, teaching plans, or other items that document growth in thinking. Over time, one would expect to see increased sophistication in the questions asked in patient care situations, increased attention to context, greater reflection of one's own actions or decision making, identification of more subtle assumptions being made in various situations, more thorough self-evaluations, and so on. Thus, a wide variety of evidence can be used to assess the learner's critical thinking.

Conclusion

Promoting critical thinking skills is not a goal that can be accomplished in one course or one learning experience, or through the efforts of a single teacher. Indeed, efforts designed to help learners grow in their critical thinking abilities must be integrated throughout an *entire* program or experience, and the focus must be on continual learner growth over time, not on perfection at a single point in time. In addition, *all* teachers must make a commitment to investing the energy to make it happen.

The strategies that are likely to promote critical thinking require that educators become facilitators of learning. They must share their thinking with learners, let learners know when they don't know something, and role model critical thinking in all circumstances, including classrooms, clinical settings, advisement and counseling sessions, meetings, their own writings, interactions with individuals in other departments, professional presentations, and so on.

"It is difficult, perhaps impossible for [learners] to develop critical thinking when the [educator] is doing all the thinking" (Kurfiss, 1989, p. 42). In addition to being professors of nursing, therefore, we need to be "professors of thinking" (Kurfiss, 1989, p. 41), and we need to teach for thinking.

It is expected that learners whose educational experience truly focuses on helping them become critical thinkers will participate more in class; be more willing to discuss mistakes; take greater responsibility for themselves and their continued learning; collaborate more effectively with peers, faculty, and members of other disciplines; and have fewer prejudices. Research is needed to substantiate these expectations, but these are worthwhile outcomes toward which to strive nevertheless.

"In 500 years, we've moved from a world where everything was certain and nothing changed, to a world where nothing seems certain and everything changes" (Gelb, 1998, p. 17). Students and nurses in practice who have good critical thinking skills will be better prepared to function effectively in a world "where nothing seems certain and everything changes." Educators' investment in promoting critical thinking skills would certainly seem to be worth the effort.

Case Study

A school of nursing faculty reviewed all existing standardized tests for critical thinking and did not feel that any of them measured critical thinking in a way that fit with the school's philosophy and definition of critical thinking. The faculty believe that critical thinking is discipline specific and that in nursing, critical thinking must be measured in a nursing context. So, they developed a one-page health care scenario with questions designed to elicit critical thinking. They administered the scenario to a group of students and asked a faculty committee to assess the results. The faculty members evaluated each paper, with widely varying results. Papers that were considered to be good examples of critical thinking by one faculty member were considered average or poor examples by other faculty members.

1. Did the health care scenario tool lack validity or reliability?
2. What could account for the widely varying faculty evaluations?
3. Since the school had a definition of critical thinking, shouldn't that have helped faculty to be more uniform in their judgments?
4. How could this faculty proceed to rework the tool (or the process) to make it a better measure of critical thinking?

Critical Thinking Exercises

1. Many employers of nurses say they want all nurses they hire to be critical thinkers. They rate critical thinking among the most desirable skills for their employees. Is it realistic to expect that all nurses will have highly developed critical thinking skills? If a nurse has good problem-solving skills, might that be enough to make her or him a valued employee?
2. In teaching nurses to always question assumptions, identify false premises, judge the validity of inferences, and question judgments, is there danger that we encourage them to be too "critical" and "judgmental" in a negative sense? Why or why not?
3. "The use of Microthemes as a teaching strategy is not applicable in a medical/surgical nursing course or a pathophysiology course because there are no controversial issues in these types of courses." Do you agree or disagree with this statement? Why?
4. You are teaching young diabetic patients how to manage their self-care. You realize they need a certain amount of critical thinking ability in order to manage their diabetes well in the long run. How can you assess whether these youngsters have those abilities?

Ideas for Further Research

1. Interview staff development educators to find out what critical thinking skills they are looking for in new nursing graduates.

2. Compare the critical thinking definitions used in various schools of nursing. What are the commonalities and differences? To what extent are the tools they use to measure critical thinking consistent with their definition?

3. Using a standardized test, measure critical thinking in a group of nursing students. Then look for variables that correlate with the critical thinking scores. (For example, grade point average, clinical laboratory grades, standardized leadership test scores, etc.)

REFERENCES

Abegglen, J., & Conger, C. O. (1997). Critical thinking in nursing: Classroom tactics that work. *Journal of Nursing Education, 36*(10), 452–458.

Alfaro-LeFevre, R. (1999). *Critical thinking in nursing: A practical approach* (2nd ed.). Philadelphia: Saunders.

Alfaro-LeFevre, R. (2001). *Nursing critical thinking indicators (CTIs).* Unpublished document, *rozalfaro@aol.com.*

Bandman, E. L., & Bandman, B. (1995). *Critical thinking in nursing* (2nd ed.). Norwalk, CT: Appleton & Lange.

Barrow, R. (1990). *Understanding skills: Thinking, feeling and caring.* London, Ontario: The Althouse Press.

Bass, B. M. (1990). *Bass & Stogdill's handbook of leadership: Theory research & managerial applications* (3rd ed.). New York: Free Press.

Beyer, B. K. (1985). Improving thinking skills: Defining the problem. *Phi Delta Kappan, 65*(7), 486–490.

Bloom, B. S. (1953). Thought-processes in lectures and discussions. *Journal of General Education, 1,* 160–169.

Bowers, B., & McCarthy, D. (1993). Developing analytic thinking skills in early undergraduate education. *Journal of Nursing Education, 32*(3), 107–114.

Brookfield, S. D. (1987). *Developing critical thinkers: Challenging adults to explore alternative ways of thinking and acting.* San Francisco: Jossey-Bass.

Brookfield, S. (1993). On impostorship, cultural suicide, and other dangers: How nurses learn critical thinking. *Journal of Continuing Education in Nursing, 24*(5), 197–205.

Burns, J. M. (1978). *Leadership.* New York: Harper Torchbooks.

Colucciello, M. L. (1997). Critical thinking skills and dispositions of baccalaureate nursing students— A conceptual model for evaluation. *Journal of Professional Nursing, 13*(4), 236–245.

Cross, K. P. (1981). *Adults as learners.* San Francisco: Jossey-Bass.

Daley, B. J., Shaw, C. R., Balistrieri, T., Glasenapp, K., & Piacentine, L. (1999). Concept maps: A strategy to teach and evaluate critical thinking. *Journal of Nursing Education, 38*(1), 42–47.

de Tornyay, R. (1990). Encouraging risk-taking by creating trust (Editorial). *Journal of Nursing Education, 29*(2), 51.

Dressel, P., & Mayhew, L. B. (1954). *General education: Exploration in evaluation* (Final Report of the Cooperative Study of Evaluation in General Education). Washington, DC: American Council on Education.

Ennis, R. H. (1985). A logical basis for measuring critical thinking skills. *Educational Leadership, 43*(2), 44–48.

Ennis, R. H. (1989). Critical thinking and subject specificity: Clarification and needed research. *Educational Researcher, 18*(3), 4–10.

Ennis, R. H. (1990). The extent to which critical thinking is subject-specific: Further clarification. *Educational Researcher, 19*(4), 13–16.

Facione, N. C., & Facione, P. A. (1996). Assessment design issues for evaluating critical thinking in nursing. *Holistic Nursing Practice, 10*(3), 41–53.

Facione, P. A. (1990). *Critical thinking: A statement of expert consensus for purposes of educational assessment and instruction* (The Delphi Study Report of the American Philosophical Association). Millbrae, CA: California Academic Press.

Facione, P. A. (1992). *The California Critical Thinking Skills Test (CCTST): College level.* Millbrae, CA: California Academic Press.

Facione, P. A., & Facione, N. (1992). *The California Critical Thinking Dispositions Inventory (CCTDI).* Millbrae, CA: California Academic Press.

Fairfield University School of Nursing. (1997). *Self-study report to the National League for Nursing Accrediting Commission.* Fairfield, CT: Author.

Ford, J. S., & Profetto-McGrath, J. (1994). A model for critical thinking within the context of curriculum as praxis. *Journal of Nursing Education, 33*(8), 341–344.

Gelb, M. J. (1998). *How to think like Leonardo DaVinci.* New York: Delacourte Press.

Grafton, S. (1992). *"I" is for innocent.* New York: Fawcett Crest.

Gryskiewicz, S. S. (2000). Creating turbulence. *Association Management, 52*(1), 46–51.

Hager, P. (1990). Non-generalizability theses in recent philosophy of education. Paper presented at the 10th Annual International Conference on Critical Thinking and Educational Reform (August 4–8, 1990). Rohnert Park, CA: Sonoma State University.

Halpern, D. F. (1994). Critical thinking: The 21st century imperative for higher education. *The Long Term View, 2*(3), 12–16.

Hanford, G. (1994). The danger of fragmentation. *Educational Vision, 2*(1), 6–7.

Johnson, D. W., & Johnson, R. T. (1989). Critical thinking through structured controversy. *Educational Leadership, 46*(8), 58–64.

Kemp, V. H. (1985). Concept analysis as a strategy for promoting critical thinking. *Journal of Nursing Education, 24*(9), 382–384.

Kramer, M. K. (1993). Concept clarification and critical thinking: Integrated processes. *Journal of Nursing Education, 32*(9), 406–414.

Krejci, J. W. (1997). Imagery: Stimulating critical thinking by exploring mental models. *Journal of Nursing Education, 36*(10), 482–484.

Kurfiss, J. (1988). *Critical thinking: Theory, research, practice, and possibilities* (ASHE-ERIC Higher Education Report, No. 2). Washington, DC: Association for the Study of Higher Education.

Kurfiss, J. G. (1989). Helping faculty foster students' critical thinking in the discussion. In A. F. Lucas (Ed.), *The department chairperson's role in enhancing college teaching* (pp. 41–50). (New Directions for Teaching and Learning, No. 37). San Francisco: Jossey-Bass.

Lipman, M. (1988). *Critical thinking—What can it be?* (Resource Publication Series 1, No. 1). Montclair, NJ: Institute for Critical Thinking, Montclair State College.

McDonald, M. E. (2002). *Systematic assessment of learning outcomes: Developing multiple-choice exams.* Sudbury, MA: NLN Press/Jones & Bartlett.

McPeck, J. E. (1981). *Critical thinking and education.* New York: St. Martin's.

Miller, M. A., & Malcolm, N. S. (1990). Critical thinking in the nursing curriculum. *Nursing & Health Care, 11*(2), 67–73.

National Council for Excellence in Critical Thinking. (1992). *Proceedings of the 12th Annual International Conference on Critical Thinking and Educational Reform (August 9–12, 1992)* (pp. 197–203). Rohnert Park, CA: Center for Critical Thinking and Moral Critique, Sonoma State University.

National League for Nursing. (2001). *Critical thinking in clinical nursing practice/RN*. New York: Author.

National League for Nursing Accrediting Commission. (2001). *Accreditation manual and interpretive guidelines by program type for post secondary and higher degree programs in nursing*. New York: Author.

Norris, S. P. (1988). Research needed on critical thinking. *Canadian Journal of Education, 13*(1), 125–137.

Paul, R. (1990). *Critical thinking: What every person needs to know to survive in a rapidly changing world*. Rohnert Park, CA: Center for Critical Thinking and Moral Critique, Sonoma State University.

Paul, R. (1992). Why critical thinking? Why now? *Critical Thinking, 1*(1), 3.

Paul, R. (1993). *Critical thinking: How to prepare students for a rapidly changing world*. Santa Rosa, CA: Foundation for Critical Thinking.

Paul, R. (1994a). Overcoming the addiction to coverage. *Educational Vision, 2*(1), 11.

Paul, R. (1994b). What are intellectual standards? *Educational Vision, 2*(1), 10.

Paul R., & Elder, L. (1995). The art of Socratic questioning. *Critical Thinking, 3*(1), 16.

Paul, R., & Elder, L. (1996). Socratic questioning within subject domains. *Academic Excellence,* Winter 1996, 14.

Pederson, C., Duckett, L., & Maruyama, G. (1990). Using structured controversy to promote ethical decision making. *Journal of Nursing Education, 29*(4), 150–157.

Perkins, D. N. (1985). Postprimary education has little impact on informed reasoning. *Journal of Educational Psychology, 77,* 562–571.

Perry, W. G. (1970). *Forms of intellectual and ethical development in the college years: A scheme*. New York: Holt, Rinehart & Winston.

Scheffer, B. K., & Rubenfeld, M. G. (2000). A consensus statement on critical thinking in nursing. *Journal of Nursing Education, 39*(8), 352–360.

Scriven, M. (1990). Foreword. In J. McPeck (Ed.), *Teaching critical thinking: Dialogue and dialectic*. New York: Routledge.

Sternberg, R. J. (1985). Critical thinking: Its nature, measurement, and improvement. In F. R. Link (Ed.), *Essays on the intellect*. Alexandria, VA: Association for Supervision and Curriculum Development.

Vinten, S. A., & Ellett, M. (2001). Extending group learning to dyad testing. Paper presented at the National League for Nursing Education Summit 2001, September 20–23, 2001, Baltimore, MD.

Watson, G., & Glaser, E. M. (1964). *Critical thinking appraisal*. Orlando: Harcourt, Brace, Jovanovich.

Watson, G., & Glaser, E. M. (1980). *Watson–Glaser Critical Thinking Appraisal manual*. New York: Harcourt, Brace & World.

13

Clinical Teaching

Clinical teaching is a complex enterprise. It is so complex that few researchers have tackled the issues that need to be addressed. Little of our present clinical teaching is grounded in research but rather is grounded in tradition, common sense, and feasibility. We don't really know, for example, how many hours of clinical experience are needed for undergraduate nursing education, for graduate education, for orientation of new staff nurses, or for teaching ancillary staff. We have little empirical evidence of which model of clinical education yields the best results. Within each clinical model, we don't know the best student–teacher ratio or how much supervision is actually needed, or whether quantity of patient assignments is more important than quality of assignments. We don't know the relative effectiveness of written assignments for clinical students (Barnard & Dunn, 1994; Oermann, 1996b).

It is the complexity of the clinical setting that makes research so difficult. There are so many variables that are difficult to control: the severity of patient illness, widely varying settings, differences in nursing and educational personnel, variable staffing patterns, and varied student motivation and preparation, to name a few. Yet it is the same complexity that makes the clinical setting such a rich learning environment. Until there is more research to guide us, we must function with the empirical evidence we do have and base our actions on the collective wisdom brought to us by more than a century of recorded clinical teaching experiences.

Purpose of the Clinical Laboratory

What kind of learning takes place in a clinical setting? What are the real purposes behind having learners spend time in clinical agencies? Some of the answers are apparent, some we can only make educated guesses about.

It seems obvious to expect theory and practice to come together in the clinical laboratory. Learners should have the opportunity to apply the theoretical concepts, rules, and propositions they have learned in the classroom. A proposition like "Frequent change in body position helps prevent decubitus ulcers" can be tested with a variety of patients to see how and under what conditions it holds true. Learners not only test the proposition but learn when to apply it, and they practice the techniques of implementation (Dunn, Ehrich, Mylonas, & Hansford, 2000). The proposition becomes more than a memorized fact; it takes on life and meaning as it is applied to real patients. Learners see how this one piece of information fits into the whole picture of patient care in a more realistic way than they ever could in a classroom.

It is in the clinical laboratory that many skills are perfected. Complex psychomotor skills may be practiced initially in a skills laboratory, but to be mastered, they often require a live rather than simulated situation. For example, learners can practice colostomy care endlessly in a simulation lab, but they will never become experts until they work with a variety of patients who have different stomas and different skin conditions and contours, using varied equipment.

Infante (1985), in her study of the clinical laboratory, noted that the opportunity for observation is an essential element of clinical learning. The skill of observation can be taught in simulated situations, but learners need repeated experience observing patients in changing circumstances so that they know what to look for in changing situations.

Problem-solving and decision-making skills are also refined in the clinical laboratory. Students should learn the basics of these skills prior to entering the clinical setting. The ultimate practice in decision making and problem solving, however, is done in patient settings with many interacting variables and constantly changing circumstances. Learners need practice using these cognitive skills under the guidance of an educator and other professional staff in real-life settings (Fothergill-Bourbonnais & Higuchi, 1995).

Learners also gain organization and time management skills in clinical settings (Gaberson & Oermann, 1999). Again, no simulation can prepare students as well as the live laboratory when it comes to organization. It is in real clinical practice, with the help of the instructor, that learners find how to organize all the data that bombards them, all the requests made of them, and all the intellectual and psychomotor tasks they must perform. They learn to set priorities by having repeated practice in doing so in complex situations. It is in the clinical laboratory that the skill of delegation is practiced and truly learned.

Cultural competence is a skill that can be learned well in the clinical laboratory (Gaberson & Oermann, 1999). Learners may know a lot of theory about how to approach clients from different cultures, but they become comfortable and more expert with cross-cultural care when they care for culturally diverse clients. The educator may plan student assignments with cultural exposure in mind.

Finally, learners of nursing become socialized in the clinical laboratory (Chan, 2002). They learn which behaviors and values are professionally acceptable or unacceptable. They learn about professional responsibility. The clinical laboratory is a place where consequences for one's actions are readily apparent and accountability is demanded. The knowledge and skills students have learned become integrated into a nursing role. They begin to see staff as role models, and they have opportunities to interact with members of other disciplines on a professional level. Some nursing students have expressed the belief that developing a sense of team membership was one of their most important goals in the clinical laboratory (Dunn et al., 2000). Students also learn how to relate to patients professionally and gain a patient's perspective of illness that leads to more caring behaviors (Fothergill-Bourbonnais & Higuchi, 1995).

For all of these reasons, learners need to spend time in clinical settings, and educators need to learn how best to use that time.

Misuse of the Clinical Laboratory

As Infante (1985) points out clearly, the clinical laboratory has historically been misused at all levels of nursing education. Nursing students, for instance, have been sent to the clinical setting to gain work experience rather than to achieve educational objectives. Clinical objectives should be as clear and specific as those for the classroom or skills laboratory. Objectives should focus on the application of knowledge and skills more than they do on learning the future employee role.

Misuse of the clinical setting also occurs when novices are given too much responsibility for patient care. Expecting too much from fledgling learners causes anxiety, instructor fatigue, and increased chance of errors. Learners should not be functioning independently in situations with relatively high levels of risk. They should be providing care in circumstances for which they are well qualified and for which they have had preliminary guidance. Objectives for beginning learners should be quite limited, focusing on specific processes of care. It is only after specific components of care have been practiced that the learner is able to integrate previous learning and provide total care.

A third way in which the clinical laboratory is misused is when learners are supervised and evaluated more than they are taught. Educators who talk about "supervising" learners in the clinical laboratory may be revealing an unconscious attitude toward student activity. They may be expecting learners to "perform" rather than to "practice." A certain amount of supervision must take place, but the emphasis should be on teaching and guiding, with the understanding that mistakes will be made. One study conducted by Wilson (1994) found that nursing students "were constantly aware that the instructor was evaluating them" (p. 84). In situations where this belief is true, learners are at a real disadvantage, because they probably cannot do their best job of learning when they know they have to simultaneously perform for an evaluation. Evaluation of clinical performance must be separated from practice time.

Models of Clinical Teaching

Several ways of structuring clinical experiences for learners have been described in the literature. In the traditional and best-known model in nursing education, instructors accompany groups of 8 to 12 learners to a clinical agency and assign the learners to patients. Although the staff of the agency retains primary responsibility for the care of the patient, the learners usually provide total patient care during the time they are in the agency. The instructor chooses patient assignments that correlate with the theoretical material being taught in the classroom simultaneously, to the extent possible. The educator works as closely as possible with each learner, although, with so many to attend to, and emergencies popping up periodically, some of the learners get minimal attention on a particular day. I can recall some of my days as a clinical instructor when I was ashamed to say that other than conference time, there was at least one student that I had not seen or taught at all. Another problem with this model is the fact that if the educator is employed by a college or university, she or he is a guest in the agency and may struggle with lack of staff trust and a feeling of separateness from the unit (Paterson, 1997). Also, agency staff can feel overwhelmed with having so many learners on a unit at one time (Furst, 1997).

Some newer models of clinical education have been used with some success. Infante (1985) developed a model that relies heavily on keeping nursing students in a skills laboratory until they are proficient with skills. They are then sent to the clinical area and are assigned to practice specific psychomotor and other skills. They are not assigned to total patient care until late in the curriculum. For example, students may be studying physical assessment and practicing it in a college laboratory until they demonstrate proficiency. They then attend the clinical setting where they practice part or all of the assessment skills, without providing any other care to the patient. An instructor may or may not be present when each student is present in the clinical setting, since times and days of laboratory sessions may not be the same for all students; preceptors are present in some cases. Obviously, the clinical agency must be willing to accept students when the educator is not present. Infante's model was tested in one nursing program with positive outcomes (Infante, Forbes, Houldin, & Naylor, 1989).

Packer (1994) has suggested a different approach. She contends that more information about clinical practice should be taught in the classroom before learners go to the clinical area. Thus, she proposes a clinical nursing course to be taught in the classroom, with small groups of students that would permit a lot of interaction with the teacher. Case studies and questioning would be heavily used to apply nursing theory, and students would, with guidance, propose nursing care approaches and discuss the alternatives, possible outcomes, and financial, organizational, or ethical ramifications. In the course of discussion, the educator would guide the learners to think about setting priorities, time management, working with an interdisciplinary team, delegation, and professional communication. Packer hypothesizes that after taking such a course, students would be more self-confident and better able to handle clinical situations in the real world. She also believes that reality shock would be reduced on entering the work world if such an approach were taken. There is no mention of this model's being tested. These first two models are proposed for undergraduate nursing students but could be adapted to other groups.

A variety of preceptorship models have been explored in the literature and in practice. Research on effectiveness and satisfaction for participants has been very positive so far (Brehaut, Turik, & Wade, 1998; Melander & Roberts, 1994; Oermann, 1996b). In a traditional preceptorship, a student is taught and supervised by a practicing nurse employed by a health care agency while an educator oversees the process and indirectly supervises the student. This type of preceptorship has been used for the clinical education of undergraduate and graduate nursing students, newly graduated nurses, refresher course nurses, and ancillary staff. There are newer collaborative teaching models in which clinical teaching associates (CTAs), who are employed by a health care agency, collaborate with educators in teaching small groups of students. The educator is more involved in the teaching process than in traditional preceptorships, with the staff preceptor, educator, and student forming a learning triad (Melander & Roberts). When the CTA model is used, educators are present for some or most of the learners' clinical time.

One variation of the CTA model is explained by Hunsberger and colleagues (2000). In their approach, designed for a two-day clinical experience, the CTA takes the lead on the first day with orientation to the unit and to the clinical assignment for a small group of students and the educator. The CTA focuses heavily on psychomotor skills that day. Both the CTA and the educator attend and share leadership in the postconference. On the second day, the educator takes over the teaching and supervisory role. This model relieves some of the stress on the educator, who does not know the patients well on the first day, and taps the expertise of the staff nurse in teaching psychomotor skills.

More on Preceptorships

The impetus for development of preceptorships has arisen from several factors. Faculty and staff development educators have agreed over the years that something should be done to bridge the gap between students' experience in academia and the realities they encounter when taking their first professional position (DeLong & Bechtel, 1999). Preceptorships increase clinical experience for students and expose them to more of the realities of the work world, which should reduce reality shock. College faculty have long sought a model of clinical teaching that would allow students to have more time and attention from a teacher than in the traditional clinical teaching model. Preceptorships afford this attention, thus potentially increasing the learning during clinical time (Beeman, 2001). College and university faculty also struggle with the multiple and growing roles they must fulfill in academia. The increased emphasis on research and publication alone precludes faculty from spending the time in clinical practice that is needed to keep skills at the expert level (Hunsberger et al., 2000). The result is many faculty members who teach in the clinical area but who feel insecure with their skill level. Preceptorships allow students to learn from practitioners with a high skill level while still being guided by faculty who have a wealth of knowledge.

Although there are real benefits to the preceptorship model, some educators perceive barriers as well (Beeman, 2001). Some faculty members fear that staff preceptors do not really have the time to supervise students, which could lead to serious errors. They believe that because preceptors do not know the school's curriculum very well, there will not be adequate correlation between theory and practice. Finally, there is the realistic fear that eventually the health care agencies will say they must charge for preceptor time (which already occurs with some nurse practitioner preceptors).

Some of the perceived barriers to successful preceptorships can be avoided by providing good preceptor orientation programs. Table 13–1 outlines the essentials of a comprehensive program of preparation. Health care agencies usually absorb the cost of releasing staff to attend the orientation, and faculty or staff development educators provide the teaching.

The roles of educator and preceptor must be clearly delineated if the preceptorship is going to work well. The educator is responsible for overseeing the educational experience and is ultimately responsible for student learning outcomes. He or she must introduce the preceptor to the learning objectives, to specifics about the course, and to methods of student evaluation. The educator must meet periodically with the preceptor (lunch meetings work well) to talk about the student learning needs and student progress, as well as to talk about any problems that may have cropped up. The educator meets with the students in conference on a regular (often weekly) basis to be sure the students are making connections to the curriculum and to help them see the "big picture" about how their experiences fit into the wider world of nursing. If clinical logs or journals are required, the educator reads them and gives feedback. The educator shares responsibility for evaluation and grading along with the preceptor (Nehls, Rather, & Guyette, 1997).

The role of preceptor is that of orienting students to the agency, assigning students to patients, teaching patient care, asking questions to be sure learners understand what they are

TABLE 13-1 Components of a Comprehensive Orientation for Preceptors

1. Purpose and expected outcomes of the clinical education of learners
2. Overview of the school curriculum as it relates to the clinical experience
3. Skills that can be expected of learners entering the preceptorship
4. Principles of adult learning
5. Common errors made by students and common misconceptions
6. Roles and responsibilities of the preceptor, the educator, and the student
7. Interactions with learners and relationship with educators
8. Introduction to course syllabi
9. Planning learning experiences
10. Clinical teaching strategies
11. Overview of evaluation procedures and measuring instruments
12. Legal implications of working with learners

Sources: Beeman, R. Y. (2001). New partnerships between education and practice: Precepting junior nursing students in the acute care setting. *Journal of Nursing Education, 40*(3), 132–134; Daigle, J. (2001). Preceptors in nursing education—Facilitating student learning. *Kansas Nurse, 76*(4), 3–6; Melander, S., & Roberts, C. (1994). Clinical teaching associate model: Creating effective BSN student/faculty/staff nurse triads. *Journal of Nursing Education, 33*(9), 422–425; and Oermann, M. H. (1996). A study of preceptor roles in clinical teaching. *Nursing Connections, 9*(4), 57–64.

doing, and evaluating student learning (Oermann, 1996a). Ohrling and Hallberg (2001) studied preceptors' perceptions of what they do for learners and found two major themes: *sheltering students while learning* and *facilitating students' learning.* In the arena of sheltering, they believed it was important to protect students from situations too difficult for them, to prevent their not being successful, and to assess their competence. Facilitating learning was accomplished by using a variety of teaching strategies, conversing with students, demonstrating skills for them, and talking them through various situations.

The relationship between preceptor and learner is an important variable in the success of the enterprise. When preceptors are selected by an agency, it is important that the criteria be more than "a warm body" (Daigle, 2001). The preceptor must be an experienced nurse who will be a good role model and must be someone who has good interpersonal skills and who wants to be a preceptor. Strong interpersonal skills are essential since the relationship must be based on mutual respect, trust, open communication, and encouragement (Bittner & Anderson, 1998). Without this kind of relationship, learning may be impaired.

Recruiting preceptors is not always easy. When talking to prospective preceptors, the benefits and rewards of the role should be explained. Some health care agencies include preceptorships as one of the criteria for climbing the clinical ladder to a higher category of staff nurse. Educational institutions reward preceptors with perks like titles, certificates or letters of appreciation, library privileges, and invitations to recognition events (Lyon & Peach, 2001). Preceptors also report intrinsic rewards like personal satisfaction from sharing their expertise with students and professional stimulation resulting from students' questions. Although there are times when preceptors could work faster without student teaching responsibilities, preceptors also report that at times an extra pair of hands are a big help (Beeman, 2001).

Preparation for Clinical Instruction

To ensure a positive learning experience for learners, whether they are undergraduate students, graduate students, refresher course nurses, or ancillary nursing staff, educators must do a lot of planning before clinical instruction begins. If the educational institution is not part of a health care system, clinical agency sites must be chosen. If the educator is part of the staff development department in an agency, clinical units within the agency must still be identified. Selection of clinical sites must be done methodically. You must consider the learning experiences that are available there. Will it be possible to obtain clinical experiences that correlate with theoretical content? Will learners have a variety of experiences? Is there enough room around the nurses' station or office for learners to use patients' charts? An often-overlooked aspect of the learning experience is the availability of role models for learners. Research has demonstrated that clinical educators are role models for learners (Wiseman, 1994), but so are staff in the agency (Gaberson & Oermann, 1999). What are the educational credentials and experience levels of the staff who will serve as these role models, and are they receptive to having learners on their unit?

If the college or university is not part of the health care system, contracts must be drawn up between the school and the clinical agency. It is sometimes the educator's role to gather data that will lead to a written contract. These data include the availability of the clinical unit for certain days and weeks and the availability of conference space, parking, and locker space. The contract also includes the maximum student–faculty ratio, evidence of completion of health records for students and faculty, and evidence of malpractice and general liability insurance for students and faculty.

Once arrangements have been made for clinical units, the educator should set up a meeting with the agency staff that will be involved with the education process. That may include a staff development educator, unit manager, or head nurse. At that meeting, the expectations of both parties can be discussed and actual implementation of the learning experience can be worked out. This is the appropriate time to share clinical learning objectives with the manager or head nurse. If the staff are familiar with the learning objectives, they can assist learners in meeting them.

After these arrangements have been made, the educator can proceed with the final preparation for clinical instruction. This last step involves making specific assignments for learners on a weekly or daily basis (if the learners are not working with preceptors). Staff input can be invaluable in planning assignments. Staff members usually know the patients and families better than the educator does. If the staff are aware of the learning objectives, they can direct the instructor to suitable assignments. In addition, educators and learners together may choose assignments. In some cases, especially with students who are nearing completion of their educational program, students may choose their own assignments, in consultation with the staff.

Even if learners are not involved in choosing their assignments, they may be held responsible for clinical preparation. A visit to the clinical agency may be required so that the learner can research the assigned patient's chart and perhaps meet the patient and/or family. Programs that do not require the learner to go to the agency prior to the clinical laboratory experience may still expect preclinical planning. The arrangements in this case often involve the instructor gathering data from the chart and passing it on to the student (McCoin & Jenkins, 1988). The learner (if a professional nursing student) is usually expected to research the medical and nursing diagnoses, lab tests, and medications and to develop a preliminary plan of care.

Goldenberg and Iwasiw (1988) conducted an investigation of the criteria used by educators in selecting students' clinical assignments. Not surprisingly, the three most important criteria used in the selection process were "students' individual learning needs, patients' nursing care needs, and matching of patients' needs with students' learning needs" (p. 260). In some cases, students' learning needs may be met just as well if they are double-assigned to the same patient (Oermann, 1996b). In these cases, each student may take a different role (for instance, one student may give the bulk of the patient care, and the other student may give medications and document care); if there is a great deal of care for a complex case, they may share equally in the workload. Wierda and Natzke (2000) describe another method of pairing students on the same assignment, but in overlapping shifts.

Conducting a Clinical Laboratory Session

After all the careful preparation by educators and learners, the clinical laboratory session begins. For many instructors, the day starts with a group preconference.

Preconferences

During the preconference, planning of patient care continues. Learners usually share some of the results of their research from the previous day. Tentative nursing diagnoses are discussed, and the assigned learner can discuss possible nursing interventions with the other learners and the instructor. This is a good time to answer students' questions about their assignments and to try to alleviate their anxieties. Preconference time may also be used to help learners organize their day and prioritize the care they must give.

If time is available, all students can discuss their patients in some depth. If time is limited—and it usually is—the educator might select just a few patients who typify the focus of the day's objectives. For example, if the objectives revolve around fluid and electrolyte balance, the teacher might have a learner with a surgical patient discuss the patient's fluid balance and the accompanying nursing responsibilities. Another learner with a patient who has congestive heart failure could present the identified fluid problems in that case. The other learners should be able to transfer some of the information to their own assigned patients.

The Practice Session

Following the preconference, the learners begin their practice for the day. The structure of the practice session may vary a great deal. For example, each learner may be providing some degree of care to one or more patients and may be reporting directly to the educator for all questions and needed help. Staff nurses, in this case, only get involved when learners give them report at the end of the practice session. In another type of structure, learners may work closely with staff nurses who answer many routine questions and provide some assistance and supervision, while the educator spends time with those learners who are in situations calling for intense teaching and guidance. Third, there are, as already explained, preceptorships with several variations of that structure.

Regardless of the structure of the practice session, a variety of teaching methods can be used. Scavenger hunts are sometimes used to help orient learners to the clinical unit. Learners are given a list of places and equipment they need to locate. This activity helps nervous novices expel some energy and do something educationally useful at the same time.

Combinations of strategies like demonstration with explanations, asking and answering questions, and coaching techniques can be used. Questioning can be used to assist learners in developing problem-solving and decision-making skills. Coaching strategies can be used to help learners set goals for themselves, to guide learners through psychomotor skills, and to help them refine their thinking processes (Grealish, 2000).

In a study by Krichbaum (1994), student learning (baccalaureate students) was significantly related to preceptor behaviors like using objectives, providing for practice, asking questions, giving feedback, and displaying concern for the learner's progress. This is the only comprehensive study to date that has looked at the effectiveness of clinical teaching behaviors.

OBSERVATION ASSIGNMENTS

Observation assignments have been used routinely in clinical education. The value of observation opportunities is supported by Social Cognitive Theory, which expresses the importance of observation in the learning process. Learners may be assigned to observe nurses or other professionals performing various aspects of health care that learners usually cannot perform. Learners might be placed, for instance, in an endoscopy room or cardiac catheterization lab for a few hours of observation. Given some guidelines to channel their observations, they usually find this a valuable experience. If they can be paired off with nurses whom they can both observe and question, the learning experience may be even better.

NURSING ROUNDS

Some nurse educators use nursing rounds as a pedagogical strategy. This technique works well with students and with graduate nurses. It involves a group of learners and their instructor visiting patients to whom the learners are assigned. Before entering a patient's room, the assigned learner briefly informs the group about the patient and the diagnosis. Once in the room, the same learner interacts with the patient while others observe as much as they can about the patient and the environment. The instructor may point out the use of certain equipment or procedures. All other discussion takes place in the corridor after the visit or in a postconference (Sedlack & Doheny, 1998; Skurski, 1985).

The purpose of nursing rounds is to expose learners to additional nursing situations and to encourage them to consult each other in planning and evaluating care. Nursing rounds provide many opportunities to apply classroom theory to patient situations and to compare and contrast patient care. Postconferences become more meaningful when learners have met many or all of the patients being discussed. There is, however, a real concern about possible violation of patient privacy during nursing rounds. Patients must be asked for permission for the group to visit, and every effort must be made to keep patient information confidential.

SHIFT REPORT

Enabling the learners to listen to or give a shift report is a useful teaching strategy. Yurkovich and Smyer (1998) identify shift report as a unique time for learning. Whether the shift report is live or taped, it is a way for students to learn the uniqueness of nursing communication and is a means of professional socialization.

LEARNING CONTRACTS

Learning contracts are a useful way to structure and guide learning in the clinical setting. A learning contract can be defined as a written agreement between instructor (or supervisor) and learner spelling out the learner's outcome objectives (Chan & Wai-tong, 2000). In addition to the learning objectives, the learning resources needed to achieve them, the learning experiences planned, a timeline, and an evaluation plan are included (Renner, Stritter, & Wong, 1993). Learning contracts have been used successfully in undergraduate and graduate education, for RN to BSN students, for new staff during orientation, for staff on a clinical ladder, and for patient education (Hiromoto & Dungan, 1991; Kreider & Barry, 1993; Lowry, 1997; Waddell & Stephens, 2000).

The way a learning contract might work in staff development is as follows. Each staff member may have slightly different learning needs and interests. Therefore, each nurse develops a learning contract with the staff development educator. It may include learning objectives related to organizational abilities, communication skills, psychomotor skills, pharmacology, disease-related knowledge, patient teaching, or any nursing skill. The role of the educator is to consult with the learner in the development of the objectives; to make resources such as literature, equipment, and role models available; and to validate achievement or arrange for it to be validated by someone else. Validation may be done by observing skill performance (live or videotaped), evaluating written work or oral presentations, or validating attendance at meetings. When used in academic settings, validation may result in a grade being given. Table 13–2 gives an example of a part of a learning contract for a new staff nurse during orientation.

WRITTEN ASSIGNMENTS

There are a number of written assignments for clinical learning that can yield measurable outcomes. The individualized nursing care plan is a standard teaching device. Care plans help

TABLE 13–2 Sample Learning Contract for a New Staff Nurse During Orientation

Learning Objectives	Resources Needed	Activities and Accomplishments	Means of Validation
Improve communication skills with families of dying patients.	1. Literature search 2. Assignment of terminally ill patients	1. Analyze the essential elements of communication in this scenario. 2. After talking with families, recount the conversation with the preceptor.	Instructor will evaluate the therapeutic adequacy of the conversation.
Correctly perform colostomy care.	1. Procedure manual 2. Practice in skill lab 3. Assignment to patient with a colostomy	1. Perform the skill in the skill lab. 2. Perform the skill on a patient with supervision of the preceptor.	1. Instructor will evaluate performance in the skill lab. 2. Preceptor will evaluate performance with the patient.

learners think like a nurse, in that they use problem-solving techniques to address patient problems, and they use their knowledge of the interdisciplinary health care team as a resource.

Clinical logs or journals may also be assigned to meet certain learning objectives. "Writing journals in clinical placements is one way in which students can create a dialogue with their teacher and reflect upon and explore their clinical experiences in the context in which these experiences occur" (Holmes, 1997, p. 489). Learners use the reflection process to relate their clinical learning to prior learning, to make sense of what they have seen and felt in the clinical setting, and to think critically about their experiences. Variations of journals or logs can be adapted to various levels of students. For instance, with beginning students, the emphasis may be on the expression of feelings and exploration of their motivation. More advanced students may be asked to relate their journal entries to nursing theories or to the nursing literature, or they may be asked to generate research ideas from their own observations. Whether journals should be used as graded assignments is a controversial issue. Some educators believe that grading a journal reduces its value as a means of self-expression and creativity (Holmes, 1997). Other educators believe journals that require certain factual information, as well as feelings, can indeed be graded as a measure of learning.

Rather than use the journal technique, some educators ask students to write brief critical thinking exercises following their clinical laboratory sessions. Armstrong and Pieranunzi (2000) describe a Critical-Thought Paper that they required of students in a psychiatric nursing rotation. This exercise asks the student to identify key problems and issues for the patient, to identify underlying assumptions that the patient and the student bring to the situation, the meaning of these issues for the patient and student, and therapeutic approaches the students used.

A mundane assignment that is used frequently is the student-generated drug card (Morgan, 1991). Students are required to look up each drug their patient is receiving and to write all the pertinent information on an index card. Since there are many published drug cards today, student-generated cards seem difficult to justify, although some educators think the process of writing the information helps to lodge it in the student's memory.

POSTCONFERENCES

Discussions with educator colleagues over the years have confirmed my belief that clinical postconferences are one of the most challenging arenas for nurse educators. The challenge arises from several sources. First, postconferences are often unstructured seminars that allow for creativity but that can dissolve into meaninglessness. Second, the conference is usually held at the end of a physically and emotionally draining practice session. Third, a few learners in each clinical group seem to believe that they learned everything that could possibly be learned during their practice time and feel that a postconference is just a boring postmortem session.

Postconference time is an ideal opportunity for pointing out applications of theory to practice, for analyzing the outcome of hypothesis testing, for group problem solving, and for evaluating nursing care (Letizia, 1998). To make the most of the opportunity, the educator should have objectives in mind for the session. However, it is also an opportunity to let learners take the lead in determining much of the direction of the conference (Letizia, 1998; Rossignol, 2000).

The least creative use of the clinical postconference is simply having each learner report what was done for his or her patient. No critical thinking is engendered by this approach, and learners find it boring. Instead of having each learner report during this time, it would be preferable to begin with just one or two learners' experiences, with the other participants asking questions and contributing to the discussion by comparing and contrasting their own experiences, and everyone brainstorming the solving of problems.

The primary topic for discussion should fit in with the laboratory objectives. If the purpose of the clinical lab is to gain experience with ways of promoting respiratory function, the conference should revolve around that objective in some way. For instance, a learner who cared for a patient with postoperative atelectasis might be asked to describe the course of hospitalization, the pathophysiology, and related nursing care. A profitable discussion and question-and-answer session could then follow to allow learners to think about why preventive care for atelectasis was not given or why it didn't work. They could be led to talk about the corrective care that was given and to evaluate its effectiveness. The educator could channel the discussion to include information on the cost of this complication in physical, emotional, and financial terms. Rossignol (2000) suggests that educators should take the role of *coaches for cognition* during conferences, monitoring the thinking level of the learners and attempting to raise it through higher-order questions. Questions at the upper end of Bloom's Taxonomy (see Chapter 7) challenge students and stimulate them intellectually.

In addition to these opportunities to stimulate critical thinking, educators should encourage learners to analyze ethical issues related to patient care. Time should also be allowed for learners to air their feelings about nursing in general or their clinical experience in particular. When feelings are expressed, the educator can take the role of listener and supporter, while the group of learners often find that this kind of sharing builds group cohesiveness (Letizia & Jennrich, 1998). Postconferences are a means to help socialize learners into the world of nursing and are another opportunity to get them to think like a nurse.

Evaluating Learner Progress

Clinical evaluation of learners has been studied little, written about extensively, and talked about excessively. In spite of all the attention given to the subject, evaluation remains a difficult, subjective, time-consuming, and often puzzling chore. It is usually the least favorite task of nurse educators, yet it is inescapable.

Learners in the clinical area need the feedback and judgment of their work that evaluation gives them. They need to know how they are doing at one level before progressing to the next. Educators must evaluate learners to determine how well they are meeting objectives and to certify that they are safe practitioners.

Nurse educators should keep in mind that no one has yet devised a way to render totally objective judgments about people's behavior. However, a lot is known about evaluation principles and practices. This knowledge helps to demystify the clinical evaluation process and to make it more scientific and perhaps less distressing.

Choices to Be Made Regarding Evaluation

Before beginning the process of evaluation, the individual educator or group of educators must make several philosophical and practical choices: Should the evaluation be formative or summative? Should it be norm referenced or criterion referenced? What type of grading system should be used? What behaviors should be evaluated?

FORMATIVE AND SUMMATIVE EVALUATION

Formative evaluation is the ongoing feedback given to the learner throughout the learning experience. This continuing evaluation process helps the learner identify strengths and weaknesses and meet the learning objectives efficiently. It prevents learners from being surprised at the end of the learning experience with a judgment about their performance for which they were not prepared. Formative evaluation may be graded or nongraded.

Summative evaluation, as it sounds, is a summary evaluation given at the end of the learning experience. The purpose is to assess whether the learner has achieved the objectives and is ready to move on to the next experience. Summative evaluation results in a grade of some type being given.

Clinical evaluation in nursing almost always involves summative evaluation. It may also include formative evaluation, whether formal or informal. The wise nurse educator provides formative feedback even if the school or agency does not require it. Learners have a right to know how they are progressing in their clinical work, and educators can protect themselves against charges that they violated due process of law if they can prove that a learner was kept apprised of clinical progress or lack of it. The evaluative information may be given on an incident-by-incident basis, daily, or weekly.

Formative feedback may be given orally or in writing. If it is given orally, the instructor should also keep notes about what transpired. Written feedback is often more valuable because the learner can take time to read and absorb the information and the educator can keep a copy for future reference.

Written formative evaluation notes are often called *anecdotal records* or *clinical progress notes.* Tomey (2000) advocates recording observations of what the learner says or does including the date, a description of the incident, and comments. Such notes provide a longitudinal view of learner progress and become one source of data for a summative evaluation. Keeping detailed weekly records of a learner's clinical experience is time consuming, yet without such data, formative or summative evaluation is dependent on the instructor's memory, a fallible tool at best. Lacking such written documentation, the instructor who is called on to justify a summative evaluation is on shaky ground.

NORM-REFERENCED AND CRITERION-REFERENCED EVALUATION

In *norm-referenced* evaluation, a learner is compared with a reference group of learners, either those in the same cohort or in a norm group. Evaluation and grading are therefore relative to the performance of the group. An evaluation process in which a student's behavior is characterized as "below average," "average," or "above average" or in which grades are distributed on a normal curve is norm referenced. See Figure 13–1 for an example of a portion of a norm-referenced evaluation tool. One problem involved in using the norm-referenced system is that unless the evaluation tool is specific about what "average" behaviors are like, the process may be unreliable. One teacher's idea of average performance may be vastly different from another teacher's.

Criterion-referenced evaluation is that which compares the learner to well-defined performance criteria rather than comparing him or her to other learners. A criterion-referenced evaluation tool defines the behavior expected at each level of performance (Cottrell et al., 1986). See Figure 13–2 for an example of a portion of a criterion-referenced evaluation tool. Many educators believe criterion-referenced evaluation to be fairer that norm-referenced evaluation. Learners are informed of the behaviors expected of them in order to pass or

	Below Average	Average	Above Average
	(1 point)	(2 points)	(3 points)

Criteria:

1. Communicates therapeutically with patients.

2. Provides appropriate explanations to families of patients.

FIGURE 13-1 Example of a Portion of a Norm-Referenced Evaluation Tool

achieve a certain grade, and they either attain that level of performance or not. Grading is less subjective when criteria are spelled out and each learner is held to that standard.

In working with a variety of educators and supervisory groups, I have found that clinical evaluation is often a mixture of both norm- and criterion-referenced approaches. Criteria for acceptable performance may be listed, but before making a final judgment about a grade, the instructor mentally compares the learner to others in the cohort. This comparison may result in a change in grade. For instance, Sharon seems to meet all the behavioral criteria for a B grade. But I have just given a B to Sam, and I think that Sharon should not receive as high a grade as Sam because of some subtle differences in their performance. So, I go back and reduce Sharon's grade to a B–. Some educators think this kind of flexibility in evaluation is justifiable and necessary; others view it as a travesty of the whole system of criterion-referenced evaluation.

GRADING SYSTEMS

The issue of grading also enters the picture when choices are being made about various systems of evaluation. The two most common options for grading are assigning letter grades and using a pass/fail or satisfactory/unsatisfactory approach. Many educational institutions require that letter grades be given in all courses, so faculty are forced to arrive at letter grades whether they are using norm-referenced or criterion-referenced methods.

Rines (1963) strongly asserted that clinical grades should always be given on a pass/fail or satisfactory/unsatisfactory basis since "human behavior of any description is much too complex to permit such fine discriminations" as required in assigning numerical or letter grades (p. 17). Many educators have been influenced by Rines's work and agree that letter grades are impractical and unfair when judgments about behavior are involved.

Criteria:	POINTS
1. Communicates therapeutically with patients (Select one):	
a. Communicates only when absolutely necessary. Information provided is sometimes accurate. Does not engage in active listening.	(1)
b. Communicates on a social level. Information given is accurate. Actively listens to patient concerns.	(2)
c. Actively listens and responds to patient concerns in a professionally helpful and accurate way.	(3)

FIGURE 13-2 Example of a Portion of a Criterion-Referenced Evaluation Tool

Criterion-referenced evaluation especially lends itself to the pass/fail system. Criteria describing minimally acceptable behaviors can be written, and the learner either performs at that level or does not. The teacher does not have to agonize over several gradations of behavior.

Faculty who work in schools that require letter grades have found ways to incorporate pass/fail clinical grading into the system. A common method used when theory and clinical practice are combined in one course is to give letter grades for the theory portion of the course and pass/fail for the clinical component. The total course grade is the theory grade as long as the student receives a pass for clinical work. If the student fails the clinical portion, a failing grade is given for the course regardless of the theory grade earned.

Another issue to be considered is the point at which students should be graded for clinical work. Educators in schools of nursing should be clear about when they are teaching and when they are formally evaluating and grading performance. In many cases, anecdotal data collected in the first or second clinical session finds its way into the final evaluation. There is no clear-cut evaluation period near the end of the clinical practice experience.

The most dramatic way to cure this problem is to institute an end-of-course performance examination. Woolley, Bryan, and Davis (1998) describe a system of evaluation with a final one-day summative clinical examination based on the New York Regents College performance examination. Such examinations, however, are labor intensive and require extensive scheduling.

If an end-of-course evaluation period is not feasible, some other means must be found to separate teaching/learning time from evaluation/grading time. At the very least, the first half of the clinical experience should be strictly learning time and the last half would then produce data that contribute to the final grade. Nongraded formative evaluation can go on throughout the entire semester so learners are aware of how well they are doing.

Behaviors to Be Evaluated

The components of clinical evaluation tools vary from one school or agency to another and may differ with each clinical specialty. Educators must decide which general areas and which specific behaviors should be observed and evaluated. Nevertheless, certain basic ingredients appear in most evaluation tools. The following areas of performance are usually evaluated:

- Use of the nursing process
- Use of health-promoting strategies
- Psychomotor skills
- Organization of care
- Maintaining patient safety
- Ability to provide rationale for nursing care
- Ability to individualize care planning and intervention
- Therapeutic communication
- Ability to work with a professional team
- Professional behaviors like following policies, being on time, maintaining confidentiality, and being accountable for one's own actions
- Written documentation of care

In some cases, individual behaviors may be defined as critical elements in the evaluation process. That is, if safety were designated as a critical element, failure to demonstrate safety in patient care during the examination or evaluation period would constitute a failure of the examination or evaluation (Woolley, Bryan, & Davis, 1998).

Sources of Evaluation Data

Information about learner behavior comes from sources other than just instructor observation. Direct observation by instructors produces most of the data, but other sources should be used to give a balanced picture of performance.

Patients who have been cared for by the learner can be asked some broad questions that will elicit data—for example, "How was your day, Mrs. C?" or "Is there anything else the student (or nurse) could have done for you, Mr. L?" It is helpful to validate this input with the learner to get both perceptions of the behaviors.

Learner self-evaluation is a good source of data. Self-evaluation is never an easy task, but learners should be taught how to do it. A survey by Abbott, Carswell, McGuire, and Best (1988) revealed that both learners and educators believed self-evaluation to be important, but the learners felt that self-evaluation was more threatening than the instructor's evaluation. Learners may evaluate themselves on the same tool as that used by the educator, or they may provide their data in a personal interview or by means of a diary or log.

Data may also be gathered from agency staff. Formal evaluation is seldom sought from staff members unless they are serving as preceptors. Informal input, however, can be valuable because the staff may see the learner functioning in situations when the educator is absent. This information, good and bad, can also be shared with the learner.

Finally, written work submitted by the learner can be evaluated and incorporated as part of the clinical grade. Nursing care plans, teaching plans, critical thinking papers, and so on, can all be used as clinical evaluation data as long as they meet the objectives of the clinical experience.

etween Educator and Learner

ve data collected, whether on a formative or summative basis, should be
writing with the learner. Conferences should be held with the learner at
ough and then at the end of the evaluation period. The content of the con-
based on the information in the anecdotal records and the rating scales or
are used. Positive feedback must be given along with the negative. Specific
ritical incidents that are highly indicative of the learner's typical performance
ted out. The more specific and concrete the educator can be, the more the
efit from the evaluation. For instance, negative information can be given in

, you have great difficulty implementing the nursing process. You need to
develop skill in selecting appropriate nursing interventions for your patients."

2. "Anna, in planning care for your patients, you have had difficulty in selecting the appropriate interventions that meet their specific needs. For example, when you cared for Paul, the 10-year-old with cerebral palsy, you tried to involve him in a game that was inappropriate for someone with his level of disability."

The second example provides better feedback for the learner. The more specific examples an instructor can give to back up a generalization, the more the learner will understand and the less likely the instructor will be accused of being unfair.

If a learner is doing poorly, the educator should call him or her in for frequent conferences and keep a record of those meetings. In addition to pointing out strengths and weaknesses, the instructor should work with the learner to develop a plan for improvement.

Clinical Evaluation Tools

The instrument or tool used for clinical evaluation should meet the following specifications:

1. The items should derive from the course or unit objectives.
2. The items must be measurable in some way. It must be possible to collect substantiating data.
3. The items and instructions for use should be clear to all that must use the tool.
4. The tool should be practical in design and length.
5. The tool must be valid and reliable (Carpenito & Duespohl, 1981).

Relatively few clinical evaluation tools in use today have been formally tested for reliability and validity. If they have not been tested, educators cannot be sure that the instruments they are using are measuring what they want to measure, and they aren't certain that the outcome would be the same if different teachers used the tool to evaluate the same learner.

Three interesting tools that appear in the literature that have been tested for reliability and validity are the rating scales by Bondy (1983, 1984), the Community Family Nursing Clinical Evaluation Tool by Hawranik (2000), and the Clinical Evaluation Tool by Krichbaum, Rowan, Duckett, Ryden, and Savik (1994). Bondy developed a five-point rating scale. The five points reflect criterion-referenced levels of competency. The beauty of the scale is that it can be applied to any clinical setting with its unique learning objectives. Hawranik's tool contains items on the nursing process and professional growth and leadership and could be used in evaluating students in most home-health settings. The Clinical Evaluation Tool by Krichbaum and colleagues is generic enough that it could be used in almost any clinical experience. It covers items on health promotion, nursing process, safety, scientific knowledge, multicultural care, therapeutic relationships, and professional behavior. These tools can be used or adapted for academic or staff development settings.

The validity and reliability of an evaluation tool or a system of evaluation is not important just because a grade may hinge on it, but because the professional future of a nurse may depend on it. A summative evaluation of clinical performance may determine a nursing student's ability to stay in nursing school, a refresher nurse's freedom to reenter the profession, or a staff nurse orientee's likelihood of holding a position in an organization.

Issues of fairness and justice enter the picture, too. The educator is in a position of power over the learner. Therefore, the learner should receive *due process* in all aspects of evaluation and its outcome. Due process includes the consistent application of fair criteria based on evidence and professional judgment (Scanlan, Care, & Gessler, 2001). Educators must take clinical evaluation very seriously and do all they can to be sure the process is clear, understandable to the learners, and professionally justifiable.

Working with learners in the clinical laboratory is a hectic, demanding, and sometimes anxiety-producing experience. Yet, it is also the aspect of teaching that often brings the greatest satisfaction and reward.

CASE STUDY

As a clinical supervisor, you are responsible for conducting yearly performance evaluations of your staff. Your agency provides a competency-based measurement tool, but most aspects of the actual conduct of the evaluation are left up to you.

1. What decisions must you make before conducting the evaluation?
2. How will you collect the data you will need for the evaluation?
3. How will you respond if a staff member disagrees with some aspect of the evaluation?
4. If a staff member receives an unsatisfactory evaluation, what are the possible next steps, and how are they determined?

CRITICAL THINKING EXERCISES

1. Should you place learners in a clinical setting that has less-than-desirable staff role models? What are the risks and how could they be mitigated?
2. Conducting nursing rounds with a large group of learners poses threats to patient privacy and confidentiality. What guidelines could you put in place to protect privacy and confidentiality?

3. What are the sources of learner stress in the clinical setting? How can they be reduced? Can this stress ever have a positive aspect?

4. Some educators believe they should have a collegial relationship with learners in the clinical setting. What would be the benefits and drawbacks of having more than a traditional teacher–learner relationship?

IDEAS FOR FURTHER RESEARCH

1. How much time does a clinical instructor spend with each learner during a clinical experience? How much time do preceptors actually spend with their preceptees?

2. What role model behaviors are educators looking for in staff nurses? What role model behaviors do learners perceive in staff nurses? In preceptors?

3. Conduct an experiment. Compare learning outcomes for a group of senior nursing students in a traditional model of clinical teaching with a faculty member versus a preceptor model.

4. In a home-health setting, compare learning outcomes for students assigned to a few long-term cases versus students making many single-visit contacts with patients.

REFERENCES

Abbott, S. D., Carswell, R., McGuire, M., & Best, M. (1988). Self-evaluation and its relationship to clinical evaluation. *Journal of Nursing Education, 27*(5), 219–224.

Armstrong, M. A., & Pieranunzi, V. (2000). Interpretive approaches to teaching/learning in the psychiatric/mental health practicum. *Journal of Nursing Education, 39*(6), 274–277.

Barnard, A. G., & Dunn, S. V. (1994). Issues in the organization and structure of clinical education for undergraduate nursing programs. *Journal of Nursing Education, 33*(9), 420–422.

Beeman, R. Y. (2001). New partnerships between education and practice: Precepting junior nursing students in the acute care setting. *Journal of Nursing Education, 40*(3), 132–134.

Bittner, N. P., & Anderson, A. (1998). The preceptoring map for RN-to-BSN students. *Journal of Nursing Education, 37*(8), 367–372.

Bondy, K. N. (1983). Criterion-referenced definitions for rating scales in clinical evaluation. *Journal of Nursing Education, 22*(9), 376–382.

Bondy, K. N. (1984). Clinical evaluation of student performance: The effects of criteria on accuracy and reliability. *Research in Nursing and Health, 7,* 25–33.

Brehaut, C. J., Turik, L. J., & Wade, K. E. (1998). A pilot study to compare the effectiveness of preceptored and nonpreceptored models of clinical education in promoting baccalaureate students' competence in public health nursing. *Journal of Nursing Education, 37*(8), 376–380.

Carpenito, L. J., & Duespohl, T. A. (1981). *A guide for effective clinical instruction.* Wakefield, MA: Nursing Resources.

Chan, D. (2002). Development of the clinical learning environment inventory: Using the theoretical framework of learning environment studies to assess nursing students' perceptions of the hospital as a learning environment. *Journal of Nursing Education, 41*(2), 69–75.

Chan, S. W., & Wai-tong, C. (2000). Implementing contract learning in a clinical context: Report on a study. *Journal of Advanced Nursing, 31*(2), 298–305.

Cottrell, B. H., Cox, B. H., Kelsey, S. J., Ritchie, P. J., Rumph, E. A., & Shannahan, M. K. (1986). A clinical evaluation tool for nursing students based on the nursing process. *Journal of Nursing Education, 25*(7), 270–274.

Daigle, J. (2001). Preceptors in nursing education—Facilitating student learning. *Kansas Nurse, 76*(4), 3–6.

DeLong, T. H., & Bechtel, G. A. (1999). Enhancing relationships between nursing faculty and clinical preceptors. *Journal for Nurses in Staff Development, 15*(4), 148–151.

Dunn, S. V., Ehrich, L., Mylonas, A., & Hansford, B. C. (2000). Students' perceptions of field experience in professional development: A comparative study. *Journal of Nursing Education, 39*(9), 393–400.

Fothergill-Bourbonnais, F., & Higuchi, K. S. (1995). Selecting clinical learning experiences: An analysis of the factors involved. *Journal of Nursing Education, 34*(1), 37–41.

Furst, E. A. (1997). Student-to-student preceptorships: A preliminary report. *Journal of Nursing Education, 36*(6), 278–281.

Gaberson, K. B., & Oermann, M. H. (1999). *Clinical teaching strategies in nursing.* New York: Springer.

Goldenberg, K., & Iwasiw, C. L. (1988). Criteria used for patient selection for nursing students' hospital clinical experience. *Journal of Nursing Education, 27*(6), 258–265.

Grealish, L. (2000). The skills of coach are an essential element in clinical learning. *Journal of Nursing Education, 39*(5), 231–233.

Hawranik, P. (2000). The development and testing of a community health nursing clinical evaluation tool. *Journal of Nursing Education, 39*(6), 266–273.

Hiromoto, B. M., & Dungan, J. (1991). Contract learning for self-care activities. *Cancer Nursing, 14*(3), 148–154.

Holmes, V. (1997). Grading journals in clinical practice: A delicate issue. *Journal of Nursing Education, 36*(10), 489–492.

Hunsberger, M., Baumann, A., Lappan, J., Carter, N., Bowman, A., & Goddard, P. (2000). The synergism of expertise in clinical teaching: An integrative model for nursing education. *Journal of Nursing Education, 39*(6), 278–282.

Infante, M. S. (1985). *The clinical laboratory in nursing education* (2nd ed.). New York: Wiley.

Infante, M. S., Forbes, E. J., Houldin, A. D., & Naylor, M. D. (1989). A clinical teaching project: Examination of a clinical teaching model. *Journal of Professional Nursing, 5*(3), 132–139.

Kreider, M. C., & Barry, M. (1993). Clinical ladder development: Implementing contract learning. *The Journal of Continuing Education in Nursing, 24*(4), 166–169.

Krichbaum, K. (1994). Clinical teaching effectiveness described in relation to learning outcomes of baccalaureate nursing students. *Journal of Nursing Education, 33*(7), 306–316.

Krichbaum, K., Rowan, M., Duckett, L., Ryden, M. B., & Savik, K. (1994). The clinical evaluation tool: A measure of the quality of clinical performance of baccalaureate nursing students. *Journal of Nursing Education, 33*(9), 395–404.

Letizia, M. (1998). Strategies used in clinical postconference. *Journal of Nursing Education, 37*(7), 315–317.

Letizia, M., & Jennrich, J. (1998). Development and testing of the clinical post-conference learning environment survey. *Journal of Professional Nursing, 14*(4), 206–213.

Lowry, M. (1997). Using learning contracts in clinical practice. *Professional Nurse, 12*(4), 280–283.

Lyon, D. E., & Peach, J. (2001). Primary care providers' views of precepting nurse practitioner students. *Journal of the American Academy of Nurse Practitioners, 13*(5), 237–242.

McCoin, D. W., & Jenkins, P. C. (1988). Methods of assignment for preplanning activities (advance student preparation) for the clinical experience. *Journal of Nursing Education, 27*(2), 85–87.

Melander, S., & Roberts, C. (1994). Clinical teaching associate model: Creating effective BSN student/faculty/staff nurse triads. *Journal of Nursing Education, 33*(9), 422–425.

Morgan, S. A. (1991). Teaching activities of clinical instructors during the direct client care period: A qualitative investigation. *Journal of Advanced Nursing, 16*(10), 1238–1246.

Nehls, N., Rather, M., & Guyette, M. (1997). The preceptor model of clinical instruction: The lived experiences of students, preceptors, and faculty-of-record. *Journal of Nursing Education, 36*(5), 220–227.

Oermann, M. H. (1996a). A study of preceptor roles in clinical teaching. *Nursing Connections, 9*(4), 57–64.

Oermann, M. H. (1996b). Research on teaching in the clinical setting. In K. R. Stevens (Ed.), *Review of research in nursing education* (pp. 91–126). New York: NLN.

Ohrling, K., & Hallberg, I. R. (2001). The meaning of preceptorship: Nurses' lived experience of being a preceptor. *Journal of Advanced Nursing, 33*(4), 530–540.

Packer, J. L. (1994). Education for clinical practice: An alternative approach. *Journal of Nursing Education, 33*(9), 411–416.

Paterson, B. L. (1997). The negotiated order of clinical teaching. *Journal of Nursing Education, 36*(5), 197–205.

Renner, J. J., Stritter, F. T., & Wong, H. D. (1993). Learning contracts in clinical education. *Radiologic Technology, 64*(6), 358–365.

Rines, A. (1963). *Evaluating student progress in learning the practice of nursing* (Nursing Education Monograph). New York: Teachers College, Columbia University.

Rossignol, M. (2000). Verbal and cognitive activities between and among students and faculty in clinical conferences. *Journal of Nursing Education, 39*(6), 245–250.

Scanlan, J. M., Care, W. D., & Gessler, S. (2001). Dealing with the unsafe student in clinical practice. *Nurse Educator, 26*(1), 23–27.

Sedlack, C. A., & Doheny, M. O. (1998). Peer review through clinical rounds. *Nurse Educator, 23*(5), 42–45.

Skurski, V. (1985). Interactive clinical conferences: Nursing rounds and education imagery. *Journal of Nursing Education, 24*(4), 166–168.

Tomey, A. M. (2000). Testing techniques—Performance assessment. *Nurse Educator, 25*(2), 59–60, 98.

Waddell, D. L., & Stephens, S. (2000). Use of learning contracts in a RN-to-BSN leadership course. *The Journal of Continuing Education in Nursing, 31*(4), 179–185.

Wierda, L. F., & Natzke, C. (2000). Students' collaborative clinical experience. *Journal of Nursing Education, 39*(4), 183–184.

Wilson, M. E. (1994). Nursing student perspective of learning in a clinical setting. *Journal of Nursing Education, 33*(2), 81–86.

Wiseman, R. F. (1994). Role model behaviors in the clinical setting. *Journal of Nursing Education, 33*(9), 405–410.

Woolley, G. R., Bryan, M. S., & Davis, J. W. (1998). A comprehensive approach to clinical evaluation. *Journal of Nursing Education, 37*(8), 361–366.

Yurkovich, E., & Smyer, T. (1998). Shift report: A time for learning. *Journal of Nursing Education, 37*(9), 401–403.

14

Assessing and Evaluating Learning

Assessing and evaluating learning are just as important as the teaching process. If we teach but have no way of knowing if people are learning, we may find that, without knowing it, we have wasted a lot of time. So, it is worth our while to focus on how and when to assess and evaluate learning.

In this chapter, a distinction will be made between assessment and evaluation of learning. I will use the term *assessment of learning* in the sense of formative feedback that is done simply to find out what and how well people are learning what we teach, without any intent to give a grade. The term *evaluation of learning* will be used to include the process of measuring the extent of learning and assigning a grade. Evaluation may incorporate formative and summative feedback. Evaluation of learning that takes place in the clinical laboratory will not be included in this chapter since it appears in Chapter 13.

Classroom Assessment

Since the 1980s, many educators have been using *Classroom Assessment Techniques* (CATs). CATs are in-class, anonymous, short, nongraded exercises that provide feedback for both teacher and learner about the teaching/learning process (*Classroom Assessment Techniques*, 1997). The purpose of the techniques is to provide the teacher with quick and timely feedback about the effectiveness of his or her teaching and the state of student learning. As Angelo and Cross (1993) have stated so aptly, "Instructors who have assumed that their students were learning what they were trying to teach them are regularly faced with disappointing evidence to the contrary when they grade tests and term papers" (p. 3). If you wait until an examination or project is given and graded in order to obtain feedback about learning, it is often too late. By that time in a course, the learner may be so far behind, so confused, or so misinformed that there isn't time to undo the damage. Administering a CAT every so often gives you an idea of how things are going while there is still time to make adjustments in teaching or to give the learners the help they need while it is still effective.

The advantages of using CATs are many. They include:

- Gaining insight into student learning while there is still time to make changes
- Demonstrating to learners that the teacher really cares if they are succeeding
- Building rapport with learners
- Spending only short amounts of time to gain valuable information
- Using the flexibility of CATs to adapt to the needs of individual classes
- Helping learners to monitor their own learning
- Gaining insight into your own teaching

The disadvantages of using these assessment techniques are that although they take little time, they do take some class time away from other activities; they can be overused to the point of frustration of the learners; and they do provide some negative feedback for the educator. Do not use CATs if you don't want to know that you aren't perfect. They are likely to point out weaknesses in your teaching process or in your style.

It is important to include the learners in all aspects of the CAT process. The CAT gives the learners feedback about their own individual learning. They should be given feedback in the next class as to the primary findings from the entire group. Including learners in this way shows them that you are serious about adjusting your teaching or enhancing their learning. The entire process can convince students of the effectiveness of assessment.

Many CATs have been identified in the literature. There are many more yet to be discovered or already in use by teachers but not yet published. Even the techniques that are published have been adapted for use in individual classrooms, so that there are multiple permutations of each technique. Following are descriptions of the most commonly used techniques.

One-Minute Paper

This CAT is probably the most commonly used. It is often called just *Minute Paper*. This technique is used in the last two or three minutes of the class period. Ask the learners to write down, on a half-sheet of paper, answers to the following two questions: "What was the most important thing you learned today?" and "What important point remains unclear to you?" (Angelo & Cross, 1993). The purpose of the CAT is not just to find out if there are points that need to be reemphasized or clarified, but also to help learners develop metacognitive, analysis, and synthesis skills.

There are many possible variations in the wording of the two questions and in the exact nature of the questions. For example, Martin (1999) suggests that in courses using high technology, including distance learning courses, you might ask "How did the technology improve your understanding of the topic, or how did it confuse you?"

Don't be discouraged if the class takes a time or two before they become comfortable with answering the questions and become truly analytical about the process. The Minute Paper is a very quick way to obtain essential information about the effectiveness of your class.

Muddiest Point

The Muddiest Point is another very popular assessment technique. It was first used by Mosteller (1989) at Harvard University. It is very simple and quick to use.

Simply ask the learners, "What was the muddiest point in today's class?" The information the teacher gains from this exercise will help not only the learners in the class, but also future learners. The teacher discovers which areas learners struggle with the most and finds better ways to deal with the content in the future.

During the subsequent class, the teacher should report back on the top few muddiest points. An interesting finding is that there are usually not more than two or three unclear points identified in any particular class (Martin, 1999). This CAT is especially useful for introductory-level courses and for totally new content.

Directed Paraphrasing

The classroom assessment technique of *Directed Paraphrasing* requires learners to put into their own words something they have just learned. This technique can be used in the classroom, as an out-of-class assignment, or with patient teaching. It provides valuable feedback into learner understanding and ability to translate information.

Directed Paraphrasing is especially useful for nurses because in their work they will often have to translate medical information into layman's terms, so it is a skill worth learning (Angelo & Cross, 1993). When asking nurses or nursing students to paraphrase a segment of information, you may specify the group for whom they are translating. For example, you may ask them to paraphrase something in a way that would be understandable to a person with low literacy or to a six-year-old child.

Application Cards

Application Cards are another technique especially useful for nursing. After you have taught an essential principle, theory, or body of information, and before you talk about how this information can be applied to the real world, ask the learners to take a few minutes and write on an index card at least one possible application of this content (*Classroom Assessment Techniques*, 1997).

You can then quickly read the responses, if the group is small, and share the best ones with the class, or you can shuffle the cards and give them out to the class and have the learners read those they feel are good examples of applications. This CAT obviously helps learners to apply the theoretical material they are being taught and also helps them to see immediate relevance of what they are learning.

Background Knowledge Probe

The *Background Knowledge Probe* has a slightly different application from the previous CATs. It is used before teaching new content to discover what the learners already know about the material. It is, in a sense, an ungraded pretest. You can hand out a few written questions for students to fill in or choose the answers, or you can write the questions on the board or transparency and have the learners write the answers on their paper. Emphasize the fact that this is not an attempt to embarrass anyone, but a useful tool for directing the rest of your teaching. Remember that CATs are anonymous, so this is not a traditional pretest, but rather an assessment of what the entire group knows.

Report the results to the class, but more importantly, use the results to guide your subsequent teaching. This CAT can save any teacher a lot of grief, because as Enerson, Plank, and Johnson (1994) state, "discovering that your students' background and preparation are at odds with your expectations can throw even the best planned lesson or syllabus off-track."

Misconception/Preconception Check

Many learners come to the study of a topic with incorrect preconceptions or misconceptions that they have developed over the years. The *Misconception/Preconception Check* helps to expose these mistaken ideas that may hinder learning. Learners must be made aware of these preconceived notions and then led to understand how those notions do not fit with the truth (Enerson, Plank, & Johnson, 1994).

When you prepare to use this CAT, think about misconceptions you have heard about in the past. This will be the start of your questions for the learners. For example, many people have misconceptions about mental illness. You could ask a few questions such as, "Can people who are clinically depressed become less depressed by trying very hard to feel happier?" "Can people who are mentally ill function well in society?" You could then ask, "How did you come by the information you gave for the first two questions?" Sharing the answers from the class and then discussing them can be a powerful way to begin the study of various mental illnesses.

Self-Confidence Surveys

Course-Related Self-Confidence Surveys allow learners to express their possible lack of confidence in learning certain content or skills. Learners may be self-confident in many areas but feel insecure in some. For example, nursing students and refresher course nurses may feel very confident with psychomotor skills but lack confidence in dosage calculations. Getting confidence levels out into the open helps learners focus on improvement and teachers to focus on assignments that will build confidence (Angelo & Cross, 1993).

Using this CAT may involve developing a short survey with five or six questions and a Likert-type measurement scale. For instance, you may ask a question like, "How confident do you feel in converting fractions to decimals?" The accompanying scale may have four categories: Very confident, Somewhat confident, Not very confident, and Not confident at all. Focusing on confidence levels rather than doing a background knowledge check helps the learner to see the educator's concern with not just learning, but the learners. Martin (1999) suggests that this CAT is extremely useful when learners must deal with technology that may intimidate them, such as in a distance learning course, or in using computers as a learning tool.

There are many other classroom assessment techniques that can be found in the literature. Table 14–1 lists more CATs that may be of use to nurse educators. In addition to these, be creative and find other ways to anonymously assess student learning or teacher effectiveness. Angelo and Cross (1993) give good advice about actually using CATs, and they are worth mentioning here.

- If a published CAT doesn't appeal to you or fit with your style, don't use it.
- Don't make the use of CATs a burden. Use them only when they can enhance the learning process.

TABLE 14-1 Additional Classroom Assessment Techniques

Technique	Description
Empty Outlines	Following a class, the instructor hands out an empty or partially empty outline of the content and asks students to complete it in a short amount of time. It helps learners recall the main points of the class.
One-Sentence Summary	Ask learners to identify the answers to "Who does what to whom, when, where, how, and why?" at the end of the class. Then they write a sentence that summarizes this key information. It assesses knowledge and ability to summarize key points.
Student-Generated Test Questions	Have learners write a few test questions (at home) for the class and answer them. This gives insight into what content students see as important, their knowledge of the answers, and what they consider fair questions. You may actually use some of the questions on an exam.
Group Work Evaluation	Use a questionnaire to obtain students' reactions to group work (cooperative learning). This helps both students and teacher to identify early problems in the group process and plan interventions.
Assignment Assessments	After assignments are completed, ask learners to assess the value, and pitfalls of the assignments, and how they can be improved as learning devices.
How Am I Doing?	Early in the course, ask learners to answer a few questions about how well you are teaching and meeting their learning needs. You may use some of the same questions you would ask at the end of the course, but doing so earlier gives you time to make desired changes.

- Don't use a CAT in class until you have tried it on yourself.
- Allow a little more time than you actually think you will need to administer a CAT.
- Be sure to give learners feedback on the CAT results.

No doubt, some classroom assessment techniques can also be used as graded assignments (Peterson & Stack, 1998). Can you see how Directed Paraphrasing, One-Sentence Summary, or Application Cards could be used as graded assignments? They could be either freestanding assignments or part of an examination. For example, if one of your objectives is for learners to be able to transfer knowledge to new situations, it would be appropriate to design an assignment around the learners' ability to think of real-world applications of content they have learned and to flesh them out in some detail.

Classroom assessment techniques can also be applied in all areas of nursing education: patient education, staff development, and academic teaching. When teaching an asthmatic about his condition, why not use the Muddiest Point to assess understanding? When teaching an in-service program on universal precautions, you could use the Background Knowledge Probe or the Misconception/Preconception Check. When teaching undergraduate students about the pathophysiology of immune disorders, you could use Empty Outlines or a One-Sentence Summary. You may plan to use these techniques when you are originally planning your classes, or when you are in the middle of a class and sense that there is a problem with understanding, you may use them spontaneously. The entire CAT process is extremely flexible.

Evaluation of Learning

All nurse educators need to know methods of evaluating learning. Whether you are evaluating patient teaching, what staff have learned from an in-service program, or what students have learned in an academic course, the concepts of evaluation remain constant.

Evaluation methods should be based on learning objectives. Objectives might be evaluated by giving a test of some sort, a behavioral evaluation, or a graded assignment. In the next part of this chapter, the focus will be on developing and scoring tests. Behavioral evaluation was covered in Chapter 13, and assignments are discussed in Chapter 3.

Good tests are devised after careful thought and planning, either before a course begins, or at least well before examination time. They should test the achievement of course objectives logically and systematically. Good exam planning involves some type of test blueprint or table of specifications. A *test blueprint* is a chart that spells out the content (behaviors, objectives) and the level of knowledge to be tested. The blueprint can be highly specific or rather general, according to the teacher's preference. At the very least, it should contain the content or objectives to be measured, a taxonomy of levels of learning to be assigned to the content or objectives, and the numbers of questions or relative weight to be given to each area. Table 14–2 is an example of a test blueprint for a 50-item test on oxygenation.

You might wonder why the decision was made to include 50 items on the test and how the test writer decided on the proportion of questions in each row and column. Every test should be viewed as a sampling process. That is, out of the universe of facts, skills, and understandings that learners are supposed to gain, an examination can test only a small portion. The educator must decide how large the sample should be and what information deserves to be sampled. The idea behind sampling, of course, is that performance on this sample of test items implies a similar grasp of the whole body of information taught. The challenge is in selecting or creating a representative sample. The test blueprint aids in making that systematic and logical sampling choice.

The decision on the number of items to include depends on such factors as amount of material taught, types of test questions used, and amount of time available for testing. A rule of thumb is that a high school- or college-level learner should be able to answer one multiple-choice question, three fill-in type questions, or three true–false questions per minute

TABLE 14-2 Test Blueprint for Unit on Oxygenation

Content	Level of Knowing			
	Comprehension	Application	Analysis/Synthesis	Total Items
Principles	2	2	2	6
Factors Affecting	3	3	4	10
Pathophysiology	3	3	4	10
Assessment	1	4	5	10
Nursing Measures		5	5	10
Evaluation of Care		2	2	4
Total Items	9	19	22	50

(Gronlund, 1998). In general, the larger the sample of questions, just as in the research process, the more reliable the test.

The decision on the levels of knowing depends on the nature of the content and the level of the learner. In the blueprint in Table 14–2, Bloom's Taxonomy is used (see Chapter 3) but only four of the levels of knowing are used. This is because the knowledge level was considered too basic for this audience (nursing students) and the evaluation level is difficult to test with multiple-choice questions, which are going to be used for this examination. In a practice profession like nursing, test questions should be heavily weighted at the higher levels of knowing. It is not enough for a nurse or nursing student, for example, to be able to recall facts; there must be understanding, application, and analysis of information.

The types of test questions that can be used are undoubtedly familiar to you. They include multiple-choice questions, true–false questions, matching items, and essays. Tests may consist of a single type of question or a combination of types, as long as the objectives are being measured at the desired levels of learning. Developing good test questions is an art as well as a science and cannot be fully taught in a single chapter of a text such as this. However, I will give an introduction and overview of each type of question. Skill in writing test items can be developed in graduate courses, in-service courses, or by reading and applying information from test and measurement textbooks. However, keep in mind that it is a skill that develops over time.

Multiple-Choice Questions

Nursing examinations are often written in the multiple-choice format. There are several reasons for this fact. One is that although they are challenging to create, they are easy to score and can be scored by computer. Another reason is that licensure and certification examinations are multiple-choice tests, and therefore educators want learners to be familiar with questions like the ones that they will be taking on these exams.

Some people have criticized heavy dependence on multiple-choice questions in nursing tests because they think you cannot test the highest levels of knowing by this means and you cannot test critical thinking abilities (Masters et al., 2001). Morrison and Free (2001) have made the case that as long as multiple-choice items require multilogical thinking (i.e., knowledge of several facts to be applied to a clinical situation), they are testing critical thinking and they can be written at the application level or higher.

To demonstrate the differences in questions written at varied levels of Bloom's Taxonomy, see the following three examples. The first tests comprehension, the second application, and the third evaluation:

1. Which parameter is it most important for a nurse to report when implementing postural drainage?
   a. Frequency of oral hygiene
   b. Number of times the patient coughed
   c. Amount of sputum expectorated
   d. Change in respiratory depth
2. An immobilized alert patient is developing atelectasis. What should the nurse do first with this patient?
   a. Oral suctioning
   b. Postural drainage

    c. Pursed-lip breathing

    d. Coughing and deep breathing

  3. An orthopneic patient is placed in high Fowler's position. What data would indicate the need to reassess the situation and maybe reposition the patient?

    a. Coughing and expectoration

    b. Inability to rest

    c. Decreased use of accessory muscles

    d. Increased chest expansion

Questions such as these test the intended level of knowing only if the exact information in the question has not already been taught in class. For example, if a teacher who taught that patients developing atelectasis should benefit from coughing and deep breathing, but not from suctioning, postural drainage, or pursed-lip breathing were to use the second question, the item would be testing recall of information at the knowledge level, not application. Because only the teacher knows what was taught and how it was presented, it is only he or she who can determine for sure what level of knowing the questions are really testing.

    A multiple-choice question has two parts. The question itself is called the *stem*. The possible answers or solutions that follow are called the *options*. The correct option is termed the *answer,* and the incorrect options are called the *distracters*. The stem can be worded as a question or as an incomplete statement. Beginning item writers may find it easier to write actual questions, but either format is acceptable (Masters et al., 2001). In either case, the stem should clearly state the problem and make sense in itself without the reader having to look at the options to find out what is being asked. Here is an example of a multiple-choice item with the stem worded as a question:

    Which phrase best defines atelectasis?

    a. A collapse in a portion of a lung

    b. Fluid in the lung

    c. Fluid in the pleural space

    d. Outpouchings in the bronchial walls

Here is a multiple-choice item with the stem written as an incomplete statement:

    Atelectasis can best be defined as

    a. a collapse in a portion of a lung.

    b. fluid in the lung.

    c. fluid in the pleural space.

    d. outpouchings in the bronchial walls.

Note that the punctuation in the options is grammatically consistent with the stem. In the first item, there is no need for a period at the end of the options because they are not complete sentences. In the second item, each option completes the sentence. Therefore, the options are not capitalized, and each option ends with a period.

    The stem should be as short as possible while still conveying the ideas clearly. Try to minimize the amount of reading that the learner has to do while taking the test. Any information that is not needed in order to answer the question should be removed. Also, the stem should include any words that might be redundant in the options. For instance, if each option starts with "It is a . . .," it would be better to add those words to the stem or change the stem to reduce the length and redundancy of the options. An illustration of this point is:

What is lung surfactant?

a. It is the external lining of the lung.

b. It is a lipoprotein substance in the alveoli.

c. It is an abnormal fluid accumulation.

d. It is the black color that results from smoking.

It would be better to reword this question to say:

"Surfactant" in the lung refers to

a. the external lining of the lung.

b. a lipoprotein substance in the alveoli.

c. abnormal fluid accumulation.

d. the black color that results from smoking.

Negatively stated stems should be avoided unless they test for important points. Negative terms in the stem tend to make questions more confusing. A question such as "Which phrase does NOT define atelectasis?" would be poor because of the focus on the negative. What would be the point of asking learners to focus on an incorrect definition? It would make sense, though, to ask a negative question if it were important for a nurse *not* to do something. For instance, To prevent infection when inserting an intravenous catheter, a nurse should never . . .

Another way to handle negative questions is to write them in the "except" format, such as: All of these statements define atelectasis EXCEPT . . .

Although these kinds of questions are not recommended, it may be difficult to test some material without resorting to them at times. When they are used, the word *except* should be placed near the end of the stem and should be capitalized or underlined.

The number of options that follow the stem may vary. There is no magic in having four options, although that is the usual pattern. Adding a fifth option decreases the chance of a learner's guessing the answer correctly, but sometimes it is so difficult to find plausible distracters that it is better to have only three options rather than make up nonsense distracters (Oermann & Gaberson, 1998; Thorndike, 1997).

Distracters should be realistic. They are most attractive when they are based on common misconceptions that learners have about the topic. Nonsense distracters should never be used, and *all of the above* or *none of the above* should be used sparingly. The *all of the above* option serves to make an item more difficult. *None of the above* should be used only in cases similar to those calling for a negative stem, in which it is important for the learner to know that avoiding certain practices or procedures is crucial.

A few more rules govern the writing of options. First, they should be grammatically consistent with the stem, both to use good style and to avoid giving unwanted clues. Too often inconsistency occurs only in the distracters, leaving the answer sticking out as clearly right because it fits best grammatically. Here is an example of a grammatically inconsistent item:

The presence of moderate acetone in a patient's urine indicates that

a. fats are being burned for energy.

b. when blood sugar is very high.

c. ACTH levels are sometimes elevated.

d. it means protein is being metabolized.

Here is the same item made grammatically consistent:

> The presence of moderate acetone in a patient's urine indicates that
> **a.** fats are being burned for energy.
> **b.** blood sugar is very high.
> **c.** ACTH levels are elevated.
> **d.** protein is being metabolized.

A second rule is that options should be fairly short and about the same length. It is easy to fall into the trap of making the correct answer longer than the distracters to include enough information to make sure that it is clearly true. If you have to write a longer answer, increase the length of the distracters as well.

Third, options should be placed in logical order, if one exists. If the options are numbers, place them in ascending or descending order. If single-word terms are being used, place them in alphabetical order. Ordering the options reduces reading difficulty for the learner.

Fourth, avoid the use of qualifying terms, such as *always, sometimes, usually,* and *never.* People who have become test-wise know that words like *all, always,* and *never* in the options probably indicate false statements. Words like *sometimes, usually, often,* and *generally* are often found in true statements. You can use these words as long as they don't give away the correct answer.

Finally, be sure to alter the positions of the correct answers in a series of multiple-choice questions. Teachers who are not aware of this point often tend to make *b* or *c* the correct answer, and students catch on to that fact very quickly. The correct answer should be evenly distributed among the letters *a, b, c,* and *d,* and the same letter should not appear more than two or three times in a row.

True–False Questions

True–false questions are designed to test a learner's ability to identify the correctness of statements of fact or principle. They are limited to testing the lowest levels of knowing, knowledge and comprehension, and thus have limited usefulness in tests for nurses or nursing students. They may be useful in evaluating patient learning or ancillary staff learning. One of the weaknesses of true–false questions is that the learner has a 50/50 chance of guessing the right answer. However, if enough true–false questions are included, the chance of guessing being of significant help decreases (Oermann & Gaberson, 1998).

When writing true–false items, make sure that you word the statement so that it is clearly true or false. For example, the following item is ambiguous and not clearly true or false:

> (T F) Diabetics who test their blood sugar four times a day have fewer complications than those who don't.

The answer to this question is "True" in many cases, but "False" in others. Learners would probably label this a tricky question. To make this item unequivocally "True," it should be worded:

> (T F) Insulin-dependent diabetics who test their blood sugar four times a day and take appropriate insulin have fewer complications than those who don't.

The rewording makes this item longer than desirable. It is best if the item contains only one idea. This one contained two main ideas. If a true–false item gets too long, it might be better to use another type of question.

As in the case of multiple-choice questions, avoid the use of qualifiers such as *always* or *never,* which tend to be found in false statements, and *sometimes* or *often,* which tend to appear in true statements (Thorndike, 1997).

There are variations of true–false questions that may be of even greater usefulness. One variation is to ask the learner to give a rationale for why the item is true or false. Another modification is to ask the learner to rewrite false statements to make them true.

Matching Questions

Matching questions test knowledge, the lowest level of knowing. They are useful in determining if learners can recall the memorized relationships between two things such as dates and events, structures and functions, and terms and their definitions. Matching questions are easy to construct and to score, but because they test only recall, they should be used sparingly.

Matching questions are set up as two lists, with the premises usually on the left and the responses on the right. All items in the list should be homogeneous—all related to one topic or concept. The number of responses should exceed the number of premises so the learner cannot answer just by the process of elimination. The instructions should indicate whether a response can be used more than once. A matching question is usually set up in the following way:

> Match the medication administration abbreviation on the left to its meaning on the right. Place the appropriate letter in the space in front of the abbreviation. Each response can be used only once or not at all.
>
> _____ **1.** a.c.   **a.** of each
> _____ **2.** o.s.   **b.** every hour
> _____ **3.** gtt.   **c.** by mouth
> _____ **4.** p.o.   **d.** before meals
> _____ **5.** q.h.   **e.** drops
>   **f.** left eye

Double matching items can be designed to increase the level of difficulty, as in the following (Carlson, 1985):

> In the spaces on the left place the letters A, M, or H to identify the measurement system in which the abbreviation belongs. In the spaces on the right, place the letter of the accepted equivalent.
>
> A = apothecaries'   _____ **1.** dr.   _____   **a.** 15 gr.
> M = metric   _____ **2.** oz.   _____   **b.** 1000 cc
> H = household   _____ **3.** T   _____   **c.** 4 cc
>   _____ **4.** Kg.   _____   **d.** 100 Gm.
>   _____ **5.** L.   _____   **e.** 30 cc
>   _____ **6.** Gm.   _____   **f.** 15 cc
>   **g.** 2.2 lb.
>   **h.** 4 dr.

Lengthening the lists of items can also increase the level of difficulty. One potential problem exists with lengthening the lists, however. Students may be using computerized answer sheets to record their answers. Most answer sheets have only five spaces for answers, so if the matching items go beyond "e," there is no place to record the answer. Being aware of this limitation can save frustration for the students and the teacher at the time of test administration.

Essay-Type Questions

Although short-answer and essay questions are valuable measurement tools, they are probably not used enough in nursing education. They are time consuming for test takers to answer, thus limiting the amount of knowledge sampling you can accomplish in a short time. They are also time consuming to score. On the other hand, essay-type questions lend themselves to testing the highest levels of knowing, especially analysis, synthesis, and evaluation.

Short-answer questions, sometimes termed *restricted response* items, place limitations on the type of response requested (Oermann, 1999). For example:

Explain in a few sentences why patients with lymphoma are susceptible to infection.

Describe three major pathological processes involved in multiple myeloma.

List two infection prevention measures a nurse should teach a patient who is going home with an ileal conduit.

Short-answer questions fit well with case study formats, also. You can provide a brief case study followed by several short-answer questions based on the case. This is a nice way to test problem-solving skills (Conyers & Ritchie, 2001).

Full essay questions are sometimes called *extended response* questions (Oermann, 1999). They permit the test taker to select all pertinent information, organize it as desired, and express the thesis in a clear manner. Here is an example of an extended response essay question:

Compare and contrast two theories of death and dying, and describe how the nurse's role in supporting a dying patient might differ depending on which of the theories the nurse subscribes to.

Scoring of extended response essays is a challenge. Unless clear guidelines are used, reliability is difficult to achieve. There are two approaches to scoring these items. One is a point method, the other is a rubric method (Brookhart, 1999). In the point method (also called the analytic method), the instructor lists the elements that must appear in the answer and assigns points to these elements depending on their importance. In the above item example, considering that the entire essay is worth 20 points within the entire examination, the elements and points might look like this:

1. Compares two theories, covering all the important components. (5 pts.)
2. Contrasts the theories, pointing out major differences. (5 pts.)
3. Describes several aspects of the nurse's role. (5 pts.)
4. Contrasts the nurse's role as it depends on the two theories. (5 pts.)

The instructor would probably give partial credit within each of these four elements, if only some of the element was included. Points may also be allocated to elements like grammar and creativity, if so desired.

TABLE 14-3 Holistic Scoring Rubric for an Extended Response Essay Question

Score	Descriptors
5	Thesis is clear and defensible. Arguments or positions are logical. Facts necessary to the thesis are included and are accurate and relevant to the thesis. Writing style is clear and organized. Grammar, word usage, and spelling are correct. Demonstrates originality of thought or creativity.
4	Thesis is clear and defensible. Arguments or positions are logical. Most necessary facts are included and all are accurate and relevant. Writing style is clear and organized. Grammar, word usage, and spelling have some minor flaws. Some evidence of originality of thought or creativity.
3	Thesis is clear and defensible for the most part, but at some points may show some weakness. Arguments or positions are usually logical, but may show some minor flaw in logic. Some supporting facts are inaccurate or irrelevant. Writing style is generally clear and organized, but significant grammar, word usage, or spelling errors exist. Little evidence of originality or creativity.
2	Thesis is unclear or arguments or positions are weak. Supporting facts are often inaccurate or irrelevant. Writing style lacks clarity and organization at times. Significant grammatical, word usage, and spelling errors exist. No originality or creativity.
1	Thesis is missing or arguments are illogical. Facts are missing or inaccurate. Writing style is unclear or disorganized. Significant grammatical, word usage, and spelling errors exist.

The rubric system of scoring includes qualitative rating scales and is sometimes termed the holistic method of scoring. This system is most useful if the teacher is just as concerned about the overall quality of the answer and the writing style as he or she is about the facts that are included in the essay. The learner is evaluated on whether the points of the argument are clear, logical, and defensible; whether the writing is clear, organized, and grammatically correct; and whether the relevant facts are included. A holistic scoring rubric for an extended response essay could look like the one in Table 14–3. The teacher decides (somewhat subjectively) which description in the rubric best matches the essay. It is very helpful for learners if rubrics such as this are shared with them before the test is given.

Test Item Analysis

Objective test items can be subjected to item analysis that provides data about the worth of the items—specifically, their level of difficulty and ability to discriminate between test takers who know the material and those who don't. Item analysis can be done quickly with a computer and appropriate software. In the absence of a software program, the educator can calculate both item difficulty and item discrimination quite easily.

Item Difficulty

It is useful to calculate item difficulty because questions that are very easy or very difficult may not serve any useful purpose. Teachers should generally try to write questions that are moderately difficult; that is, on a moderately difficult question, the difficulty score would fall midway between 100 percent correct responses and the chance level of getting a correct response (50 percent for true–false, and 25 percent on four-option multiple-choice). So, for an optimum true–false question, 75 percent of the learners should get the correct answer, and for an optimum multiple-choice question, around 60 to 65 percent of the learners should get the correct answer (Oermann & Gaberson, 1998).

Item difficulty is defined as the proportion of test takers that answer the question correctly. It is calculated by dividing the number of people who got the item right by the number who took the test (Thorndike, 1997).

$$\text{Difficulty Index} = \frac{\#\ \text{correct}}{\#\ \text{total test-takers}}$$

The resulting fraction (converted to a percentage) provides an estimate of difficulty, with the higher percentages indicating easier questions.

Item Discrimination

Item discrimination is an estimate of the usefulness of an item in differentiating between learners who did well on the whole test and those who performed poorly. In other words, a discriminating question is one that learners who did well on the rest of the test got right but learners who didn't do well on the test got wrong. The process for calculating item discrimination involves ranking the test papers from highest to lowest scores and choosing the top 25 to 30 percent and the bottom 25 to 30 percent. If you had 50 test papers, you would select the top 13 to 15 papers and the bottom 13 to 15 papers. If papers 13 and 14 both had the same score, you would include both in the sample. Next, for each group and each objective test question, you would tabulate the number of people who selected each option. Your final tally for a multiple-choice question might look like this:

Question 1

	a	b	c	d
Highest 13	1	3	9*	0
Lowest 13	3	5	2*	3

In looking at this chart, you can see that 9 of the 13 test takers in the highest group got the correct answer (c), while only 2 in the lowest group got it right. Obviously, the item is discriminating. You can do one more calculation to arrive at a *discrimination index* (Thorndike, 1997). Subtract the number of people in the lowest group who got the item right (RL) from the number in the highest group who got it right (RH) and divide by half of the sample size (½ n). The formula appears like this:

$$\text{Discrimination Index} = \frac{RH - RL}{\frac{1}{2}n}$$

In the case of our hypothetical test:

$$\text{Discrimination Index} = \frac{9 - 2}{13} = .54$$

This number (.54) is an average discrimination index. The index ranges from −1.00 to +1.00, with the higher the value the better the discrimination of the item. A negative index indicates that more people in the highest group got the question wrong than those in the lowest group. Such questions are flawed in either content or format and should be reworked before using again. Likewise, questions that are too easy should be adjusted before using again. Items with a discrimination index of .40 and higher are generally considered to be good items (Oermann & Gaberson, 1998).

An item analysis serves two purposes. It helps the teacher give more valid scores on the exam being analyzed, and it enables him or her to build a file of well-constructed test items for future use.

It should be obvious by now that test writing is a time-consuming task that warrants a lot of attention. Because so much hinges on grades, educators must be careful to ensure that grades are a true and fair indication of learning that has taken place. It is possible to use test items that have been written and published by others. Test banks designed for use by educators accompany many textbooks. When using test banks, however, be aware of certain pitfalls. Many of the items are written at the lowest levels of knowing, and many contain violations of generally accepted item-writing principles (Masters et al., 2001). If you use a test bank, be careful to adjust the items as needed to meet your test blueprint and principles of good item writing.

Evaluating Patient Learning

There are not many cases in which you will be able to evaluate patient learning by means of a written test. There generally is little time to do so, nor would many patients look favorably on having to take a written test. It may be possible to ask a few true–false questions in writing or orally, but that may be all you can do. There are a few other techniques that give you some feedback about patient learning, although they are admittedly not comprehensive. One is to ask the person to read a pamphlet or fact sheet summarizing what you have taught and to underline the important information. That technique gives you some idea about whether the person understands and can prioritize the information you have covered. You can also interview the person and, through discussion and questioning, elicit information about understanding (Foster, 1987).

The fact that obtaining valid and reliable indicators of patient learning is difficult does not mean you have to abandon the attempt. The most important outcome of patient teaching is generally a change in patient behavior related to health care practices. For example, you may teach a new mother about bathing a newborn, and she may be able to repeat back what you have said and answer your questions, but the ultimate test of whether learning has taken place is whether the mother bathes the newborn safely and correctly. So, return demonstration can give you valuable evaluation data if you have taught a skill. You may also, over time, be able to collect physical evidence of the effectiveness of patient teaching. For instance, hemoglobin A1c blood values can provide feedback on long-term glucose control in a diabetic you have been teaching. Serum drug levels indicate whether patients have been taking prescribed drugs regularly (Foster, 1987). For legal and accreditation purposes, you must find a way to document not only teaching, but also some evidence of what the patient has learned.

Assessing and evaluating learning consumes a lot of time and requires expertise. Nevertheless, the process is worthwhile if we can determine that our teaching is effective and our learners have really learned.

Case Study

You are teaching a class for 10 infection control nurses from your geographic area on insect-borne diseases. Although these are experienced nurses, this information is quite new to them and you want to be sure they are learning as you go along.

1. What Classroom Assessment Techniques would be most appropriate to use: Muddiest Point, Student-Generated Test Questions, Application Cards, or Self-Confidence Surveys?
2. What would be the advantages and disadvantages of using each of these CATs with this population?
3. If you use Application Cards and no one comes up with good applications, what is this feedback telling you?
4. Develop a new CAT that would be appropriate for this class.

Critical Thinking Exercises

1. What are some things that could go wrong in using Classroom Assessment Techniques, and how could you prevent them from happening?
2. Compare and contrast two CATs: Misconception/Preconception and Background Knowledge Probe. What are the advantages of each?
3. How might you assess or evaluate problem-solving skills among new graduates?
4. In evaluating patient learning, how can you tell the difference between failure to learn and lack of interest in applying learning?
5. In conducting research, we are taught not to use measurement instruments unless they have demonstrated reliability and validity. Does this principle apply to measuring classroom learning? Why or why not?

Ideas for Further Research

1. Compare the use of two different CATs like Muddiest Point and One-Minute Paper in two different sections of the same class. Which CAT yielded the richest data?
2. Survey faculty in academic or staff development settings regarding their use of CATs.
3. If you are using objective examinations, test them for reliability and validity.

4. Find out if there are any significant differences when conducting item discrimination analysis when you use the upper and lower 25 to 30 percent of the papers or if you use only 15 percent of the upper and lower groups. (If fewer papers were just as good, it would make hand calculation of item discrimination more efficient.)

REFERENCES

Angelo, T. A., & Cross, K. P. (1993). *Classroom assessment techniques.* San Francisco: Jossey-Bass.

Brookhart, S. M. (1999). *The art and science of classroom assessment: The missing part of pedagogy.* ASHE-ERIC Higher Education Report (Vol. 27, No. 1). Washington, DC: The George Washington University, Graduate School of Education and Human Development.

Carlson, S. B. (1985). *Creative classroom testing.* Princeton, NJ: Educational Testing Service.

Classroom assessment techniques. (1997). Retrieved November 14, 2001, from Indiana University Web site: *http://www.indiana.edu/~teaching/sfcats.html.*

Conyers, V., & Ritchie, D. (2001). Case study class tests: Assessment directing learning. *Journal of Nursing Education, 40*(1), 40–42.

Enerson, D. M., Plank, K. M., & Johnson, R. N. (1994). *An introduction to classroom assessment techniques.* Retrieved November 14, 2001, from The Pennsylvania State University Web site: *http://www.psu.edu/celt/CATs.html.*

Foster, S. D. (1987). Evaluating patient learning. *MCN, 12*(2), 131.

Gronlund, N. E. (1998). *Assessment of student achievement* (6th ed.). Needham Heights, MA: Allyn & Bacon.

Martin, M. B. (1999). *Classroom assessment techniques designed for technology.* Retrieved June 4, 2001, from Middle Tennessee State University Web site: *http://www.mtsu.edu/itconf/proceed99/Martin.htm.*

Masters, J. C., Hulsmeyer, B. S., Pike, M. E., Leichty, K., Miller, M. T., & Verst, A. L. (2001). Assessment of multiple-choice questions in selected test banks accompanying text books used in nursing education. *Journal of Nursing Education, 40*(1), 25–31.

Morrison, S., & Free, K. W. (2001). Writing multiple-choice test items that promote and measure critical thinking. *Journal of Nursing Education, 40*(1), 17–24.

Mosteller, F. (1989). The "Muddiest Point in the lecture" as a feedback device. *On Teaching and Learning: The Journal of the Harvard–Danforth Center, 3,* 10–21.

Oermann, M. (1999). Developing and scoring essay tests. *Nurse Educator, 24*(2), 29–32.

Oermann, M. H., & Gaberson, K. B. (1998). *Evaluation and testing in nursing education.* New York: Springer.

Peterson, J., & Stack, C. (1998). A Minnesota story: A system approach to classroom assessment and research. In T. Angelo (Ed.), *Classroom assessment and research: An update on uses, approaches, and research findings* (pp. 67–77). San Francisco: Jossey-Bass.

Thorndike, R. M. (1997). *Measurement and evaluation in psychology and education* (6th ed.). Upper Saddle River, NJ: Prentice Hall.

Index